DATE DUE

WITHDRAWN

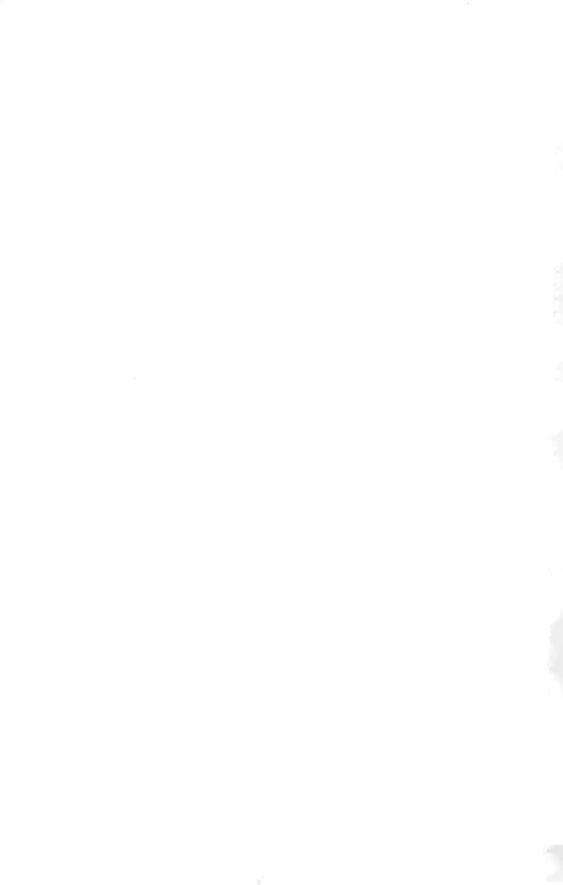

# MEDICARE AND MEDICAID AT 50

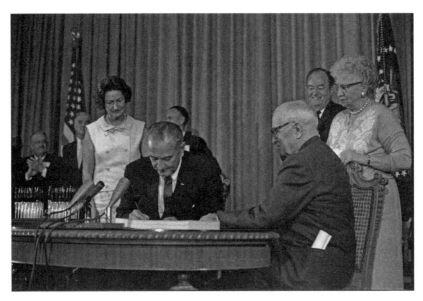

President Lyndon B. Johnson signing Medicare and Medicaid into law on July 30, 1965 at the Harry S. Truman Library in the presence of former President Truman, former First Lady Bess Truman, Vice President Hubert H. Humphrey (right), and First Lady "Lady Bird" Johnson (left).

# MEDICARE AND MEDICAID AT 50

## AMERICA'S ENTITLEMENT PROGRAMS IN THE AGE OF AFFORDABLE CARE

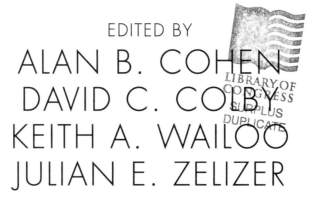

EDITED BY

ALAN B. COHEN

DAVID C. COLBY

KEITH A. WAILOO

JULIAN E. ZELIZER

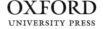

OXFORD
UNIVERSITY PRESS

# OXFORD
UNIVERSITY PRESS

Oxford University Press is a department of the University of
Oxford. It furthers the University's objective of excellence in research,
scholarship, and education by publishing worldwide.

Oxford    New York
Auckland    Cape Town    Dar es Salaam    Hong Kong    Karachi
Kuala Lumpur    Madrid    Melbourne    Mexico City    Nairobi
New Delhi    Shanghai    Taipei    Toronto

With offices in
Argentina    Austria    Brazil    Chile    Czech Republic    France    Greece
Guatemala    Hungary    Italy    Japan    Poland    Portugal    Singapore
South Korea    Switzerland    Thailand    Turkey    Ukraine    Vietnam

Oxford is a registered trademark of Oxford University Press
in the UK and certain other countries.

Published in the United States of America by
Oxford University Press
198 Madison Avenue, New York, NY 10016

© Oxford University Press 2015

Library of Congress Cataloging-in-Publication Data
Medicare and Medicaid at 50 : America's entitlement programs in the age of affordable care / edited by
Alan B. Cohen, David C. Colby, Keith A. Wailoo, and Julian E. Zelizer.
p. ; cm.
Includes index.
ISBN 978–0–19–023154–5
I. Cohen, Alan B., editor.    II. Colby, David C., editor.    III. Wailoo, Keith, editor.
IV. Zelizer, Julian E., editor.
[DNLM: 1. Medicaid—history.    2. Medicare—history.    3. Health Policy—history—United
States.    4. History, 20th Century—United States.    5. History, 21st Century—United States.
W 250 AA1]
RA412.4
368.4′200973—dc23
2014042846

1 3 5 7 9 8 6 4 2
Printed in the United States of America
on acid-free paper

*Rashi Fein*
*1926–2014*

*This volume is dedicated to the memory of Rashi Fein, PhD, Professor of the Economics of Medicine, Emeritus, at the Harvard Medical School. Rashi, our longtime friend and colleague, passed away on September 8, 2014.*

*He was closely affiliated with the Robert Wood Johnson Foundation Scholars in Health Policy Research Program for more than 20 years, serving as chair of the National Advisory Committee for eight years (1994–2002). He cared deeply about fostering the development of young scholars.*

*For more than six decades, from positions in the public, private, and academic sectors, he was a prominent participant in health policy efforts, including the development and early implementation of the Medicare and Medicaid programs. His chapter in this volume is a fitting capstone to a stellar career in academia and public service, and we are grateful to have his wisdom grace these pages.*

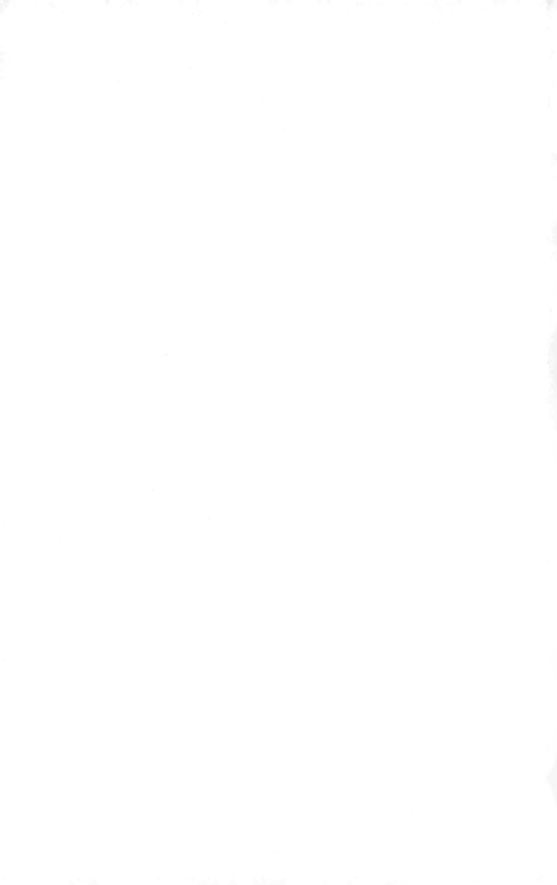

# CONTENTS

## CONCLUSION: THE WORLD THAT MEDICARE AND MEDICAID MADE 333
*Alan B. Cohen, David C. Colby, Keith A. Wailoo, and Julian E. Zelizer*

# INTRODUCTION

## *MEDICARE, MEDICAID, AND THE MORAL TEST OF GOVERNMENT*

ALAN B. COHEN, DAVID C. COLBY, KEITH A. WAILOO,
AND JULIAN E. ZELIZER

The political struggles over President Obama's 2010 healthcare reform law, the Affordable Care Act (ACA), opened a contentious new chapter in the already tumultuous 50-year history of Medicaid and Medicare. The ACA's promise to overhaul American health care, expanding health insurance to 48 million uninsured Americans who lacked private health insurance and were not eligible for Medicare or Medicaid, angered some as a "government take-over of medicine," even as it excited others about progress in improving the public's health. The law promised to create a new system of health insurance exchanges to provide citizens with the best coverage options available. But because the ACA was also built into a pre-existing system of programs and policies, the law cast a large and worrisome shadow. By proposing to compel states to expand Medicaid coverage dramatically and mandating that individuals pay a penalty if they did not purchase insurance, the law worried many Americans—among them governors and attorneys general (prompting 28 states to file lawsuits to strike down portions of the law). For many of America's elderly, these intense political and legal debates surrounding the ACA created confusion and sowed seeds of anxiety about the future of the other government program they had grown to depend upon—Medicare.

From the moment that President Obama proposed to take on healthcare reform, his opponents insisted that the initiative posed a grave threat to Medicare beneficiaries. Medicare would be cut, they said, as part of the new program. Supporters of the ACA (from Congressional Democrats to AARP) and the White House rebutted the charge, aware of the political damage carried by the accusation. Separating myth from fact, the *U.S. News and World Report* reassured seniors that Medicare was not being replaced by "Obamacare." Any changes would be modest; for example, some higher-income Medicare beneficiaries should expect to pay more for medications after the ACA was implemented.[1] Calming anxious Medicare beneficiaries about Medicaid expansion, the Medicare.gov website explained, "Medicare isn't part of the Health Insurance Marketplace established by ACA...you'll still have your same benefits and security you have now."[2] Seniors could still expect the same security they had come to cherish.

But their worries, stoked certainly by ACA opponents but also by the very talk of reform, spoke volumes about the powerful role of Medicare and Medicaid in American life, as well as the anxieties generated about how these two programs would interact with each other and with whatever new ACA programs were developed. Nothing symbolized the complexities, stakes, and confusions of the moment better than when, in 2009, a South Carolina man insisted to Republican Congressman Robert Inglis, "Keep your government hands off my Medicare!" Inglis tried to explain that his Medicare health care was government health care, "but he was having none of it"—a sign of the intensity of individual ownership that many people associate with the benefit.[3] Both Medicare and Medicaid were iconic parts of the American social insurance system, but both were vulnerable, albeit in different ways. The assertion that the ACA and its Medicaid expansion would harm Medicare beneficiaries played one group against the other, and one set of vulnerabilities (lack of health insurance) against the other (health security of the elderly). Why this claim had such charged resonance is one among the many themes in this volume.

The two signature programs were born as part of the Great Society in 1965, but with different origins, evolutions, and philosophies guiding them. Medicaid began as a welfare program for a segment of the poor—highly stigmatized and contentious. Most policymakers saw the program as an inconsequential development, added to the Social Security Amendments of 1965 by House Ways and Means Chairman Wilbur Mills only as a stratagem to stifle conservatives' proposing it as their alternative to Medicare. As a program where each state matched its own dollars with federal funds in order to provide care for poor women and their children, governors and legislators were wary from the start about the federal bargain. Medicaid's fate would depend heavily on how debates over welfare and poverty unfolded between states and the federal government. In 1969, 12 states had not yet joined the program. But by 1977, only one held out—Arizona. In 1982, more than a decade after the law was passed, it too would adopt the program, with a waiver of some federal requirements.

Medicare began very differently; from the start, it was a federal entitlement program through and through. If Medicaid was considered a minor program, legislators celebrated Medicare as the single most important expansion of health care in the twentieth century. Funded in large part by payroll taxes designated specifically for the program in the paychecks of working Americans, this healthcare plan was not stigmatized as a welfare giveaway. As with Social Security, Americans came to see the benefits as earned—as government returning to them contributions they had made through their Social Security taxes. Some saw this as a right to health care. From the start, then, what each program symbolized to Americans differed dramatically. For the 50 years since their creation, the question of what each reflected about the nation's commitments to its citizens, and what beneficiaries in each might win or lose under any new reforms, had sweeping implications.

In many ways, the debates surrounding the ACA clarified Americans' understanding of its complex healthcare system; but in many ways, the ACA debates spread confusion about Medicare, Medicaid, and how they affected one another. The pages ahead help to explain this complicated landscape by telling the story of Medicare and Medicaid together—their inception in the 1960s, their 50-year evolution and expansion, their wide impact on the states and the country, and how the changing fortunes of these two signature programs, in turn, changed the nation. These stories are often told separately, as if insuring the elderly as a social commitment stands apart from insuring people in poverty; yet 50 years ago, the elderly were a major part of the face of poverty in America. The volume, therefore, brings together leading scholars, writers, and policymakers from multiple disciplinary perspectives to analyze the questions that have long shadowed these programs, and to clarify many of the lingering confusions about whether reform in one realm helps or harms the other. In the pages ahead, we ask these questions: What was the original Medicare and Medicaid vision, and how did it change? What have been their key accomplishments and failures? How and why have both programs expanded in the five decades since their creation—and with what political, social, financial, and legal ramifications? And why, despite their growth, did there remain a pressing need for new reforms to extend health insurance to those lacking private health insurance and not eligible for Medicare or Medicaid? Apart from clarifying confusions in the wake of the ACA and Medicaid expansion, the fiftieth anniversary of both programs in 2015 provides an additional reason to take a deep and studied breath—and to look critically at their history and development, and to gather lessons for the future.

When the two programs are pitted against each other in today's ACA debates, one irony stands out about healthcare reform in our time. In earlier decades, advocates for healthcare reform and expanding health insurance saw Medicare, not Medicaid, as the model to follow in reaching universal health coverage. Medicare was to be the building block for future expansions, with health insurance for the elderly only a first step toward that larger goal. By 1972, Medicare had expanded to include disabled individuals and individuals with kidney failure. For advocates of national reform, these were steps two and three: a natural progression, extending the benefits of Medicare outward to other populations. But Medicare reform in later decades shifted course—leaning heavily toward preserving the program as a program *for* the elderly, rather than extending its generous commitment to others. This trend, as well as the new climate of budget-cutting and fiscal conservatism, as we shall see, has had the effect of sealing off Medicare beneficiaries from other groups, making them protective of their own benefits, wary of expansion to other groups, and creating expectations that both advanced and hindered later reform efforts.

In the meantime, Medicaid (which was in 1965 the "poor person's program") was also being transformed—its coverage slowly expanding in ways the early architects never imagined. As Lawrence Brown and Michael Sparer wrote a decade ago, "Medicare is the preferred reform model because, so the axiom held, poor people's programs [like Medicaid] are poor programs—not only inequitable but also politically precarious."[4] Yet they found that it was Medicaid—a program that began as a meager anti-poverty measure and still carried the "weighty cultural burden of welfare medicine"—that had grown incrementally over the decades, increasing eligibility and inching toward a middle-class entitlement in the face of America's stubborn resistance to universal healthcare coverage. In 2014, Medicaid had become the largest single source of healthcare coverage in the United States, covering 66 million people,[5] including low-income children, pregnant women, and adults; Medicare, by comparison, covered 52 million Americans.[6] With ACA implementation and new enrollments, Medicaid's numbers could grow by tens of millions in 2015 and 2016, particularly if hesitant states choose to adopt the law's Medicaid expansion.[7] Whether or not this will be the new path to universal coverage only time will tell.

What is it that seniors were afraid of losing? Medicare, like Medicaid, had enlarged well beyond the early 1965 vision, creating an expansive blanket of health security. Traditional Medicare (Parts A and B, signed into law by President Lyndon Johnson over strong Republican opposition) covered hospital stays and home health visits (A), and doctors' office visits and outpatient visits (B). Thirty years later, Part C, Medicare+Choice, was added as a conservative spin to the program as part of a balanced budget deal in 1997. Reflecting a new political environment friendly to privatization, Medicare+Choice gave beneficiaries the option of enrolling in private insurance plans with some enhanced benefits and savings, but also with some constraints. Then in 2003 came Medicare Part D, supported by Republican President George W. Bush and passed by a Republican Congress that established a new prescription drug benefit for the elderly and restructured Part C as "Medicare Advantage." Beneficiaries worried about losing all of these benefits built up over the years as the ACA was implemented and as Medicaid expanded.

In this fraught and contentious environment filled with myth, confusion, vulnerability, and political accusations, it becomes especially crucial to understand the relationship between these two programs—their disparate philosophies, their distinct historical trajectories, their dramatic changes over time, and the underlying social commitments they reflect.

Divided into five parts, the volume begins by examining the original vision and actors and events shaping the march to enactment in an era when—much like today—partisanship dominated Washington, D.C. Examining the intentions of the planners, the political and social underpinnings of these programs in Lyndon Johnson's Great Society, and the role of the president, Congress, and other forces in shaping the trajectory of both programs, Julian Zelizer exposes a political contentiousness that bears some resemblance to our current fractious political environment. In this case, the contentiousness produced programs that proved to be remarkably durable rather than fragile. David Barton Smith explores how the civil rights movement impacted the implementation of Medicare and its commitment to the ideal of equal health opportunity. Rashi Fein offers reflections on the challenges of implementation based on his experience in federal government—serving on the staff of President Kennedy's Council of Economic Advisers, working with the Acting Secretary of Health, Education, and Welfare (Wilbur Cohen) as chair of the Medical Assistance Advisory Council to secure resources for and to mold the Medicaid program, and sitting on the boards of trustees of two different healthcare organizations observing these programs from a distance. Jonathan Oberlander and Theodore Marmor (who also had worked with Wilbur Cohen) examine why Medicare did not expand into universal coverage as its architects had wanted and anticipated, and how Medicare became separated from the goal of national health insurance as Medicare spending rose, as the political environment shifted rightward, and as budgetary politics grew heated in the 1980s and 1990s.

Part II focuses on the early years of program implementation, and how (despite ongoing controversy) the programs became integral to the nation's political fabric, remaking societal values and relationships, altering individuals' expectations about government, and influencing the political environment more broadly. Between 1965 and 1980, issues of race, aging, shifting demographics, rising costs, and shifting public opinion about health and social welfare reshaped the programs. Jill Quadagno reveals how Medicaid began as a program for the very poor and gradually became a benefit reaching into the middle class and became the fourth largest program in the federal budget, even as the program retained aspects of its poor law legacy. The chapter explores how this transformation came about—as the benefits of the program expanded to cover 20 percent of the population today, it also became the primary payer for 63 percent of skilled nursing facility residents. Sara Rosenbaum next argues that the courts were a major player in this transformation. She examines how the rise and fall of a liberal judiciary, and not Congress, buttressed the idea of Medicaid as an entitlement, driven by litigation around the very meaning of "entitlement." A close analysis of judicial intervention, the chapter explains how judicial decisions effectively created the modern legal understanding of the Medicaid program. Mark Schlesinger concludes with insight on Medicare's social impact over five decades—that is, how the program changed elders' self-perceptions, empowering them to become a potent constituency with a unitary social identity. With these changes in the political identity of seniors came new challenges, from policymakers struggling to harness their proposals and plans to Medicare's growing influence on its beneficiaries' social identities.

Part III turns to the 1970s and 1980s, when rising costs and the rightward turn in American politics pushed Medicare and Medicaid in new directions. Surprising developments emerged during this period, even as the programs continued to expand. By the 1980s, Mark Peterson observes, Medicare had become American "bedrock," so precious and important to its elderly constituency that it was considered the new "third rail" of politics (a phrase previously reserved only for Social Security). His chapter explores how the Republican takeover of Congress in the 1990s and the "Gingrich revolution" that followed, with new concerns about fiscal solvency, altered the "untouchability" of Medicare. Uwe Reinhardt examines another response to Medicare's fiscal growth: how the program revolutionized payment to healthcare providers, beginning in 1984 with prospective payment for hospitals using DRGs (diagnosis-related groups), followed by prospective payment for physicians using RBRVS (resource-based relative value scale) methods in 1992, and more recently with other experiments in cost containment. It was Medicare, he argues, not the private sector that proved capable of innovative reform. Frank Thompson then tells the story of how governance of Medicaid changed in this era, as entrenchment forced changes in the power of the states to shape the program. Although Congress had designed the program, now congressional entrepreneurship, and a trend toward executive branch federalism in the Clinton administration and waivers giving latitude to the states were transforming Medicaid programs in new directions. Yet, despite these retrenchment efforts, the embattled program saw four periods of growth. Andrea Campbell concludes this part of the volume by tracking public opinion and examining how US citizens retained broad support for Medicare and Medicaid from 1965 to 1994, even as they expressed waning confidence in some of the programs' features. Those attitudes, Campbell argues, bolstered and stabilized the programs through tumultuous times.

Part IV returns to the question of how the programs relate to each other in the context of the ACA and examines how an expansive array of stakeholders (from nursing homes to pharmaceutical companies and hospitals) has come to depend on the programs. But even with the passage of the ACA, new challenges appear on the horizon. Keith Wailoo argues that the history of Medicare and Medicaid expansion suggests an enduring appeal of "big government," and that, beneath the rhetoric, there have been overwhelming forces driving Republicans and Democrats alike to embrace expansion. From the 1970s to the 1990s, and up to the current ACA era, the private sector has come to depend on Medicare and Medicaid funds—a fact that points to future expansion. Judith Feder sees long-term care coverage as the "missing piece" in the Social Security Amendments of 1965, and argues that its exclusion from national reforms has led to Medicaid becoming (by default) the primary funding source for long-term care. As a result, middle-class individuals today must spend down their private assets in order to qualify for Medicaid long-term care coverage. Jacob Hacker concludes this part of the volume by considering the relationship between Medicare and the medical-industrial complex that it helped to build over the past 50 years, and how Medicare's initial passive pricing (which made the program a "servant" to this complex) shifted so that today Medicare (through greater assertiveness regarding cost) has become the "master." As cost control becomes increasingly important in US health care, Hacker explores the implications of this "master-servant" relationship for the future of American healthcare costs, health care, and healthcare politics.

Part V takes a retrospective look at Medicare and Medicaid in the age of the ACA, drawing lessons from the 50-year history. Seeing Medicare as a major reference point in American political history, James Morone and Elisabeth Fauquert contrast the very brief "Medicare moment" of 1965 (with its embrace of massive social and political change, pressing concern about inequality, and values of egalitarianism) against the political, economic, and social ideals of later eras as neoliberal concerns about the functioning of markets and economic growth predominated. Only this shift could explain how two Democratic presidents, Bill Clinton and Barack Obama, promoted the market-based expansions at the center of ACA health insurance reforms. Paul Starr looks back at this sweep of history as well, exploring how policies become entrenched, enabling them to resist attempts to change or undo them and to survive transfers of congressional or executive power. His observations help explain the resistance of Medicare beneficiaries to further reforms, for he argues that what becomes entrenched may undermine, as well as advance, the original goals of a policy, becoming a matter more of regret than of satisfaction. Starr asks: Will the ACA become entrenched in the same way? Will it become an object of regret? Or will the ACA become entrenched in a degraded form?

A final chapter by the editors Alan Cohen, David Colby, Keith Wailoo, and Julian Zelizer reviews this history but also looks ahead, asking: What parts of this history are most important for charting the course ahead?

At the entrance lobby to the Hubert H. Humphrey Building in Washington, visitors are welcomed by the words of the former Vice President:

> The moral test of a government is how that government treats those who are in the dawn of life—the children; the twilight of life—the elderly; and the shadows of life—the sick, the needy, and the handicapped.[8]

When those words were uttered at the building's dedication in 1977, more than a decade had passed since Medicare and Medicaid enactment, but debate about their high cost had already grown intense, testing the nation's commitment to continue on the same path. Our goal in the pages ahead is to provide a richer portrait covering the birth of the programs, the politics behind their creation and development, their place in US health care over time, and analysis of the moral and political commitments that underpin them. Our chapters focus on the diverse viewpoints that combined to create policy, the evolving challenges, and the people affected by reform debates. Looking back, we ask whether Medicare and Medicaid today, greatly altered since the 1970s, still meet the moral test of government articulated by Hubert Humphrey. Looking ahead, we ask: What does the future hold for Medicare and Medicaid in a dynamically changing healthcare system undergoing major reform? Should the nation's commitment to each program, both politically and financially, be expanded or reduced? And what should policymakers, citizens, beneficiaries, and others bear in mind about the values and commitments undergirding these programs as they chart a course for the future? A close look at the fraught and contentious past can, and should, guide the way forward.

## Notes

1. Andrea Adleman, "Will Obamacare Affect Medicare? Myths and Facts," *US News and World Report*, August 13, 2013, http://health.usnews.com/health-news/health-insurance/articles/2013/08/19/will-obamacare-affect-medicare-myths-and-facts.

2. Medicare.gov (The Official U.S. Government Site for Medicare), http://www.medicare.gov/about-us/affordable-care-act/affordable-care-act.html.

3. As Inglis later noted, "I had to politely explain that 'Actually sir, your health care is being provided by the government.... But he wasn't having any of it." Philip Rucker, "Sen. DeMint of S.C. is Voice of Opposition to Health-Care Reform," *Washington Post*, July 28, 2009, http://www.washingtonpost.com/wp-dyn/content/article/2009/07/27/AR2009072703066.html?sid=ST2009072703107.

4. Lawrence D. Brown and Michael S. Sparer, "Poor Progress: The Unanticipated Politics of Medicaid Policy," *Journal of Health Politics, Policy and Law* (2003) 22, no. 1: 41.

5. http://www.medicaid.gov/AffordableCareAct/Medicaid-Moving-Forward-2014/Downloads/April-2014-Enrollment-Report.pdf.

6. http://www.cms.gov/Research-Statistics-Data-and-Systems/Statistics-Trends-and-Reports/MedicareEnrpts/index.html?redirect=/medicareenrpts/.

7. "Medicaid Moving Forward," Henry J. Kaiser Family Foundation, http://kff.org/medicaid/fact-sheet/the-medicaid-program-at-a-glance-update/. By the end of calendar year 2014, a Congressional Budget Office report estimated that another 7 million people more would be "enrolled in Medicaid and CHIP than would have been the case in the absence of the ACA." They predicted that 11 million more people (both those who had been eligible before for Medicaid and CHIP but also those newly eligible under the law) would sign on in 2015, bringing the total covered to nearly 25 million. They based their estimate on the premise that "more states will expand Medicaid eligibility." Congressional Budget Office, "Updated Estimates of the Insurance Coverage Provisions of the Affordable Care Act, April 2014," p. 11, https://www.cbo.gov/publication/45231.

8. Remarks at the dedication of the Hubert H. Humphrey Building, November 1, 1977, *Congressional Record*, November 4, 1977, vol. 123, p. 37287.

# MEDICARE AND MEDICAID AT 50

# PART I

# ORIGINS, VISION, AND THE CHALLENGE TO IMPLEMENTATION

Crafted during the tumultuous 1960s, Medicare legislation had been long debated and long planned; by contrast, Medicaid was a last-minute legislative concoction by Democrats, a small expansion of a pre-existing poverty program meant to ward off support for a watered down Republican alternative. Medicare was a national healthcare entitlement for the elderly; Medicaid was a federal-state partnership to aid a small segment of the poor. Advocates for the programs saw them as setting the stage for a broader array of national health insurance plans; detractors saw a nation moving perilously toward socialism.

The chapters in this section examine the vision, origins, and early implementation of these two programs in an era when-much like today-political fractiousness dominated. In Chapter 1, Julian Zelizer describes how and why these programs emerged from contentious times, and how the lack of consensus in Congress forced lawmakers to design programs that proved to be resilient and capable of dramatic expansion. David Barton Smith, in Chapter 2, examines how their passage at the height of the Civil Rights era meant the incorporation of civil rights ideals in their implementation, and how this convergence left a continuing legacy. Rashi Fein, in Chapter 3, offers the perspective of a policymaker who participated in the early design and implementation years. His analysis focuses on the pitched battles over Medicaid fees paid to physicians and the ways in which the politics of the poverty program diverged from that of the federal entitlement, Medicare. Finally, in Chapter 4, Jonathan Oberlander and Theodore Marmor examine just how different Medicare's trajectory has been from what its architects imagined in 1965, and how the ensuing political calculations and economic battles of the 1970s and 1980s undermined the view that Medicare would be a first step toward universal health coverage.

# THE CONTENTIOUS ORIGINS OF MEDICARE AND MEDICAID

## JULIAN E. ZELIZER

Recent discussions about the passage of the Affordable Care Act (ACA) displayed a marked nostalgia in comparing the political battle over President Obama's signature program to the struggle over Medicare and Medicaid in 1965. Pundits have pointed to a variety of aspects of modern politics—from the polarization of the political parties to the visceral anger among Tea Party Republicans toward anything that President Obama does—to explain why the president had so much trouble passing what looks like, in historical perspective, a moderate program. "The current debate," noted Brookings economist Henry Aaron, "is an order of magnitude more intense, dishonest, and verging on indictable than was the case with either of those two programs."[1] The same factors have been said to account for the ACA's difficult path to implementation, compared to the speedy one-year rollout of Medicare.

These claims about the origins of these programs have important implications for their futures. Some have expressed fear that the contentious origins of the ACA make it less likely that the program will survive over time. According to this outlook, programs with thin political support at the outset will encounter only stronger opposition in the years to come.[2] Yet the history of Medicare and Medicaid suggests a story with a different ending. The conventional wisdom gives a mistaken impression of the politics of the 1960s and the political foundation of our two largest national healthcare programs. Although it is true that the Social Security Amendments of 1965—the legislation that created both of these healthcare programs—passed on a bipartisan vote, the political struggle in these years was equally, if not more, contentious.

The argument that Medicare and Medicaid were built in a calmer atmosphere rests on two myths about this earlier period.[3] The first is that Washington once worked much better than it does today. Leaders from the more functional Congresses of the 1960s understood how to produce bipartisan compromise, while those of today do not. The second myth is of the strength of liberalism in the 1960s. The political marginalization of conservatives meant that liberals—whose ideas shaped the polity and whose leaders shaped the political world—could obtain support for the programs they desired.

It turns out that neither of these myths is accurate. Uncovering what's wrong with them goes a long way toward explaining how and why the federal government took on responsibility for health care in the 1960s after several false starts in previous decades. It also explains why that responsibility was, and remains, limited, even after the passage of the Affordable Care Act.

The first myth, about the way that Washington worked, doesn't make sense from the perspective of the period. The years leading up to the passage of Medicare and Medicaid saw the publication of a vast literature in the social sciences and journalism about the dysfunctional state of Washington. Then, too, Congress was the broken branch of government.

Whereas the problem today centers on the divisions between the political parties, bipartisanship itself posed a threat in the early 1960s. Bipartisan alliances between Southern Democrats and Midwestern Republicans on the key committees lay at the root of what one liberal senator, Joseph Clark, called the "Sapless Branch" of government. Since the late 1930s, Southerners had controlled a disproportionate number of committee chairmanships. In the House, these committee chairs formed a conservative coalition with Midwestern Republicans that blocked liberal legislation from ever reaching a vote on the floor. In the Senate, conservatives could rely on the filibuster (which then required 67 votes to end) if liberals somehow succeeded in sneaking a bill to the upper chamber. Liberals had watched bills such as anti-lynching legislation persistently die a procedural death at the hands of conservatives who used these tactics.

The Southern Democrats held this coalition together. Their power in Congress had forced liberalism to make huge compromises from the very start of the New Deal. Programs that would potentially tamper with the racial structure of Dixie were off limits. As a result, federal programs either delegated administration to state and local governments, which could be more tightly controlled by local Southerners sensitive to race relations, or omitted residents of the South altogether.[4]

The other relevant myth holds that healthcare legislation had a relatively easy pass through the supposed high point of a liberal era in American politics. But a recent generation of historians has rediscovered the immense power of conservatism in national politics after the New Deal and through the 1970s. Influential businessmen, for instance, devoted an enormous amount of resources to conservative political organizations and elected officials throughout this time period. Grass-roots conservatism, revolving around anti-communism, gained a strong foothold throughout the nation. The nomination of Barry Goldwater as the Republican presidential candidate in 1964 revealed the strong foothold that the Right was gaining within the GOP, even if the time was not quite right for a national candidate like him.[5]

Most important, the combination of the committee process and the dominant role of Southern Democrats turned Congress into a bastion of conservatism. The resurgence of conservatism on Capitol Hill had started after the 1936 Democratic landslide, in response to President Roosevelt's proposal to pack the Supreme Court and reorganize the executive branch. The resulting conservative coalition would continue to gain strength through the next two decades.[6] During the early 1960s, liberals found themselves continually frustrated with the coalition's ability to block their proposals—ranging from federal aid to education, to civil rights, to health care.

This was the political context in which liberal Democrats had tried, and failed, to pass a national healthcare plan for almost a generation. The struggle leading up to the passage of Medicare and Medicaid had been nothing short of explosive. Before cutting Social Security became the "third rail" of politics in the 1980s and 1990s, proposing health insurance had been the third rail of politics since the 1930s. President Franklin Roosevelt, who proved to be extremely bold in pursuing a number of social and economic policies, chose to leave health insurance for another time when he pushed for the creation of Social Security, fearing that dealing with the issue of medical care would stifle support for his other programs, given the positions of the American Medical Association (AMA). "It was my original belief," Edwin Witte, director of the President's Committee on Economic Security explained, "that it would probably be impossible to do anything about health insurance in a legislative way, due to the expected strong opposition of the medical profession."[7]

The first major effort by a president to push for national health care had disastrous results for liberals. When President Harry Truman proposed such a plan in 1949 in an attempt to capitalize on his upset re-election victory against Thomas Dewey, he suffered a devastating defeat at the hands of a Congress that included a significant Democratic majority in both the House and the Senate. Truman's proposal drew the ire of the AMA, which conducted a fierce lobbying campaign that equated universal health care with socialized medicine. In the heat of the Cold War, AMA officials warned that congressional passage of a national health insurance program would destroy American medicine—allowing government bureaucrats, rather than doctors, to dictate what decisions were made in the examination room—and would open the door to other kinds of programs that would quickly undermine the free market. The AMA's counteroffensive dwarfed the typical response of a professional association: its Washington-based lobbying campaign cost more than any similar effort by other organizations until that point in history. The leadership hired the public relations firm Whittaker and Baxter to put together a state-of-the-art advertising campaign against the bill. Michigan Congressman John Dingell blasted the multi-million dollar campaign of "misrepresentation" and "slander" and "untruth" which he said will "reach proportions which may well prove dangerous not only to the cause of Health Insurance, but to every liberal committed to the idea and may even have a detrimental affect upon the Democratic Party."[8] Dingell was right.

The association also worked at the grass-roots level, flooding districts with propaganda about the proposal's dangers. The campaign popularized the term "socialized medicine" into American political dialogue, warning that the proposal would bring "medical Soviets" into the United States.

The AMA enlisted physicians to spread information to their patients and to build opposition in key districts. According to Senator Howard McGrath, who supported Truman's plan, the AMA was prohibiting physicians who supported the legislation from speaking before medial associations and they imposed a gag rule on British physicians who came to the U.S. and praised their country's health care system. "This is medical dictatorship at its worst," McGrath said.[9] The doctors found ready allies in Congress, where the conservative coalition had no appetite for this plan. Leaders showed little interest in allowing the legislation to leave the key committees. At the outset of 1950, a year in which the AMA spent over $1 million on this issue, legislators in *both* parties were terrified to vote in favor of Truman. The AMA mounted successful campaigns to defeat two proponents of Medicare, Wisconsin Representative Andrew Biemiller and Florida Democrat Claude Pepper, both Democrats. "The doctors in Florida agreed that the first three minutes of every consultation with every patient," Senator Pepper later lamented, "would be devoted to attacking socialized medicine and Claude Pepper. They were so bitter that their wives took the streets and highways. They tried [to] paint me as a monster of some sort."[10] They received strong support from conservative organizations like the American Legion, which reminded members that their veterans had fought to protect the free enterprise system that had made possible the "highest standards of medical care and the finest medical institutions attained by any major country in the world…."[11]

The legislation was dead by the end of the year. "The Democratic high command," boasted Elmer Henderson, president of the AMA, "apparently is bowing to the public's reaction against any proposal for a compulsory health insurance program."[12] The defeat was so massive and so severe that program advocates assumed it would be impossible to build support for another proposal in the near future.

By 1957, healthcare proponents had recovered enough to try again, this time with a more limited proposal. Liberals introduced a program (sponsored by Congressman Aime Forand) that would provide national health insurance to the elderly through the Social Security system. Unlike some other safety net programs that had suffered in a climate of anti-communism, Social Security had become increasingly popular in the 1950s. The benefits, which were limited to covering the cost of hospital care for a specific period, would be paid for through the Social Security tax. Liberal advocates of the plan argued that a less ambitious proposal might stand a better chance of winning support in Congress. They also hoped that targeting a part of the population generally seen as "deserving" of assistance—the elderly—might help deflect attacks. Finally, liberals anticipated that connecting their proposal to Social Security might improve its chances of success. By linking the two programs in the public imagination, proponents hoped to win public opposition to their side by counteracting AMA claims about this program being some kind of anomalous, anti-American import from the Soviet Union. It wasn't socialized medicine, proponents said, it was the healthcare version of Social Security, a program that was the law of the land. Even with the limitations that building the program into Social Security entailed, the proposal's advocates envisioned health care for the elderly as a wedge that would pry open the gates to a more ambitious program later. They predicted that if Congress passed *this* legislation, they would gradually be able to win support for a broader program that covered the entire population.

The elderly faced severe health problems. With private employment plans in the manufacturing sector constituting the fastest-growing sector of health insurance in this period,[13] the elderly were left out in the cold. Many older Americans were unable to purchase adequate coverage. The burden for their care often fell on the shoulders of their families, welfare programs, and charitable organizations. Medical breakthroughs in the 1940s and 1950s, ranging from the advent of antibiotics to revolutionary surgical procedures for the heart, had only exacerbated this problem by increasing healthcare costs. As these services grew, hospitals expanded. The number of people employed by hospitals doubled from 1950 to 1964. Because people were living longer (8.7 percent of the population was over 65 in 1961, compared to 4 percent of the population at the turn of the century), elderly people made up a larger fraction of doctors' rolls.[14] The combination of longer life spans and a renaissance in curative medicine resulted in all sorts of new expenditures. Hospitalization insurance was quickly becoming a big part of healthcare costs. And even though the elderly remained a small percentage of the patient population in hospitals, they disproportionately lacked insurance.[15]

But liberals were too optimistic about their proposal and the inevitability of reform. The forces of conservatism remained strong, firmly aligned against them. Conservatives in Congress, including Wilbur Mills, the chairman of the Ways and Means Committee, which had jurisdiction over income taxation, Social Security, unemployment compensation, and trade, warned that the passage of Medicare would threaten Social Security by forcing Congress to raise payroll taxes beyond acceptable levels (at that point 10 percent of payroll). Others repeated the AMA's claims that this new plan was just as dangerous as Truman's, even if it appeared less ambitious. And yet others, particularly from the South, voiced concerns about the possible impact of a national health insurance program for the elderly on race relations.

One strategy of opponents in Congress was to pass a more limited health-care bill, something just large enough to show government action without actually doing very much. In 1960, Chairman Mills teamed up with Senator Robert Kerr to muster support for the Kerr-Mills bill, which created a means-tested healthcare program called "Medical Assistance for the Aged." This program would be funded by the federal government and the states, and administered by the states, for "medically indigent" elderly citizens. The welfare program would cover only a small portion of the population and provide very limited coverage. It depended on the states to make it work. As Michigan Senator Pat McNamara predicted, "The blunt truth is that it would be a miracle of the century if all of the states—or even a sizable number—would be in a position to provide the matching funds to make the program more than just a plan on paper."[16] Forand blasted the legislation as a meaningless bill that conservatives had used to try to stifle his proposal, but it nevertheless passed as the short-lived Medical Assistance for the Aged Program.

The election of Democrat John F. Kennedy in 1960 raised the hopes of liberals. The Massachusetts Senator had indicated in his campaign that he supported a national program to provide health care to the aged, which the media started to call "Medicare" (to the frustration of the administration, which feared that the label would cause the elderly to expect coverage of doctors' bills as well). Legislative sponsors again offered a version of the 1957 bill in Kennedy's first year in the White House. When Kennedy put forth the proposal, the conservative *Chicago Tribune* published a headline that read, "Assail Medicare as a Hoax."

The Kennedy administration mounted an uncharacteristically intense public relations campaign to promote the legislation. Ivan Nestigen, an official from the Office of Legislative Liaison, had convinced the president to be more outspoken about Medicare. He worked with a broad coalition that included the AFL-CIO, the National Council of Churches, and the American Public Welfare Association to create public pressure for reform. The administration coordinated with local groups of elderly citizens who organized protests in favor of the bill, and the Department of Health, Education, and Welfare (HEW) distributed information supportive of the proposal. A shift in public opinion followed, with a majority of voters supporting Medicare by the summer of 1962.

The campaign for Medicare extended well beyond the White House. The coalition behind Medicare included liberal legislators in the House and Senate who had entered into office during the 1950s and had been pushing for a wide-ranging program of liberal domestic policy for several years without much success.

A network of organizations with a mass membership basis formed a second part of the liberal coalition that would back Medicare in the 1960s. These organizations, which especially drew strength from organized labor and the civil rights movement, had partnered to push legislation designed to broaden access to the middle class and to provide more Americans with security from risk. In 1961, the AFL-CIO created the National Council of Senior Citizens for Health Care, the organization that would become the most visible lobbying force behind the Medicare legislation. Organized labor provided the Medicare cause with huge grass-roots support and connected the idea to social movement politics. Given organized labor's estimated membership at the time, which reached 30 percent of the workforce, it had substantial clout in Congress. Local Democratic officials helped out as well. The Democratic powerhouse in the Midwest, Chicago Mayor Richard Daley, instructed his precinct captains to conduct a petition drive to support the bill. "We've listened to charges of socialized medicine," Daley said, "under Franklin D. Roosevelt and Harry Truman, and now we're hearing it under John F. Kennedy."[17]

A rally and fundraiser attended by President Kennedy at Madison Square Garden in May 1962 marked the high point of this campaign. Approximately 17,500 people packed the Garden to watch the president—the last event in a public relations blitz that included over 30 smaller rallies that the AFL-CIO had organized in different parts of the nation to build support for the program—while an additional 2,500 sat outside in the scorching 90-degree heat just to listen to what he had to say. In a speech that was broadcast on national television and radio to 20 million people (smaller rallies were held in 45 other cities), Kennedy rebutted every argument that had been made by his opponents and called for immediate action: "This bill serves the public interest. It involves the Government because it involves the public welfare.

The Constitution of the United States did not make the President or the Congress powerless. It gave them definite responsibilities to advance the general welfare, and that is what we are attempting to do." The point of the rally was not so much to sway legislators, which many White House officials doubted could be accomplished through this kind of tactic, but rather to promote health care as an issue for the midterms, and even possibly for their 1964 presidential campaign. The speech was poorly delivered and uninspiring, one of Kennedy's least impressive, and failed to win much praise.

Even if the speech had been another Gettysburg Address, liberals could not simply steamroll their ideas through Congress. Once again, conservatives held their ground. The president of the AMA warned that the administration's Medicare proposal, which the organization again called "socialized medicine," was dangerous. The bill, he said, "would lower medical care, for it would introduce into our system of freely practiced medicine the elements of compulsion, regulation, and control." The AMA spent close to $100,000 to rent the Garden two nights after Kennedy's rally, and they purchased airtime on 190 television stations to respond to Kennedy's speech, calling the plan a "cruel hoax and a delusion." The plan would give insurance to millions of Americans who did not need it, said Dr. Edward Annis, who spoke from an empty Madison Square Garden (where viewers could still see the banners from Kennedy's rally),[18] and would destroy the private insurance system. Kennedy's plan, he warned, would "put the Government smack into your hospitals."[19]

The AMA doubled its spending, replicating the campaign that it had conducted against President Truman, but now spending even more money and sending out even more representatives to scare legislators off from voting for a bill. AMA officials blitzed congressional districts, making it clear that it would cause trouble for any legislator who was even thinking about voting yes for the plan. Members of the House remembered what had happened to Biemiller and Pepper in retaliation for their support of health care in 1950. The association visited senators and representatives in Washington to remind them that the AMA would make it worth their while to oppose the legislation. During the 1962 midterm campaigns, AMPAC, the political arm of the association, raised and donated $7 million to key players in the House, including all the relevant players on the House Ways and Means Committee.

The AMA organized a sophisticated operation involving the wives of association physicians. Enlisted participants held coffee klatches, which appeared informal but were in fact carefully orchestrated, with women in the local community. Over refreshments, the sponsors outlined all the dangers posed by the Medicare proposal and explained how socialized medicine remained a very real threat. At a key moment, the hostess played a recording by Ronald Reagan, a well-known conservative who had made a name for himself as the president of the actor's union and spokesman for General Electric, in which he railed against Medicare as a serious threat to capitalism and democracy. Reagan, who would run for governor of California in 1966, mesmerized listeners with his soaring rhetoric and polished delivery. He warned, "One of the traditional methods of imposing statism or socialism on a people has been by way of medicine. It's very easy to disguise a medical program as a humanitarian project, most people are a little reluctant to oppose anything that suggests medical care for people who possibly can't afford it."

Meanwhile, the AMA continued to scare legislators by communicating directly with their constituents. The association sent posters to doctors, entitled "Socialized Medicine and You," which were to be displayed in waiting rooms; it also provided pamphlets warning patients of the risks they faced should legislation pass. The doctors also placed immense pressure on members of the American Nurses Association to reverse the organization's position in favor of the bill—"unethical pressures," according to the nursing president.[20] When in 1962 a group of doctors in New Jersey, led by Dr. Bruce Henriksen in Point Pleasant, threatened to boycott a proposed Medicare program by having hospitals refuse to treat patients whose bills would be paid for with government funds, the head of the AMA defended the statement. "At no time was any threat made or intended," argued Dr. Edward Annis, "to deny care to those in need of it. In fact, it was to defend the principles of quality medicine which prompted this action."[21]

In contrast to the AMA, the health insurance lobby tended to work behind the scenes, focusing more on interacting with and distributing information to politicians rather than members of the public. Though they were immensely influential in the legislative debate, they remained far less visible to most Americans who followed the issue.[22]

The debate followed predictable battle lines in Congress. The toughest opponent remained Wilbur Mills, who continued to express concerns that Medicare would damage Social Security. Ignoring the efforts of organized labor to pressure him at the district level, he told the Kennedy administration that he did not have the votes to pass the bill in the House. To the frustration of Medicare supporters, Mills had a solid standing in the second district of Arkansas. He was known among his colleagues for a phantom Arkansas drawl that came and went, depending on whether he was speaking to constituents or Washington lobbyists and politicians. According to the AFL-CIO's Nelson Cruikshank, Mills conveyed the feeling that "he was so completely in control of his district that it didn't make any difference to him."[23] Mills didn't really care about Kennedy's public relations campaign. In fact, it just annoyed him and made him dig in even more. "To get a vote on Medicare in the House," legislative liaison Lawrence O'Brien explained, "we had to persuade Mills, and you don't persuade Mills with a rally in Madison Square Garden."[24]

Mills refused to let the bill come up for a vote up until the time of Kennedy's death in November 1963. Kennedy watched with frustration as the proposal languished in the House. Two days before Kennedy's death, *Washington Post* columnists Rowland Evans and Robert Novak wrote, "As long as Mills keeps opposing health care financed through the Social Security system, President Kennedy's plan is doomed in the Ways and Means Committee."[25] And worse, administration vote counters agreed with Mills that the votes to pass the bill simply were not there in the House. The administration had worked with liberal legislators to try everything, from redesigning the bill to "going public." But conservative opponents held the day.

The Kerr-Mills program, meanwhile, had turned out to be a stunning failure. Three years after the Medical Assistance for the Aged program was created, only 28 states had put it into operation. States had imposed such stringent guidelines that a very small portion of the population had received any benefits—less than 1 percent of the elderly as of July 1963. The kinds of benefits provided, and associated administrative costs, varied greatly by state. Wealthier states like New York and California received a disproportionate amount of federal funds. Few states used the benefits to reach new populations; instead, most simply shifted people already on welfare into the program.[26] Liberals remained more convinced than ever that the federal government needed to create a social insurance program for health care.

As vice president, Lyndon Johnson had demonstrated a commitment to the passage of Medicare throughout Kennedy's time in office—a commitment that he redoubled the moment that he took over the presidency.

Johnson immediately began implementing plans for what became known as the "Great Society," an attempt to expand and complete the social welfare vision of the New Deal. Johnson believed health care to be integral to the Great Society and Medicare a priority.

Even while Johnson secured breakthrough legislation in civil rights and poverty, he could not win support on Medicare during his first year in office. Mills and Johnson's Social Security team went over the proposal numerous times, revising and adjusting the numbers with the intention of finding a bill that could pass the House. There had been so many congressional hearings on Medicare between 1962 and 1964 that Congress had amassed 14,000 pages of testimony.[27] Despite all the discussion and negotiations, Mills still refused to let the bill out of committee, and, like Kennedy's team, Johnson's assistants couldn't identify enough support on the House floor. When the Senate added Medicare as an amendment to Social Security legislation that the House had passed as a way to circumvent Ways and Means, Mills killed the amendment during conference committee. Mills threatened to hold up vital revenue legislation if liberals insisted on the healthcare amendment. By the end of the year, the proposal was dead in committee; everything depended on the outcome of the election. "I don't know whether we can pass it next year or not," Johnson admitted to future Vice President Hubert Humphrey.[28]

The breakthrough finally took place after the 1964 election. Republican candidate Barry Goldwater, who had the backing of the AMA, had inadvertently aided the cause of Medicare by expressing his opposition to the plan in terms that alienated large segments of the voting public. (He also made statements about privatizing Social Security.) During the campaign, Johnson used the senator's opposition to Medicare as a key example of his extremism. Many congressional Democratic candidates had also made Medicare a central theme in their campaigns, promising to vote for the legislation if they came to Washington. In one ad, called "Medicare," viewers saw a boat in the ocean as the narrator said, "On September 1, 1964, Barry M. Goldwater interrupted his vacation cruise and headed for shore in a big hurry. Destination? Washington, D.C." The narrator continued: "He arrived just in time to cast his vote." A voice said, "No." Then the narrator concluded the ad by stating, "Then he turned around and headed back. Senator Goldwater flew across the continent twice, almost 6,000 miles, to vote against a program of hospital insurance for older Americans. As he said in the *Atlanta Constitution* on January 26, 1963, 'I've got my own Medicare plan. I've got an intern for a son-in-law.' Flip answers do not solve the problems of human beings. President Johnson wants a program of hospital insurance for older Americans."[29]

Experts believed that Goldwater's opposition to Medicare had been devastating to the GOP. Not a single incumbent in either party who had expressed his or her support for Medicare was defeated.[30] "Social Security and medical care were primary issues in 1964," Ohio Republican Frank Bow acknowledged, "and the Republican response on these issues was a major factor in the disaster that befell us."[31]

The outcome of the election temporarily transformed the legislative environment in Washington. The new Congress had huge Democratic majorities in both the House and the Senate, each filled with liberals who finally had the numbers, when allied with moderates in both parties, to outflank a diminished conservative coalition. Liberals took advantage of the new conditions in the House. They reinstituted the Twenty-One-Day rule, which empowered the majority to bring a bill directly to the floor even if the House Rules Committee refused to allow it for a vote. The House also changed the party ratios on all committees, with the new Republican Minority Leader Gerald Ford offering little resistance, based on the feeling they would be rolled. The changes resulted in the placement of three more pro-Medicare legislators on the House Ways and Means Committee (Tennessee's Richard Fulton, Georgia's Phil Landrum, and Ohio's Charles Vanik).

The scale of Barry Goldwater's devastating defeat also led a helping hand to liberals. Republicans felt so deflated after the election that few were willing to be associated with right-wing conservatism. Many Republicans shifted from merely opposing Medicare to proposing alternatives that might win more support than the administration's plan.

The successes of the civil rights movement had also increased the likelihood of passing healthcare legislation. The passage of the Civil Rights Act in the summer of 1964 made racial change inevitable by, among other things, banning the provision of federal funds to segregated services. The result was that Southern legislators now had more incentive to vote in favor of new federal services for their region, even if those funds threatened white supremacy, because it was now clear that racial desegregation was going to happen anyway. Why, then, turn away federal funds?

The result was that, in the first few months of 1965, the parties entered into a partisan competition to push for health care bills after decades of gridlock. Republicans offered two alternative versions of healthcare. Scholars, including some in this volume, continue to debate whether Lyndon Johnson (Morone and Blumenthal) or Wilbur Mills (Marmor, Starr, Zelizer) deserves more credit for the final legislative product.[32] Although this is an interesting and important question, neither man would likely have achieved success without the dramatic change in the political environment signaled by the election.[33] The new numbers gave Johnson the majorities he needed, while they made further opposition within Congress almost futile.

Republicans quickly shifted course. Wisconsin's John Byrnes, the ranking Republican on the House Ways and Means Committee, proposed legislation offering federal insurance to cover the cost of physician's bills, paid for by a premium from participants matched by federal money. Another alternative, proposed by Missouri Republican Thomas Curtis, backed an AMA-drafted plan that expanded the levels of benefits in the Kerr-Mills program. By now, however, policymakers largely regarded Kerr-Mills as a failure, and they doubted that an expansion would overcome its inherent limitations. As in 1960, the primary purpose of both plans was to siphon off support for a broader social insurance program.

President Johnson urged his legislative point man Wilbur Cohen to find some kind of compromise that Wilbur Mills would be able to claim as his own. Mills and Cohen were part of a tightly bound policy community composed primarily of experts from the executive and legislative branch, as well as related interest groups. During this era, social scientific policy experts worked closely together with relative autonomy from electoral politics.[34] This was an era when technocratic expertise commanded great support, and the political process gave elites considerable room to negotiate and compromise outside the public eye.

To the surprise of nearly everyone, including Cohen, Mills did precisely this during a conference committee when he came up with the famous "three-layer cake" structure for Medicare. Part A provided insurance for hospitalization, Part B insurance for doctors' visits, and Part C expanded the original Kerr-Mills benefits. The legislation combined aspects of all three proposals currently in circulation in the House. Part C, later called Medicaid, received the least attention because its predecessor program (Medical Assistance to the Aged) has been such a catastrophic failure that few thought the new legislation would have any serious impact.

Even in these final moments of the legislative debate in March 1965, when liberalism seemed strongest and Congress appeared to be a bill-making machine, liberals agreed to significant compromises designed to placate conservatives and ensure the bill's passage. One of the most consequential of these compromises, as Uwe Reinhardt (Chapter 9) and Jacob Hacker (Chapter 14) discuss in this volume, was to allow hospitals and doctors, rather than the federal government, to determine what fees they would charge for various services.[35]

The final vote in the House likewise revealed the fragility of the emerging consensus over Medicare. The House passed the Social Security Amendments by a 313 to 115 vote on April 7; 248 Democrats and 65 Republicans voted in favor of the bill. The Republican motion to substitute the Byrnes bill in its stead lost by only 236 to 191. The margin of victory for the final package was thus much narrower than the numbers on the roll call suggest; freshman Democrats made the difference in the passage of Medicare as we know it.[36]

As with the Affordable Care Act, the administrative body responsible for implementing the new healthcare program—in this case, the Social Security Administration—encountered problems in getting the program up and running. Approximately 700,000 eligible seniors failed to sign up for coverage in the program's first year, despite being eligible. "Medicare workers in Washington are learning that door-to-door selling is a rugged job," noted one reporter for *The Washington Post*. When officials went door to door, people would not open up or they would slam the door shut right in their face.[37] As David Barton Smith explores further in this volume, some hospitals in Southern states initially refused to accept federal funds in an effort to undermine the integration of their institutions. In Massachusetts, delays in federal reimbursements left many hospitals deep in debt, forced to borrow at high interest rates so that they could pay their employees.[38]

In retrospect, the reports of trouble were greatly exaggerated. By the end of the summer of 1966—one year after Congress had built it—Medicare and Medicaid were providing benefits to millions of elderly, disabled, and poor people.

The remainder of this volume will explore the history of Medicare and Medicaid since that time. Over the past 50 years, the program has alternately benefited from political consensus and suffered as an object of partisan conflict, but still it remains. Today, Medicare and Medicaid remain huge programs that consume a substantial part of the federal budget and arguably dominate US healthcare policy.[39] A central feature of the Affordable Care Act was to open up coverage to millions of Americans through Medicaid.

Contentious origins do not inevitably produce weak programs. During the 1960s, proponents of Medicare drew on certain advantages—pressure from social movements, the availability of autonomous policymaking spaces that gave experts and elected officials room to negotiate compromises, and the power of a transformative election—to overcome long-term resistance. Instead of hindering Medicare's future, the lack of consensus in Congress forced lawmakers to design programs that proved to be both resilient and capable of dramatic expansion. It is not too early to hope that the legislative history of the Affordable Care Act may produce similarly resiliency.

NOTES

1. Allison Linn, "You Think the Obamacare Fight Is Ugly?" *CNBC*, October 1, 2013.
2. Recent work by the political scientists Charles Shipan and Forrest Maltzman has demonstrated that programs that have greater roll call opposition at the time of passage are more likely to be amended in the future. Forrest Maltzman and Charles R. Shipan, "Change, Continuity and the Evolution of the Law," *American Journal of Political Science* 52, no. 2 (2008): 252–267.
3. For an exploration and critique of these myths, see Julian E. Zelizer, *The Fierce Urgency of Now: Lyndon Johnson, Congress and the Battle for the Great Society* (New York: Penguin, 2015).
4. Ira Katznelson, *Fear Itself: The New Deal and the Origins of Our Time* (New York: Norton, 2013).
5. Kim Phillips-Fein, *Invisible Hands: The Businessmen's Crusade Against the New Deal* (New York: Norton, 2010); Lisa McGirr, *Suburban Warriors: The Origins of the New American Right* (Princeton, NJ: Princeton University Press, 2002); Donald T. Critchlow, *Phyllis Schlafly and Grassroots Conservatism: A Woman's Crusade* (Princeton, NJ: Princeton University Press, 2007). For a review of the literature on conservatism, see Julian E. Zelizer, *Governing America: The Revival of Political History* (Princeton, NJ: Princeton University Press), 68–89.
6. Ira Katznelson, *Fear Itself: The New Deal and the Origins of Our Time* (New York: Liverlight, 2013).
7. David Blumenthal and James Morone, *The Heart of Power: Health and Politics in the Oval Office* (Berkeley: University of California Press, 2009), 34.

8. John Dingell to Harry Truman, 12 October 1950, Harry Truman Presidential Library, Online Documents.
9. Press Release, 21 March 1949, Harry Truman Presidential Library, Online Documents.
10. Jill Quadagno, *One Nation Uninsured: Why the U.S. Has No National Health Insurance* (New York: Oxford, 2006), 42.
11. American Legion, Resolution, January 1950, Harry Truman Presidential Library, Online Documents.
12. "Democrats Seen Yielding on Health Bill," *The Sun*, April 19, 1950.
13. David Blumenthal, "Employers-Sponsored Health Insurance in the United States—Origins and Implications," *The New England Journal of Medicine* 355, no. 1 (2006): 83.
14. John N. Wilford, "More Doctors Devote Full Time to the Aged; Research Outlays Rise," *Wall Street Journal*, January 12, 1961.
15. Rosemary A. Stevens, "Health Care in the Early 1960s," *Health Care Financing Review* 18, no. 2 (Winter 1996): 12–22.
16. Theodore R. Marmor, *The Politics of Medicare*, 2nd ed. (New York: Aldine, 2000), 28–29.
17. Ron Grossman, "Affordable Care Act Traveled Road Similar to Medicare in 1960s," *Chicago Tribune*, September 29, 2013.
18. John Dickerson, "KennedyCare," *Slate*, November 7, 2013, http://www.slate.com/articles/news_and_politics/history/2013/11/john_f_kennedy_s_health_care_failure_jfk_and_barack_obama_s_tough_fights.html.
19. Peter Kihss, "AMA Rebuttal to Kennedy Sees Aged Care 'Hoax,'" *New York Times*, May 22, 1962.
20. James L. Sundquist, *Politics and Policy: The Eisenhower, Kennedy, and Johnson Years* (Washington, DC: Brookings, 1968), 309.
21. Ralph Chapman, "AMA Backs Rebel Doctors; Truman Hits Them," *New York Herald Tribune*, May 10, 1962.
22. Wilbur Cohen, interview with Peter A. Corning, July 20, 1966, Interview 1, Columbia University Social Security Project: Oral History (Columbia Center for Oral History, New York), 26–27.
23. Nelson Cruikshank, interview by Peter A. Corning, February 15, 1966, Interview 2, Columbia University Social Security Project: Oral History (Columbia Center for Oral History, New York), 83–89.
24. Michael O'Brien, *John F. Kennedy: A Biography* (New York: Dunne, 2005), 569.
25. Rowland Evans and Robert Novak, "He Cannot Sway Wilbur Mills on Medicare," *The Washington Post*, November 20, 1963.
26. US Senate, Special Committee on Aging, *Medical Assistance for the Aged: The Kerr-Mills Program, 1960–1963*, October 1963.
27. Sue A. Blevins, *Medicare's Midlife Crisis* (Washington, DC: Cato, 2001), 44.
28. Recording of Telephone Conversation between Lyndon B. Johnson and Hubert Humphrey, October 1, 1964, 9:46 p.m., Citation #5802, Recordings and Transcripts of Conversations and Meetings, LBJ Presidential Library, Austin, Texas.
29. "Medicare," *LivingRoomCandidate.Com*.

30. Jill Quadagno, *One Nation, Uninsured: Why the U.S. Has No National Health Insurance* (New York: Oxford University Press, 2006), 71.
31. Irving Bernstein, *Guns or Butter: The Presidency of Lyndon Johnson* (New York: Oxford University Press, 1996), 170.
32. Blumenthal and Morone, *The Heart of Power*; Julian E. Zelizer, *Taxing America: Wilbur D. Mills, Congress, and the State, 1945–1975* (New York: Cambridge University Press, 1999); Marmor, *The Politics of Medicare*; Paul Starr, "The Health-Care Legacy of the Great Society," in *Reshaping the Federal Government: The Policy and Management Legacies of the Johnson Years*, eds. Norman J. Glickman, Laurence E. Lynn, and Robert H. Wilson (forthcoming).
33. Zelizer, *The Fierce Urgency of Now*.
34. Zelizer, *Taxing America*.
35. Paul Starr, *Remedy and Reaction: The Peculiar American Struggle over Health Care Reform* (New Haven, CT: Yale University Press, 2013).
36. Sundquist, *Politics and Policy*, 319.
37. Sarah Kliff, "When Medicare Launched, Nobody Had a Clue Whether It Would Work," *The Washington Post*, May 17, 2013. Stephen Mihm, "Medicare Had Messy Rollout Too," *Bloomberg*, October 15, 2013.
38. Herbert Black, "Lag in Medicare Pay Has Hospitals in Red," *Boston Globe*, September 17, 1966.
39. Colleen Grogan and Eric M. Patashnik, "Between Welfare Medicine and Mainstream Entitlement," *Journal of Health Politics, Policy, and Law* 28, no. 5 (2003): 821–858.

...

# 2

# CIVIL RIGHTS AND MEDICARE
## HISTORICAL CONVERGENCE AND CONTINUING LEGACY

DAVID BARTON SMITH

Most accounts of the United States' civil rights struggle and the creation of Medicare treat them as unrelated stories, as if their convergence in the mid-1960s was accidental. And yet, the idea that the two most transformational events in the last century in both our troubled history of race relations and in the organization and financing of health care would take place at the same time and be unrelated makes no sense. What happened?

Few mentioned it at the time; indeed, most of the key actors had reason *not* to call attention to it. The federal government architects of the Medicare program—Wilbur Cohen, Robert Ball, Arthur Hess, and others—sought to avoid a backlash that could destroy Medicare's chances of passage as well as its implementation. Southern politicians hoping to obtain credit for getting something for their constituents convinced themselves that their districts' "racial sensibilities" would be discretely accommodated, as they always had been in the past. Hospitals welcomed the possibility of new income streams. Within hospitals, an organizational culture that stressed calm and stability encouraged administrators to understate upsetting changes to their patients, their staffs, and the communities they served. A low-key approach also served the interests of civil rights activists. Although—as we shall see—activists played a central role in the implementation of the Medicare program, their adversaries only learned about it afterward.

At a deeper level, race has always been a concealed part of the logic of "American exceptionalism" that makes the United States the only remaining developed nation lacking some form of universal health insurance coverage for all its citizens. Race—and the logic of white supremacy—is hidden in the compromise patchwork solutions, the expansion of private insurance, the creation of producer cooperative solutions in the form of voluntary Blue Cross plans, the creation of the dominant voluntary hospitals sector, the ideology of individualism, the opposition to public solutions, and the promotion of freedom of choice and free market solutions that have dominated, and continue to dominate, health care in the United States. All of these policy choices have a disparate impact on blacks and other disadvantaged minority groups. The notion of "social solidarity," so frequently invoked as an explanation of the social insurance systems of other countries, never came up as an argument for similar universal protections in the United States. Only during the civil rights convulsions of the 1960s did the notion of "being all in it together" have any salience. Medicare, in its essence, was the gift of the civil rights struggle.

The civil rights movement's gift forced the racial and economic desegregation of American hospitals. This feat generated few headlines, no film footage for the nightly news, and next to no attention from scholars. Yet, it is an important story. In many respects, what the civil rights movement and those implementing the Medicare program were able to accomplish together was the most significant legacy of both. American hospitals went from being the nation's most racially and economically segregated institutions to its most integrated. This chapter summarizes the story.

## THE OLD ORDER

Most readers, lacking memories of the medical world that existed prior to the passage of Medicare and Medicaid, take too much for granted. It's all too easy to be persuaded to feel nostalgic about the past. Much of that past was shameful.

A brutal iron law determined the amount and quality of care you received. The more money and the more private insurance you had, the more care you got. Hospital admissions, physician visits, specialty and preventive care all followed this pattern. Unfortunately, the poorer you were, and the less private insurance you had, the more likely you were to be sick and in need of care. This system, in other words, allocated care directly in relationship to income and insurance coverage and inversely in relation to need. Care tended to be rigidly segregated by income. Poor people received care in the stark charity wards of hospitals, in urban public hospitals, or in the clinics of medical schools and teaching hospitals. That involved block scheduling, wooden benches, long waits, and few of the protections that now exist for people who were then regarded, for the most part, as just research and teaching material.

Blacks were assigned to the lowest tier of this caste system of care. In the South and most border states, blacks obtained care in segregated clinics and or in private practices often outfitted with separate waiting rooms where one would wait until all the white patients in a separate, better-appointed waiting room had been seen. Hospital care in the South was rigidly segregated by race. Many hospitals excluded blacks altogether or cared for them on "colored wards," often in the basement or in an adjoining building. In large part because of this exclusion, the majority of black babies were born at home—a situation reflected in disparities in infant and maternal mortality rates.[1] Income, education, and social status made no difference for blacks trying to get access to care. Even the families of black physicians, who were growing in affluence, found themselves excluded as patients.[2]

Nor could black physicians obtain privileges at most mainstream hospitals or participate in most specialty training programs. Ironically, this exclusion insulated them from white control and thus thrust them into civil rights leadership roles in many Southern communities. Medical segregation inadvertently supplied the critical backbone of the emerging civil rights movement.

The federal government's Hill-Burton program was complicit in supporting this old order. Passed in 1946, the Act provided federal grants and loans for upgrading US hospital facilities. Obtaining these funds required assurances that the facility "will be made available to all persons residing in the territorial area of the applicant without discrimination on account of race, creed or color, but an exception shall be made in cases where separate hospital facilities are provided for separate population groups, if the plan makes equitable provision on the basis of need for facilities of like quality for each group."[3] While the Hill-Burton Act was the only federal act providing explicit support in the twentieth century for "separate but equal" Jim Crow arrangements, most other federal funding, while never explicitly acknowledging it, heavily subsidized such practices. As a Civil Rights Leadership Council report in 1961 documented, federal tax dollars flowed disproportionately from Northern to Southern states, providing a massive federal subsidy for Jim Crow practices at the expense of taxpayers in Northern states that barred such arrangements.[4]

## THE CIVIL RIGHTS ACT OF 1964 AND MEDICARE

Both the Kennedy and Johnson administrations, concluding that caution was the better part of valor, followed rather than led in the civil rights struggle. Kennedy delayed for more than two years in introducing the civil rights legislation he had promised during his campaign, allowing grass-roots civil rights activists to take the lead. He introduced his bill under duress, as public pressure mounted in reaction to the nightly news images of young demonstrators in Birmingham attacked by police dogs, battered by fire hoses, and packed into its jail. The most controversial section of the civil rights bill, Title VI, prohibited the provision of federal funds to organizations or programs that discriminated on the basis of race. Its inclusion was influenced by the Kennedy administration's belated decision to join in a federal court case, *Simkins v. Moses Cone*, that challenged the constitutionality of the separate but equal provision in the Hill-Burton program.

Upon assuming the presidency after Kennedy's assassination, Johnson began an awkward courtship of the civil rights movement. As a Southerner, he faced a special challenge as a result of the growing influence of the civil rights struggle in shaping public opinion. Johnson had to prove his civil rights credentials in a way that Kennedy never had. His skillful orchestrating of the passage of the civil rights bill, overcoming the longest filibuster in Senate history, helped assure a landslide victory in the presidential election. That victory, in turn, produced the Medicare Act.

Johnson had the full support of all the civil rights activists in both the election and the passage of Medicare—now he owed them for both. Johnson invited Montague Cobb, MD, the president of the National Medical

Association (NMA), to be the sole representative of the medical profession at the Medicare signing ceremony at the Truman Presidential Library in Independence, Missouri. The NMA, representing black physicians, had been waging a fierce battle to desegregate hospitals and their medical staffs since 1953. The organization's decision to support the bill—it was the only national medical society to do so—had widened the gulf between it and the American Medical Association.

With Johnson on their side, black medical activists saw their best opportunity yet to undo federal support for a segregated healthcare system. On paper, Title VI of the Civil Rights Act gave them precisely the leverage they needed. The Act explicitly prohibited the flow of federal funds to any institution or program that discriminated on the basis of race. So far, however, Title VI had proved to be a paper tiger. It prescribed no fines and provided no periodic reporting, subpoena powers, or, most important, resources for its enforcement. Individuals could file complaints. A complaint-driven system of enforcement, however, shifts the burden of proof onto victims, who might well fear retaliation. In the first year after the passage of the Civil Rights Act, the Johnson administration focused on encouraging voluntary compliance. As a few courageous hospitals in the South learned, this didn't work. White flight followed desegregation, punishing compliance and rewarding hospitals that flaunted the new law. In the face of hospital intransigence, the Department of Health Education and Welfare (HEW) appeared to have few options to force medical desegregation.

The unanticipated consequence of not providing HEW with adequate tools to investigate Title VI compliance was to shift control over its enforcement to the civil rights movement. The Medical Committee for Human Rights (MCHR; a group organized to provide a medical presence at civil rights demonstrations in the South), the NMA, and the National Association for Colored People's Legal Defense Fund (NAACP-LDF) all began doing volunteer field investigations of hospitals in the summer of 1965 with HEW's encouragement. They submitted more than 300 Hill-Burton Title VI complaints against hospitals, provided intelligence that would later be put to use in developing an enforcement offensive, and began a strained partnership that increasingly blurred the boundaries between activists and the federal officials enforcing Title VI in hospitals.

By December 1965, civil rights activists and top HEW officials had all come independently to much the same conclusion: the pending implementation of the Medicare program offered the best chance to make Title VI work, but only if more resources could be devoted to the effort.

The goal of developing a shared agenda got off to a rocky start. An unsuccessful effort by civil rights activists to meet with HEW Secretary John Gardner on December 7, 1965, turned into an impromptu press conference outside the secretary's office. John Holloman, representing the NMA and MCHR, and Conrad Harper, from the NAACP, accused HEW of failing to implement desegregation policy in the medical field. Medicare, they claimed, offered "a golden opportunity to wipe out discrimination in southern hospitals."[5] They pledged to enlist the support of other civil rights groups in an effort to pressure HEW. Holloman then fired off a telegram to the secretary, accusing him of freely meeting with conservative elements of the medical establishment and questioning his commitment to racial justice. That same day, the NAACP-LDF released a damning report on the failure of HEW to enforce Title VI, insisting that no Medicare funds be released to hospitals that were not in compliance.

The Johnson administration had not fully anticipated the consequences of the passage of Medicare on its civil rights responsibilities. Following the recommendation of Vice President Hubert Humphrey, Johnson had endorsed an approach in which the individual federal agencies making the funding decisions took responsibility for Title VI compliance.[6] This policy set in motion a Medicare Title VI enforcement effort with a momentum all its own. In a December 14, 1965, memo to HEW executives, Secretary Gardner began transforming this decentralized approach into a plan. "This is too important to be treated as anything less than the highest priority in our total program.... The key is adequate staffing. We must assign as large a part of our staff resources to this activity as required to assure effective administration.... The heads of each operating agency will be held responsible for meeting this requirement along with all other responsibilities."[7] Gardner had, in effect, transformed all of HEW into a civil rights enforcement agency.

Gardner's memo set Johnson's two signature pieces of legislation on a collision course. Medicare, the Civil Rights Act, or both might be destroyed in the process, but there was no turning back. The hospital Title VI certification for Medicare had, in effect, been turned over to the civil rights movement. Those responsible for the implementation of the Medicare Program and those concerned about assuring the integrity of Title VI clung to the same raft in treacherous rapids. In March 1966 they would plunge together over the falls with no bottom in sight.

THE SHORT HAPPY LIFE OF THE OFFICE OF
EQUAL HEALTH OPPORTUNITY

In February 1966, the Surgeon General's Office of the US Public Health Service created the Office of Equal Health Opportunity (OEHO) as the agency specifically responsible for certifying hospitals wishing to become Medicare providers for compliance with Title VI. It had a staff of five. More than 6,000 hospitals would have to be certified compliant by July 1966. Most hospitals in the South were noncompliant. Many in the North, though compliant on paper, in practice were not. Northern hospitals too frequently shuttled black patients to welfare wards no matter their insurance status and, in many cases, matched multiple occupancy rooms by race. Blacks who were otherwise qualified were still excluded from medical staff privileges and admission to hospital-based nursing schools in many Northern hospitals.

As OEHO had defined the stakes, those hospitals wishing to participate in the Medicare program could not just offer assurances of good intentions as of July 1, 1966. They had to be fully, genuinely, racially integrated. At the very least, the hospital had to meet the "smell test" of local civil rights groups. This had never been a part of the original game plan of those crafting the Medicare program.

Gardner appointed Peter Libassi, a key staff member of the Civil Rights Commission, as his Special Assistant for Civil Rights in January 1966. Libassi was responsible for coordinating HEW's civil rights efforts in health, education, and welfare for Gardner. Tension simmered between Libassi and the tightly knit team that had long been immersed in the intricate political, administrative, and technical details of transforming the idea of Medicare into a reality.[8] The whole implementation process had suddenly become dependent on an odd-couple partnership between the orderly, detail-oriented team of professional civil servants at HEW and a messy, chaotic, emotional, and inventive grass-roots social movement and its newly recruited activists at OEHO.

Whether by intent or accident, the design of the implementation plan was ingenious. The delegation of Title VI certification to OEHO freed the team at the Social Security Administration, led by Commissioner Robert

Ball, to develop the mechanical details of how the program would work with hospitals and physician groups. Thus Social Security officials could play "the good cops," leaving the "bad cop" job to the new office buried deep within HEW's bureaucracy. The Social Security Administration's reputation as a highly professional, apolitical agency also provided wonderful cover for the revolutionary intentions of the OEHO operation. The Social Security Administration had a large, experienced national workforce and a team of central planners widely respected by the leadership of both parties. As a result, as Ball would later reflect about the experience, "there was almost complete delegation of authority and responsibility to the Social Security Administration from higher levels. I don't think I can exaggerate the degree of this, the thought from above was: 'we are not going to try to, in any way, interfere with the agency's sole responsibility to put this in effect.'"[9] OEHO benefited from both the cover and the full delegation of certifying powers. Indeed, the insulation between the two operations was so complete that Ball never even met the OEHO's director, Robert Nash.[10]

In effect, delegating Title VI enforcement to the OEHO meant delegating it to the civil rights movement. This was hardly the only aspect of Medicare's implementation delegated to outside interest groups. Medicare borrowed its cost-based reimbursement system for hospitals from the design of Blue Cross plans, which were still essentially operated as hospital insurance cooperatives. The Joint Commission on Accreditation of Hospitals (JCAH), a voluntary organization established by hospital and medical associations, screened hospitals to ensure their compliance with Medicare's quality standards. Decisions involving costs and standards of care were routinely delegated to doctors and hospitals, the very parties, as several contributors to this volume remind us, who stood to benefit financially from the program. In fact, the Title VI certification process represented the only Medicare provider requirement delegated to broader consumer groups. OEHO was, in effect, the only broader public interest guardian at the gate to Medicare.

Delegating Title VI certification to the OEHO involved huge risks, to the point that most former OEHO staff I interviewed refused to believe that the decision could not have been made without approval and support from the top. It was one thing for HEW's secretary to reluctantly acknowledge that Title VI would be applicable to the Medicare legislation without any elaboration during its consideration in the Senate, and quite another to acknowledge what that actually meant in terms of how it would be implemented in the program. Many of these staff members believe that there had to have been a meeting between Johnson and Gardner, possibly in January or February of 1966, where "the decision" to aggressively enforce Title VI was made. I have been unable to find any record of such a meeting. Given the Johnson administration's commitment to delegating compliance with the Civil Rights Act, it is entirely possible that the process simply developed a momentum of its own and, once started, could not be stopped. In this respect, the "decision," or lack thereof, may well have been the domestic equivalent of the "decision" to escalate the war in Vietnam.

In any event, on March 4, 1966, the highest-stakes poker game in the history of federal domestic policy began. Every hospital in the country received a letter over the Surgeon General's signature describing the guidelines for compliance. The letter asked the administrator to sign and return an enclosed Assurance Form and a brief questionnaire by March 15. "We will review the questionnaires as they arrive and if any deficiencies are noted we will let you know so that you can take necessary action to correct them. Representatives of the Department of Health, Education, and Welfare will be visiting hospitals on a routine periodic basis to supplement this information and to be of further assistance in resolving any problems that may arise."[11]

Shortly before this, Gardner quietly approved the temporary volunteer transfers of staff from other parts of HEW to the OEHO. With their salaries and travel costs covered by their home agencies, these "temporary transfers" remained off the books of OEHO. They proved a source of surprise and consternation in Washington when elected officials began to hear about the inspections from hospitals in their constituencies. Anyone in HEW could request the temporary reassignment; eventually, about 1,000 volunteers transferred to the OEHO. The agency's strange ragtag army included local Social Security field managers from the South, bench scientists from the National Institutes of Health, Public Health Service nurses, pharmacists from the Food and Drug Administration, even a "medical officer from the Indian Health Service complete with an Eskimo secretary."[12]

The volunteers did not, however, represent a random slice of HEW employees. Many were already involved with the civil rights movement and saw the temporary voluntary transfers as an opportunity to incorporate their activism into their day jobs. While few of the Southern volunteers from the Social Security Administration had been active in the civil rights movement, almost all could recount troubling experiences they were powerless to stop; volunteering for the OEHO gave them an opportunity to demonstrate where they really stood on issues of racial equity. Over the summer, OEHO provided jobs for 60 similarly motivated medical students to serve on the hospital inspection teams. The volunteers, whether civil servants or medical students, and whether or not they fully understood the risks they were taking, joined to do their part to make the ideals of the civil rights movement a reality. No one had to be drafted.

The OEHO's director, Robert Nash, was the right field commander for this passionate army of volunteer bureaucrats. A Southerner and a low-profile civil servant, he reportedly told one of his recruits, "If I don't want to take on a hospital, I'll refer it to General Council for advice. Three months later they will get back to me with a reason why I should not do anything. If I want to take on a hospital, I'll just use my own lawyers and do it."[13] He, along with the volunteers that joined him, wanted to act.

Volunteers received varied levels of training; some attended hastily cobbled together two-day training sessions, while others just learned on the job. The first set of these workshops, held in Atlanta in early April 1966, provided training for about 250. A second workshop in Dallas, a month later, trained another 125 federal officials.[14] Representatives from across the civil rights movement, from the American Jewish Committee and the Anti-Defamation League to the Southern Christian Leadership Conference and the Student Nonviolent Coordinating Committee, participated as observers and consultants. The doctor-activists who had formerly criticized HEW—Hubert Eaton, John Holloman, and Charles Watts—also served as consultants. The absence of representatives from the mainstream medical and hospital trade associations is notable.

Those volunteers with experience in the civil rights movement knew what to expect, but no amount of training could have prepared the unseasoned recruits for what they encountered. They nevertheless proved, for the most part, resilient and resourceful. In some Southern towns, rental car agencies collaborated with local police to ensure that OEHO investigators received vehicles with missing paperwork; the police then arrested the drivers for possession of a stolen car.[15] Local officials made the case to investigators that people should be "free" to choose whether they would go to the previously colored or white ward or whether they would be willing to share a room with a patient of a different race. The OEHO inspectors didn't budge. The only "choice" for a hospital was whether it wanted to participate in the Medicare program, and the only "choice" for patients was whether they wanted to go to a hospital qualified for Medicare. There could be no "freedom of choice" because patients would not "choose" to desegregate a facility on their own for fear of retaliation. Everyone had to be "all in it together."[16]

Frank Weil, one of the more experienced civil rights movement recruits to OEHO in 1966, proved particularly adept at circumventing obstructionism. "I got shot at but they missed, although Hertz was somewhat miffed when I turned in a car with bullet holes."[17] When Weil suspected a hospital of doing the "HEW shuffle" (shifting patients around just for the inspection), he made the required advance notice from a phone booth around the corner. Having learned that the Louisiana Red Cross continued to segregate the state's blood supply, he made a policy decision on the spot. "I didn't know whether I really had the authority or not, I just sent a telegram to the President of the Louisiana Hospital Association that ALL the hospitals in Louisiana would not be in compliance with Title VI until the blood supply in Louisiana was integrated." It was integrated in a matter of hours.[18]

The OEHO volunteers would not have succeeded without the "invisible army" of local civil rights activists, which included hospital employees. Local allies made it impossible for a hospital to conceal any noncompliance. Investigators had to plan their meetings with these individuals carefully in advance to keep them from being fired by the hospital. One investigator recalled meeting a contact after going into the lingerie section of the town's department store to evade a police officer who was following her:

> A cop in uniform was usually unwilling to go into ladies lingerie, and you'd go down the stairs and out the back door, and your contact would take you to the meeting. There, the local NAACP or church group would meet with you and some of the black employees of the hospital. They'd go over the floor plans of the hospital with you and show you where the black lunchroom was.... You'd then go on the visit and the hospital administrator would take you on a tour. You'd go down to the basement where the black cafeteria was and he'd say, "Well, why we don't go this way," and you'd say, "No, we'd like to go this way." You'd then walk into the shabby black staff lunchroom.[19]

The investigators recruited from Southern Social Security offices often were able to gain compliance with less resistance, through some combination of

Southern charm and local connections. Southern hospital administrators frequently requested that the OEHO "do us first" as a way of indicating that they wanted to comply, but needed the Feds to take the heat.[20] From a business perspective, administrators saw segregation as a drag on operating expenses that simultaneously limited the patient population and required a duplication of staffing and equipment. Many administrators of Jim Crow hospitals therefore welcomed the pending changes. Southern investigators emphasized that no one was forcing the hospitals' actions. After all, hospital administrators had signed the Title VI assurance and had indicated their desire to participate in the Medicare program; the OEHO representatives were simply helping them fulfill this commitment. One volunteer recalled that most of the hospital administrators were the kind of people who "would make a full stop at a stop sign in the middle of the night. If they said they would do something, they would do it."[21]

Some situations required special handling. Richard Smith, MD, was assigned to put extra pressure on a Texas hospital of particular interest to President Johnson. Marshall Hospital, in Lady Bird Johnson's home county, needed to be brought into compliance. Smith, having announced his visit, found himself escorted to the hospital by a caravan of locals in pickups with shotguns. The administrator would not be budged; he insisted that the hospital would never desegregate. "Fine," Smith finally replied, "but you just tossed away $100 million in Medicare funding." A week later, Smith got a call from the chairman of the hospital's board. "The trustees have just fired the administrator and want to know what they had to do to desegregate and get the Medicare money."[22]

The transformations demanded by the OEHO went well beyond cosmetic changes. Far from just eliminating the "white" and "colored" signs on the doors and waiting rooms, hospitals had to remove opportunities for self-segregation. Doors, waiting rooms, and the flow of patients had to be rethought so that white patients could not avoid their black neighbors. The certification process was designed to change behavior, not attitudes.

The line between the civil rights movement and the OEHO had blurred. OEHO now represented an unusual and perhaps unique example of "regulatory capture," not by the industry being regulated, but by a social movement seeking to transform it. At the first training session, in April, a debate erupted over who owned and controlled the meeting. Some argued that OEHO should force the desegregation of all hospitals (the position of the civil rights groups), while others argued that the agency should focus only on those hospitals that had signed the nondiscrimination assurance and wished to participate in Medicare (the official position of the Social Security Administration).[23] In the end, since almost all hospitals ended up applying to participate, the distinction didn't matter.

## THE FINAL PUSH

For the most part, the OEHO operated in a world unto itself. Marvin Watson, the president's appointment secretary and chief political watchdog, asked for weekly reports on the hospitals certified. But other than asking for special efforts to gain compliance from hospitals in Texas that might prove politically embarrassing to the president, Watson did not interfere in the decision process. As implementation approached, these reports became weekly face-to-face meetings.[24]

By mid-spring, the OEHO had started to come under more pressure, but only in terms of getting the job done, on time, without compromising the level of compliance. In early April, Dr. Philip R. Lee, an assistant to Gardner, had a meeting with Gardner, Ball, and other senior HEW officials in which Gardner "let us know in no uncertain terms that he was not at all satisfied with the progress that had been made up to that time; that he wanted us to devote whatever resources were necessary to assure maximum compliance on the part of hospitals. . . . The Secretary was absolutely firm in his decision that we would not compromise with the requirements, the issue of civil rights was too important to compromise."[25]

In the last month before the start of Medicare, White House concerns grew that the bluff on Title VI enforcement in Medicare might not work. A staff report to the president on May 23, 1966, concluded that, while no national embarrassment from hospital noncompliance loomed, some of the Southern states posed serious problems. OEHO had only limited options: "Waive compliance for an additional time period which would obviously encourage recalcitrance, refuse certification of some of the more recalcitrant areas as a demonstration that resistance will not be allowed and, for the moment, ignore other noncompliance or ban all financial assistance to all non-complying institutions." Moreover, the report warned that Alabama Governor George Wallace, a prominent and politically powerful segregationist, was threatening to turn noncompliance into a regional cause.

The staffer recommended that "a final course of action not be determined until we are close to June 30" to give Gardner and his OEHO force as much operational room as possible.[26]

The workload and pressure on "Gardner's force" grew. "Everyone worked eighteen to twenty hours a day. We used a hotel room near Social Security just to shower and change clothes," one staff member reported.[27] Weil reported sleeping on a cot in his office.[28]

In the last few days before the beginning of the Medicare program, Johnson, some of his White House staff, and Secretary Gardner became even more nervous. Ball, meanwhile, had organized an emergency task force in HEW, complete with a situation room. A map with pins indicated possible trouble spots where a surge in admissions might overwhelm the capacity of local hospitals. A good part of the concern, as Ball put it, was to be able to "take action in anticipation of problems under Medicare arising from the application of the Civil Rights Act to hospitals."[29] About half of the hospitals in Alabama, Mississippi, Louisiana, and South Carolina had still not been certified for Title VI as of mid-June. With Johnson's support, the task force placed National Guard helicopters on standby and developed plans for transporting patients refused admission by local hospitals to military and Veterans Administration facilities.

Just a few days before the July 1 deadline, Ted Marmor, an assistant to Wilbur Cohen, the undersecretary of HEW, was one of several civil servants summoned to a meeting at the White House with Watson. "You tell your boss," Watson told Marmor, "I don't want any screw ups, no hitches! You have helicopters ready. I don't want any stories about anyone dying because they were refused hospital care!"[30] By now, as this statement makes clear, the Johnson administration was committed to desegregating hospitals. Watson could have possibly demanded that Gardner and his staff certify the hospitals. Instead, whatever misgivings they had, they braced for possible confrontation.

On June 30, 1966, on the eve of Medicare's implementation, Johnson celebrated its inauguration in a televised address: "The program is not just a blessing for older Americans. It is a test for all Americans—a test of our willingness to work together. In the past we have always passed that test. I have no doubt about the future. I believe that July 1, 1966, marks a new day of freedom for our people."[31]

Certainly the Office of Equal Health Opportunity had met the test. Approximately 3,000 hospitals had been quietly, uneventfully, and successfully desegregated in less than three months. No helicopters or backup military hospitals were needed. (While Medicare permitted the payment of "emergency" admissions to nonparticipating hospitals, and many hospitals in the South that had yet to gain Title VI approval took advantage of this, that loophole was soon closed.) A key part of national life, one involved in healing our bodies, was now involved in healing our body politic. A social institution that had lagged behind in racial integration was now leading the way.

## What Happened?

It is not a coincidence that the implementation of the Medicare Program in the summer of 1966 coincided with the high tide of the civil rights movement. They were hopelessly intertwined. Medicare, the result of a landslide election propelled by the passage of the Civil Rights Act and the civil rights movement that shadowed its implementation, was a gift of that movement. Civil rights activism had attended the birth of the Medicare and Medicaid programs, fundamentally reshaping the organization and delivery of health care in the United States.

Hospitals became the most racially and economically integrated private institutions in the nation. Within a decade, all but four or five of the once more than five hundred black hospitals had either been closed or converted to other purposes.[32] Most of the public hospitals that had exclusively served the indigent either closed or converted to facilities that also served the economic mainstream. The change happened so quickly that many did not believe it had really occurred. New black facilities that were built to replace the old ones at the end of the 1960s were slowly abandoned by their former patients and medical staffs, who were now welcomed at formerly racially or economically segregated white institutions. Racially separate waiting rooms in private physician practices disappeared, following the lead of the hospitals and the new economic power of black beneficiaries.

Economic segregation also declined within facilities. The separation of private and public inpatient accommodations, with few exceptions, no longer exists. The wooden benches and block scheduling of indigent clinics have mostly disappeared. Clinic accommodations for indigent patients are, for the most part, indistinguishable from those in private office practices.

Within a decade, the "iron law" that had governed the use of care by race and income, inversely related to need, had been turned on its head.[33] In the Medicare program, expenditures per nonwhite beneficiary gradually increased to the point where they exceeded similar expenditures per white beneficiary. Age-adjusted numbers for hospital discharges and days of care for blacks and for low-income persons now substantially exceed those of whites and high-income persons.

Between 1966 and 1980, racial and economic differences in rates of premature death (death before 65) and infant mortality (deaths before one year of age) shrank in the United States.[34] The drop was particularly notable in infant mortality and deaths due to motor vehicle accidents in the South—areas where access to hospital care because of racially exclusionary policies had been most problematic.[35] Differences since then have essentially remained unchanged. In the "new order," influenced by Title VI regulations, "differences" in health outcomes previously blamed on genetic and behavioral differences have universally become "disparities," an inequity that public officials and providers of care have a moral, if not legal, responsibility to eliminate.

There are, of course, many qualifications that make this assessment less triumphal. Several other chapters in this volume discuss the continuing struggles to provide equal access to healthcare services, even under the Affordable Care Act. Yet, that legislation also includes civil rights language, Section 1557, to address many of the limitations that have plagued Title VI enforcement in health care. It eliminates the physician and health plan exclusion and requires regular statistical reporting, reducing dependence on a complaint-based enforcement process that is often ineffective. As Title VI was for Medicare, Section 1557 is the "sleeper" provision of the ACA that no one talks about. Will it have a similar impact? A half-century ago, the combined power of the federal purse, the ideal of equal justice, and the gift of a grass-roots social movement made the power to heal, however incomplete, possible. Perhaps as a nation we still possess that power.

## NOTES

1. Albert Dent, "Hospital Services and Facilities Available to Negroes in the United States," *Journal of Negro Education* 18, no. 3 (1949): 326–332.

2. Brenda Armstrong, interview by David Barton Smith, June 27, 1996, recording available in the David Barton Smith Health Care Segregation Collection, Temple University Library, Philadelphia, PA [hereafter, DBS Collection].
3. Hospital Survey and Construction Act, 42 U.S.C. § 291e.
4. Roy Wilkins and Arnold Aronson, "Proposals for Executive Action to End Federally Supported Segregation and Other Form of Discrimination," submitted to the White House, August 29, 1961, White House Central Files, JFK Presidential Library, Boston, MA.
5. "HEW Correspondence File," December 7, 1966, Medical Committee for Human Rights Records, University of Pennsylvania, Kislak Center for Special Collections, Rare Books and Manuscripts.
6. Lyndon Johnson, "Memorandum on Reassignment of Civil Rights Functions," September 25, 1965, American Presidency Project, University of California Santa Barbara, http://www.presidency.ucsb.edu/ws/index.php?pid=27275&st=&st1=.
7. John Gardner, "Memorandum to Executive Staff, December 14, 1965," as quoted by Elaine Heffernan in *OCR Historical Record: Title VI Implementation* (unpublished manuscript, LBJ Presidential Library, Austin, TX [hereafter, LBJ Library]), 163–164.
8. Theodore Marmor, telephone interview by David Barton Smith, April 13, 2014.
9. Robert Ball, as quoted in *Reflections on Implementing Medicare, Restructuring Medicare for the Long Term Project: Study Panel on Medicare Management and Governance*, ed. Michael Gluck and Virginia Reno (Washington, DC: National Academy of Social Insurance, January 2001), 10–11.
10. Robert Ball, telephone Interview by David Barton Smith, September 15, 1998.
11. "Title VI and Hospitals," *Journal of the National Medical Association* 58, no. 3 (May 1966), 212–213.
12. Frank Weil, interview by David Barton Smith, May 26, 1995, recording available at DBS Collection.
13. Weil, Smith interview.
14. United States Commission on Civil Rights, *HEW and Title VI* (Washington, DC: 1970), 16.
15. Ruth McVay, interview by David Barton Smith, May 25, 1995, recording available at DBS Collection.
16. Marilyn Rose, "Memorandum to David Barton Smith, November 20, 1997," DBS Collection.
17. Weil, Smith interview.
18. Weil, Smith interview.
19. McVay, Smith interview.
20. Julian Suttle, interview by Barbara Berney, January 8, 2013 (Astoria, NY: BLB Productions, 2014).
21. Robert Childers, interview by Vanessa Burrows, January 4, 2014 (Astoria, NY: BLB Productions, 2014).
22. Michael Tidwell, "The Quiet Revolution," *American Legacy* 6, no. 2 (2000): 25–32.
23. Childers, Burrows interview.
24. Leo Gehrig, interview by Michael Gillette, February 13, 1990, transcript, LBJ Library.

25. Philip Lee, transcribed interview by David McComb, January 28, 1969, LBJ Library.
26. Farrus Bryand, "Memorandum to the President, May 23, 1966," White House Central Files, LBJ Library.
27. McVay, Smith interview.
28. Weil, Smith interview.
29. Ball, as quoted in "Reflections," 59.
30. Marmor, Smith interview.
31. Lyndon Johnson, "Statement on the Inauguration of the Medicare Program, June 30, 1966," *Public Papers of the Presidents: Lyndon Baines Johnson 1963–1969* (Washington, DC: Office of the Federal Register), 676–677.
32. Nathaniel Wesley, *Black Hospitals in America: History, Contributions, and Demise* (Tallahassee, FL: NRW Associates Publications, 2010).
33. David Barton Smith, *Health Care Divided: Race and Healing a Nation* (Ann Arbor: University of Michigan Press, 1999), 200–210.
34. Nancy Krieger, et al., "The Fall and Rise of US Inequalities in Premature Mortality 1960–2002," *PLOS Medicine* 5, no. 2 (2008): e46; doi:10.1371/journal.pmed.0050046.
35. Douglas Almond, Kenneth Chay, and Michael Greenstone, "The Civil Rights Act of 1964, Hospital Desegregation and Black Infant Mortality in Mississippi," MIT Department of Economics Working Paper No. 07–04 (Cambridge, MA: December 31, 2006), http://papers.ssrn.com/sol3/papers.cfm?abstract_id=961021; Haochi Zheng and Chao Zhou, "The Impact of Hospital Integration on Black-White Differences in Mortality: A Case Study of Motor Vehicle Accident Death Rates" (working paper, Department of Economics, Boston University, December 2008), http://s3.amazonaws.com/zanran_storage/artsandscience.usask.ca/ContentPages/16757159.pdf.

# 3

# THE EARLY DAYS OF MEDICARE AND MEDICAID

## *A PERSONAL REFLECTION*

RASHI FEIN

The passage of Medicare and Medicaid—officially Titles XVIII and XIX of the Social Security Act—represented the largest expansion of protection against the financial implications of ill health in American history. I witnessed these events firsthand: I had come to Washington in 1961 as a staff member to the Council of Economic Advisers (CEA) with a portfolio that emphasized "do good" programs, and stayed for the remainder of the Kennedy administration and into the Johnson administration. Those of us involved in developing and implementing Johnson's War on Poverty saw those two programs as important components of the Great Society, yet many of us wished for a more comprehensive agenda: a national health insurance program that would provide insurance protection for the entire population. While it was clear that it would take some time for such a program to gain political support, most knowledgeable observers, the so-called "health policy experts," believed that national health insurance would come into being within half a decade. Pessimists thought it might take eight to ten years.

As is now clear (and as Jonathan Oberlander and Theodore Marmor discuss in Chapter 4 of this volume), we were wrong. Medicare and Medicaid were not structured as social experiments, designed to yield information on "lessons" for the future. We can nevertheless learn from the experience of administering and financing two very different programs based on different social contracts. Medicare was a "social insurance" program designed to cover *everyone* over a certain age threshold; Medicaid was a "welfare" program based on means testing. In 1968, Wilbur Cohen, the acting secretary of Health, Education, and Welfare (HEW), asked me to chair the Medical Assistance Advisory Council (MAAC), the advisory group for administering Medicaid, including its relationship to Medicare. It soon became clear to me that the assumptions driving Medicaid, a poor people's program tied to welfare eligibility, were very different from those behind Medicare, an entitlement program involving social insurance—based on my experiences with each in various settings: as the first chairman of the MAAC; as a member of the Board of Trustees of a large teaching hospital and of a long-term care institution; as a member of the Board and chair of the technical committee of an organization dedicated to enacting national health insurance; and, finally, as a Medicare beneficiary. This chapter, therefore, is necessarily more personal than the usual academic contribution; nevertheless, my experiences are revealing of the different attitudes toward Medicare and Medicaid and the ways that those attitudes have affected the two programs.

## MEDICAID AND THE MAAC: MY EXPERIENCE AS A PUBLIC SERVANT

Many of these programs in my original CEA docket would be termed "human capital" interventions.[1] I worked with individuals who administered and evaluated programs housed in HEW, as well as in other departments (e.g., Labor and State). In the light of my later involvement with the Medicaid program, it is interesting to note that I had much greater contact with programs involving education, health care, and social security than with welfare or social and rehabilitation activities. Following my two years at the CEA, I became a Senior Fellow in the Economic Studies Program at the Brookings Institution. There, I continued my relationships with my old friends at HEW and made new friends involved in the War on Poverty through the Office of Economic Opportunity (OEO). It was here that I was first able to observe and be involved in the development of Medicare and Medicaid.

That involvement dramatically increased in April 1968 when I was appointed chair of the Medical Assistance Advisory Council, a 21-member Council that had been established under the 1967 amendments to Titles XVIII and XIX. The Council advised the secretary of HEW on matters of general policy and made recommendations for improving the administration of Title XIX, including the relationship between Medicaid and Medicare. These 1967 amendments also increased the scope of activities of the parallel Health Insurance Benefits Advisory Council (HIBAC), a similar advisory body for Medicare that had been established two years earlier. The MAAC was supposed to do for Medicaid what HIBAC was already doing for Medicare. HIBAC's membership was drawn from the hospital, medical, and other health fields, with at least one member representing the general public. In contrast, the MAAC's membership was drawn from state and local government agencies, nongovernmental organizations, and groups concerned with health. In contrast to HIBAC's single "public" member, the amendments required that a majority of the MAAC membership had to be representatives of consumers of health services.

HIBAC's existence at the inception of Medicare meant that it was actively involved in negotiating the regulations affecting Medicare. Thus, unlike the MAAC, which had been created after the adoption of many of the federal regulations impacting Medicaid, HIBAC played an important role in Medicare's early implementation. The first chair of HIBAC was my Brookings colleague Kermit Gordon, who had served as the director of the Bureau of the Budget and who later would become Brookings' president. I recall encountering him one evening in a Brookings elevator. He looked exceedingly tired and, when I expressed concern, he responded that HIBAC had been meeting to finalize its recommendations on hospital reimbursement regulations and that he felt as if he alone was "all that stood between the American Hospital Association and the gold at Fort Knox." None of the issues I encountered as chair of the MAAC would have caused me to feel that way. Gordon's successor was Charles Schultze, who also had served as director of the Bureau of the Budget and who later would become chair of the CEA. It is not false modesty on my part to suggest that my appointment as chair of the MAAC could be interpreted as proof that the MAAC was not as prestigious or important as HIBAC.

What was true of the Council chair was also true of the members. As noted in the publication *Medicine and Health* in March 1968, "Well-known health economist Rashi Fein, Ph.D., was named to head the twenty-one-member group [MAAC]. But with only a few exceptions, the members are not as well-known as Fein or most members of the more prestigious HIBAC."[2] *Medicine and Health* suggested that the difference in membership, and what it saw as HEW's failure to make use of the MAAC, meant that the secretary "didn't really want any advice in running Medicaid."

While there was some truth in *Medicine and Health's* assessment, I believe that HEW's lack of interest in the MAAC probably stemmed from contrasting attitudes toward social insurance and welfare. Medicare was a social insurance program administered by the Social Security Administration (SSA) that universally covered individuals 65 and older, regardless of income. The program represented the kind of structure that could serve as a basis for the United States to move to national health insurance. Conversely, Medicaid was a welfare program administered by the Social and Rehabilitation Service (SRS), a new HEW agency that combined services for children, the elderly, the poor, and the disabled. Although Johnson's Great Society placed great emphasis on serving the poor, the entire point of the program was to minimize, if not eliminate, poverty. Administrators viewed Medicare as the model for national health insurance and Medicaid as a necessary but temporary program for the poor. Not surprisingly, Wilbur Cohen, who helped create Social Security in the mid-1930s, felt a greater affinity to Medicare than to Medicaid. There was little question that Cohen viewed Medicare, not Medicaid, as "his baby." Were he still alive today, he would be surprised to learn that the Affordable Care Act's road to universal coverage goes through Medicaid.

The contrast between the programs also manifested itself in the federal resources available for administering them. Although states conducted much of the day-to-day operation and administration of Medicaid (especially the determination of eligibility for medical assistance), this fact alone could not explain the difference in levels of support for the programs. Shortly after the first meeting of the MAAC in August 1968, I received a copy of a memorandum from the chief of the Advisory Council Support Group that compared the larger number of staff members provided by the SSA to HIBAC with the smaller staff numbers (but more extensive responsibilities) of the MAAC.[3] This kind of staffing comparison became a constant undercurrent to the meetings of the MAAC. Later, in October 1968, I was informed about the loss of four secretarial workers who had resigned their positions or had been reassigned without replacement. All were experienced workers who felt overworked.

Nor did the agency overseeing the Medicaid program have sufficient resources to oversee the states' actions. Particularly given the racial and regional tensions in implementing Medicare and Medicaid, as described in Chapter 2 by David Barton Smith in this volume, some level of federal oversight seemed essential. And yet, the budget was so limited that staff could only visit every state with a Medicaid program once every three years. A single visit once every three years hardly enabled the federal government to assess state performance and create adequate accountability.

All of this provided evidence that the cliché "a program for the poor is a poor program" had some validity. What was not clear, however, was whether this result was inherent in the structure and design of Medicaid, or instead was a result of HEW leadership's lack of interest. This "lack of interest" may be partially explained by the bumper crop of Great Society legislation, much of which involved the expansion of or creation of new HEW programs. With an overfull plate, something had to give, and that turned out to be the oversight function of Medicaid. The complex relationship between federal and state authorities may have added to federal officials' ambivalence. The administrative structure of Medicaid, in which the federal government provided funding administered by the states, meant that, at times, critical matters fell "between the cracks."

As a consequence of what might be termed "benign neglect," the MAAC found that Council members had to develop their own agenda rather than respond to the secretary or the Medical Services Administration's requests for advice. While this maximized the Council's freedom, it also left the members feeling irrelevant. Nevertheless, the problems that the Council encountered were trivial compared with the challenges that federal authorities faced: a new program (Medicaid) competing for attention with another new program (Medicare) of far greater interest to the general public and HEW authorities; a shortage of money and personnel with which to administer the new program; and no clear lines of demarcation between federal and state responsibilities for decision-making and accountability. Senator

Paul Douglas summed up the net result: "An expert on Social Security is a person who knows Wilbur Cohen's telephone number." One can hardly imagine a similar statement in reference to Medicaid.

These early days helped set the context for the development of Medicaid and influenced the attitudes toward Title XIX. Though Medicaid was a comprehensive program that addressed the financial problems faced by different target populations, its complexity generated a good deal of misinformation and confusion. Many people—including policymakers—believed it was a program that paid for the medical care of all poor persons, not realizing that only some of the poor were recipients. Administratively, Medicaid referred to its participants as "recipients," while Medicare had "beneficiaries." Most Americans, and many state and federal officials, did not fully grasp the distinctions between the "categorically needy" and the "medically needy," nor did they understand the different rules that applied to these groups. Confusion reigned as well concerning the differences between rules applying to Medicaid and those applying to the traditional cash benefit programs with which Medicaid was associated: Old Age Assistance, Aid to Families with Dependent Children, Aid to the Blind, and Aid to the Permanently and Totally Disabled. Decision-makers also found it difficult to deal with Medicaid's unusual structure: two very different population groups, served by two vastly different parts of Medicaid. One funded medical care for persons who were defined as categorically needy (and, depending on state action, medically needy), while individuals unable to pay the fees for long-term institutional care received a very different set of benefits.

All of these issues necessarily played out in the real world of politics. Was the program costing more than Congress had anticipated because individual states (New York was often cited as an example) were setting income definitions for the medically needy in a manner that made many more individuals eligible for assistance than Congress had in mind when it enacted Title XIX? Was the program being "ripped off" by those engaged in fraud and abuse? In March 1969, for example, Washington newspapers reported that Maryland authorities had released the names of 28 physicians who allegedly had billed the Maryland Medicaid program for over $20,000 in 1968. Was the program wasting money or reaching the "deserving poor?"

One specific problem arose because of the pressure to restrain Medicaid spending. For some states, that meant adopting a fee schedule for Medicaid services that was far below that in the private healthcare market (for both insured and uninsured individuals) and also below the Medicare standard. At the beginning of the Medicaid program, some hospital administrators may have seen the replacement of what previously had been charity care with a below-market payment as a significant advance. But, once in place, the low fee schedule was difficult to amend. It dramatically reduced physicians' willingness to treat Medicaid recipients. I vividly recall a conversation from 25 years ago in which a liberal state commissioner of health who administered a Medicaid program shared his struggles with raising low physician fee schedules. He wanted to increase the fees to improve access to physician services, but was painfully aware that a large (20 percent) increase in fees would increase the state's Medicaid budget by close to a corresponding amount—an amount far in excess of what the body politic could accept. More to the point, even a 20 percent increase would not raise the fee schedule enough to significantly increase the number of participating physicians. This problem had plagued the Medicaid program virtually from the beginning, but it was not something that the secretary of HEW, the administrator of the SRS, or other federal officials had asked the MAAC to examine.

As chair of the MAAC, I met many times with Dr. Francis Land, who oversaw the Medicaid program, but I never intersected with Mary Switzer, the SRS administrator. Though the Council was supposed to advise the secretary, it received only one request from the secretary for advice on any subject. That request came on January 3, 1969 (two and a half weeks before Wilbur Cohen's last day as secretary), and may have been stimulated by my interim report submitted to the secretary a few days earlier. In his letter, Cohen stated that he would be departing on January 20, 1969, and, as if "for the record" for the incoming Nixon administration, he expressed hope that the Council would "consider several [issues] in the coming year that (were) of particular concern to me."[4] These included evaluations concerning who was receiving medical care and services, who was being left out and why, what changes in federal and state legislation should be called for to close that gap, and what administrative changes at HEW and in the various states would enhance the program. He also wished that the Council would "investigate thoroughly just what it would take for the Nation to standardize nationally such well-known inequities as eligibility consideration; types, quantity, and quality of services provided; and the use of other programs to augment Title XIX."[5] Finally, Cohen added to his rich agenda for the future by discussing the need for integrating child health services and the need for research, development, and demonstration projects.

Members of the Council had previously argued that the question of standardizing eligibility should be our number one priority, but their views could not carry the day absent any indication of interest on the part of any HEW official. Perhaps, however, this letter and its suggestions did have an impact on the next administration, which set up (though, most regrettably, without informing the MAAC) the distinguished McNerney Task Force, chaired by Walter McNerney, then president of the Blue Cross Association, to examine the Medicaid program and a number of associated questions about its administration.

The covering letter for the interim report that I submitted to the secretary made special reference to the need for more resources for the MAAC. This did not come as a surprise to Cohen, with whom I had discussed the matter a month earlier. Nevertheless, the situation had by then become even more dire: we had been informed that, at current funding levels, the Council would be able to meet only one time during the second half of the fiscal year. The secretary's proposed new activities for the Council stood in sharp contrast with his failure to recognize or refer to our need for more resources. Nor did he refer to our advice regarding 15 specific recommendations made by the Advisory Commission on Inter-Governmental Relations for Medicaid.

Today, 50 years after the enactment of Title XIX and more than 45 years after the early MAAC reports, Medicaid faces many of the same issues and problems. If anything, they have perhaps become more complicated as a consequence of the enactment of the ACA. That is not to suggest that, aside from the ACA, Medicaid has not changed over the past 50 years. It certainly has, and in many beneficial ways for specific target populations (e.g., children). Rather, it is to suggest that many structural problems that now exist were present from the beginning.

### MEDICARE AND MEDICAID: MY EXPERIENCE AS A TRUSTEE OF HEALTHCARE ORGANIZATIONS

I was invited to serve on the Board of Trustees of a Harvard-affiliated teaching hospital in the late 1960s. The dean of Harvard Medical School encouraged me to accept, on the premise that I would learn a lot if I joined and participated in board meetings and activities. Thus, I was involved with hospital administration during a period when hospital financing changed radically. I remember the general director of the hospital once saying to the board: "Before Medicare I kept a list of things the hospital needed in the drawer of my desk and while speaking with a possible hospital benefactor, I pulled the drawer out a bit and glancing at the list considered which item might be of interest to that potential 'sugar daddy.' Then Medicare came along. The list became less important. Medicare made all things possible." An even richer relative, Uncle Sam, had appeared on the scene to substitute for the sugar daddy. Certainly every hospital director still wanted—and continues to welcome—philanthropic dollars, but Medicare continues to provide the hospital's financial underpinnings. That this new attitude had a basis in reality is revealed by even the most cursory examination of changes in the sources and rapid growth of hospital receipts and expenditures.

The dean was correct: I learned a lot, especially about the impact of Medicare. I recall that, at almost every Trustee meeting, I would raise my hand at the conclusion of the financial report and offer a correction to the language used in the generally upbeat oral presentation that reported on our "profits." I suggested that the words "excess of receipts over expenditures" be substituted for the word "profits." In part, my desire to avoid the term "profit" stemmed from the battles in various states over hospital "profits," the hospital's not-for-profit status, and its non-payment of taxes. The attorney general of Massachusetts had asked hospitals to report on their community contributions, and it seemed politically inappropriate to confess to making "profits"—though these were not distributed to stockholders—while simultaneously arguing that we were a nonprofit community enterprise that couldn't pay taxes or lower its fees or charges without jeopardizing our financial stability.

But more than that was at stake. I believed that language influenced the way that hospital leaders and trustees looked at things and, consequently, our attitudes and behavior. If we talked about profits we might begin to think about maximizing them (most trustees had taken Economics 101), and it would then be a small step to think about how to price hospital services, especially nontraditional ones without a pricing history (e.g., in vitro fertilization was a new service that had opened up just such a conversation). Over time, this might conflict with the institution's ethos and mission. The fact that I intervened at meeting after meeting suggests that I fought a losing battle.

Even had we adopted my language, we could not avoid the fact that our financial structure had changed; we no longer were the hospital we had been. And so we would listen to a presentation about building an addition to the hospital and learn that, as if by sleight of hand, it wouldn't really cost anything because Medicare, the National Institutes of Health (NIH), and other organizations would end up paying for it. Most often, the expansion did not increase bed capacity, but instead provided new or improved facilities for research or treatment. Woe unto that trustee who did not understand the nature and power of indirect costs! I do not recall a single vote that rejected a possible expansion on fiscal grounds. Nor was this situation unique to our hospital.

Much of the pressure for hospital growth resulted from opportunities created by Medicare, opportunities that made it much easier to finance new bed capacity and treatment or research facilities by ensuring a "guaranteed" source of revenue. At heart, however, the issue reflects the broader, and more basic, problem of basing medical care on market models. Each entity within the medical sector operates to maximize its power, growth—call it what you will. While institutions make arguments for expansion based on their ability to care for the sick, in fact, each institution operates in its own self-interest. This is not because hospital leadership is irresponsible or selfish or prone to narrow vision. Rather, societal interest is not maximized by summing individual self-interests. Some hospitals expand and some close as a result of market pressures, but the laws of the marketplace do not guarantee that the ones that disappear are redundant, unnecessary, or poorly managed. Nor are the factors that impel expansion of a hospital the same ones that lead to the expansion of, say, a grocery store. We expect each hospital's behavior to be responsive to market pressures, even as we believe that this should not be the case for the hospital sector as a whole. That Medicare funding patterns and incentives exacerbated the basic problem can hardly be disputed. I do not believe that one can understand the US hospital sector or the federal Medicare program without understanding how hospitals changed as a consequence of the fiscal revolution associated with Medicare.

As money became "easier," and the nature of trustee discussions changed from those of mission and of "doing good" to a greater emphasis on expansion and the flow of money, a number of trustees became less interested in the enterprise, boiling down to the sentiment: "If this is what we're going to talk about, I may as well stay downtown and work on making money."

Consequently, as "doing good" discussions disappeared, there was less "feeling good," weakening the commitment that had motivated individuals to give time and effort to the well-being of the enterprise. Interestingly, this problem did *not* affect healthcare systems primarily associated with Medicaid; the sorts of facilities that depended on Medicaid payments continued to command support and interest from community leaders, including some who had become less interested in the (apparently) "rich" hospitals.

Around the same time that I observed the impact of Medicare on the Harvard-affiliated hospital, I also had the opportunity to join the Board of Trustees of a Harvard-affiliated institution that provided long-term care. This latter experience provided insight into the importance and influence of Medicaid. While the new programs represented new sources of revenue vitally important to both institutions' economic well-being, there the similarity ends. The differences between Medicare and Medicaid were large and real.

I was fortunate to serve on the Board of the long-term care facility long enough to witness new programs that brought significant changes to the institution and its resident population. Perhaps the most significant was a shift from an exclusive emphasis on institutionalizing individuals who needed long-term care to the development of housing alternatives that reduced the demand for institutionalization and, as a consequence, the waiting list for admission. This shift neither negated nor interfered with the institution's mission to care for the frailest and neediest among us. The leadership took this mission very seriously and most, if not all, board members could quote the words that lay at the heart of the institution's behavior.

But therein lay a problem. Fulfilling the mission required adequate funding, and only a small proportion of Americans could provide private funding for long-term care. Furthermore, while many individuals believed that Medicare would pay for long-term care, this was not the case. Once an individual had exhausted private resources, Medicaid became the funder of last resort. Thus, though Medicaid's image was and is that of a medical care program for the poor (especially poor children), a high proportion of Medicaid dollars goes for the long-term care of individuals who viewed themselves (and who were viewed by others) as middle-class persons. The general public does not have a good understanding of this part of Medicaid; nor do many legislators. It was, however, well understood by those associated with the funding and management of such institutions, including the state budget and finance authorities who had to deal with Medicaid, as a very large and not easily controlled state budget item.

As a member of the Long-Range Planning Committee for this institution, I could not help but be aware of the conflict between the need to diversify sources of revenue and the mission to care for the neediest among us. As a member of the Board of Trustees, I could not help but be aware of the delicacy of the negotiations between the long-term care institution that needed to receive as high a per diem payment as possible and the state budget authorities who wanted to pay as low a per diem rate as possible. Absent clear guidelines regarding reimbursement, such negotiations inevitably took on a political dimension. It was easy to imagine that the "daily rate" was determined through some technocratic process that would yield the same answer, regardless of who was paying for the patient. The reality, of course, was quite different, and helps explain why large long-term care institutions, like large hospitals and colleges, hired persons with responsibility for "governmental affairs." Like it or not—and, on balance, institutions liked it—government was a partner to their service activities.

But state government was of two minds: on the one hand, it wanted to claim credit for being a partner in public discussions of the services provided to community members; on the other, it needed to be a fiscally responsible partner in discussions of state budgets and taxes. State legislators and policymakers hoped to meet the expectations of the average voter who had a desire for the services financed by government and a desire not to pay higher taxes. In practice, this meant that long-term care institutions whose finances were heavily dependent upon state Medicaid payments faced far more pressure to contain expenditure growth than did those hospitals whose support largely came from the federal government through Medicare. Whereas one institution focused on belt tightening, the other focused on ways to expand. My simultaneous service on both boards sometimes left me spinning in circles, but I became much more knowledgeable about aspects of Medicare and Medicaid that were not revealed by the usual sources of data.

## Medicare Beneficiaries and My Experience with the Committee for National Health Insurance

I turn now to the insights I gained about Medicare as a Board member of the Committee for National Health Insurance (CNHI), one of several organizations that advocated for the enactment of a national health insurance program. Formed in 1969 under the leadership of Walter Reuther, president of the United Automobile Workers (UAW), CNHI had close ties to the labor movement. The CNHI's financial support came largely from the UAW, and its most active period spanned the years when the UAW and labor unions were at their maximum strength. As a liberal organization supporting a tax-based social insurance approach to national health insurance (what today would be called "single payer," or "Medicare for All"), it had close ties to Senator Edward Kennedy, the leading proponent of a tax-based social insurance program during the 1960s. During the Clinton presidency, the CNHI went out of existence and turned over its assets to the AFL-CIO for the promotion of the Clinton reform plan.

During my time as a CNHI Board member and chair of its Technical Committee, beginning in the early 1970s and continuing through its demise, the CNHI worked on designing various approaches to national health insurance. I recall many discussions involving Medicare beneficiaries and consideration of the ways in which Medicare benefits could be enhanced. Nevertheless, the social insurance schemes designed by the Committee excluded Medicare beneficiaries, whether for a limited period of time (three to five years) or for some lengthier unspecified period. Otherwise, CNHI's leaders feared, such a plan could never gain the support of Medicare's vast constituency (see also Chapter 7 by Mark Schlesinger in this volume). It was nevertheless clear that the Medicare population eventually would be incorporated into the national health insurance program.

How does one explain this phenomenon, especially in light of the then-prevailing assumption that the aged and disabled were supporters of liberal causes? Why was it assumed that the elderly, who recently had benefited from the enactment and implementation of Medicare and Medicaid, would not support the extension of healthcare financial protection to others? The answer lay in the realization that the elderly were enrolled in a successful program that, as they saw it, was operating effectively and efficiently. Whatever their views about national health insurance and the need to help others in theory, in practice national health insurance posed a threat. A new program might not work as smoothly; at a minimum, it would surely have some "growing pains." They furthermore understood that their voice would be weakened as they moved into a program with many more enrollees, who might have different interests and priorities than theirs. What had once seemed so easy and appealing to proponents of national health insurance—that is, building on the foundation stone of Medicare—suddenly appeared much more difficult, as the foundation stone could not be touched or built upon. The early architects of Medicare had not understood that enacting a program for a segment of the population might effectively remove that segment from the fray. Potential supporters might stand on the sidelines asking the question, "What's in it for me?" and answering with the comment, "Potential headaches and benefit cutbacks."

I do not recall any discussion of this possible phenomenon during the period leading up to the enactment of Medicare. I am not suggesting that, had Medicare proponents realized that the enactment of Title XVIII might weaken support for national health insurance, they would have shelved it, but rather that the question of how to minimize such an effect was, regrettably, not part of the political discourse. In retrospect, the phenomenon appears obvious. Incrementalism has its political advantages, but it also has its political costs.

The political status of Medicaid recipients was quite different. Those enrolled in Medicaid were less likely to vote than Medicare beneficiaries, and Medicaid recipients (whether receiving long-term care or medical services) were less likely to feel threatened by the enactment of a more comprehensive plan. Indeed, the status of the Medicaid population, combined with that of the uninsured, was the very reason to be in favor of national health insurance. There was far greater reason to believe that these groups would support a plan endorsed by Senator Kennedy.

Over the years, CNHI developed or participated in the development of numerous proposals. Though always painful, it became politically necessary to move away from a social insurance approach. The support for a Medicare-like approach was not based on an academic evaluation of the strengths and weaknesses of Medicare versus Medicaid; rather, we believed in social insurance. When it became necessary to accept a compromise and depart from the Medicare (more correctly, "improved Medicare") model, we wanted to depart as little as possible. Senator Kennedy's willingness to accept various compromises distressed us. We refused to recognize that we might have to answer the question, "How many troops do the labor movement and the CNHI have?" As a consequence, the proposals we advanced were variants on a theme of social insurance, tweaked to meet political constraints.

## MY EXPERIENCE AS A MEDICARE BENEFICIARY

I close on a final set of experiences that I have had with Medicare: as a beneficiary. I have been told that I would not be affected if Medicare disappeared because my employer offers comprehensive insurance benefits, including retiree coverage. But such a statement ignores the fact that the principle of ceteris paribus (all things being equal) does not hold in the real world: private insurance premiums would increase if Medicare did not cover a high proportion of medical costs for persons over 65 and the disabled. Absent Medicare, employers would react to higher premiums by reducing health benefits and/or shifting costs to employees.

Medicare is a valuable insurance policy that provides peace of mind as well as financial protection. It did so for me even in the years during which I did not have expensive or frequent medical encounters. Then, quite unpredictably, one year's charges exceeded the total for the previous 22 years. I benefited from Medicare not only financially, but also from the realization that my physician would not be forced to consider my ability to pay when determining how to treat me.

My care was documented in mailings (labeled "This Is Not a Bill") that listed each treatment I received, the provider's billed amount, the Medicare approved fee, the actual Medicare and supplemental insurance payment, and the balance that I had to pay. Perhaps these data were designed to make me appreciate Medicare. Perhaps the disparity between charges and actual payments would lead me to feel sorry for providers. Perhaps the mailings were supposed to help me uncover fraud, but if so, they often used unrecognizable treatment codes. The forms are ubiquitous. As a beneficiary, I wonder about their purpose.

In its relationship with beneficiaries, Medicare turns out to be like many government programs and budget expenditures: many individuals enjoy the benefits, even while being unaware of their source or that government is involved.

My recounting of these experiences is intended to remind us that Medicare and Medicaid, like all enterprises and endeavors, have operated and have been evaluated and discussed in particular contexts. These contexts were dependent on the cast of characters involved, including their attitudes and biases, as well as on extraneous events and on timing. Convenient as it may be to assume that everyone involved in the early administration of Medicare and Medicaid always demonstrated rational behavior based on objective analysis, that is simply not the case. What was true of the MAAC and the HEW leadership throughout the Johnson administration and, for a time, the Nixon administration, was also true of the relationships between Medicare and US hospitals, as well as between Medicaid and nursing homes. The same could be said for the CNHI's decisions. In some sense, they were all logical; in another sense, they were not.

Medicare and Medicaid require that we know as much as possible about the context within which they developed. We cannot fully understand this history if those who observed and participated in it are unable to provide their perspectives because of the ravages of age. It is already too late to recapture the past from all of the individuals who participated in the early implementation of Medicare and Medicaid. For various reasons, the history of the enactment of Titles XVIII and XIX attracted many scholars, but the history of the period following enactment received much less attention. Regrettably, therefore, we know less about how Medicare and Medicaid were implemented than we do about how they were enacted.

This has important implications for our present activities. Put simply, we should not wait until the fiftieth anniversary of the passage of the ACA to start collecting data on how the law is being implemented. This is not a criticism of those who are already writing histories of their participation in the ACA's creation. The histories of the future, however, will be richer and more useful if the archives, the primary sources that will be mined by future scholars, are enriched, not by accident, but by design. Health policy will evolve, but change will always be with us. Just as it is never too late to start, so is it never too early to begin.

## Notes

1. Materials referred to in this section may be found in the Rashi Fein Collection, Francis A. Countway Library of Medicine, Harvard Medical School.
2. "Medicaid and the MAAC," *Washington Report on Medicine and Health*, March 10, 1968, 1.
3. Letter from Francis L. Land, Commissioner, Medical Services Administration to Charles Cubbler, Chief, Advisory Council Support Group, August 12, 1968.
4. Letter from Wilbur J. Cohen to Rashi Fein, January 3, 1969, 1–3.
5. Letter from Wilbur J. Cohen to Rashi Fein, January 3, 1969, 1–3.

# THE ROAD NOT TAKEN

## WHAT HAPPENED TO MEDICARE FOR ALL?

### JONATHAN OBERLANDER AND THEODORE R. MARMOR

When President Lyndon Johnson signed Medicare into law on July 30, 1965, he declared, "no longer will older Americans be denied the healing miracle of modern medicine."[1] On that promise, and much more, Medicare has delivered. Over the past 50 years, Medicare has provided tens of millions of seniors with a crucial measure of financial security and access to medical care. A secure retirement would be unimaginable for most Americans without Medicare. Moreover, since 1972 Medicare has provided coverage to Americans with permanent disabilities and end-stage renal disease. Medicare, as a traditional social insurance program, has always accepted eligible beneficiaries regardless of their health status, has never charged persons with pre-existing conditions higher premiums, and has never ended coverage for persons who develop an expensive medical condition—practices all too common, until recently, in private insurance markets in the United States. Put simply, Medicare has been a reliable source of health coverage and economic security for many of this nation's most expensive, medically complex, and hardest-to-insure populations—populations who otherwise would struggle to obtain insurance.

Yet as much as Medicare has accomplished, as much impact as it has had on American health care, as much good as it has done for its beneficiaries and their families, Medicare's architects hoped that the program would become much more. They never imagined that, a half-century after its birth, Medicare would look as it does today, with seniors comprising the vast proportion of its enrollees. Medicare, they expected in 1965, would soon expand far past social insurance protection for the elderly and would evolve into a full-scale system of national health insurance for all Americans. Medicare was designed as a first step to a government-administered, universal social insurance program—what today we would call single-payer national health insurance. In short, "Medicare for All" was the reform vision, but one that was to be implemented over time.

The failure of Medicare to fulfill that aspiration raises important questions about the politics of Medicare and health reform in the Unites States. Why didn't Medicare expand into Medicare for All, as its designers anticipated? Why did Democrats, beginning in the 1970s, largely abandon the Medicare strategy? How has the separation between Medicare and broader reform shaped the policy landscape we have today, including Medicaid and Obamacare? And what role has Medicare played in health reform debates over the last half-century? Rashi Fein's Chapter 4 in this volume offers some possible explanations for these questions from the point of view of a participant. In this chapter, we offer an analysis that takes a broader view, reflecting on the changing political appetite for national health insurance in the years following Medicare's enactment.

## THE MEDICARE STRATEGY

Medicare's origins lie in early twentieth-century debates about reforming American medical care. From 1915 through the 1940s, American reformers tried unsuccessfully to follow the path of European reformers who had established various forms of social insurance programs for health expenses and sickness pay. In 1945, Harry Truman became the first US president to propose government health insurance for all Americans. Truman's surprise victory in the 1948 presidential election, combined with Democrats winning majorities in both the House and the Senate, appeared to open the window to enactment of what was then called national health insurance. But the Truman proposal never came close to becoming law, stymied by the conservative coalition of Republicans and Southern Democrats that controlled Congress, the fierce resistance of the American Medical Association (AMA), and the Cold War stigma of "socialized medicine."

After the defeat of Truman's plan, administration officials began searching for an alternative strategy. Medicare emerged as that alternative, conceived as a more pragmatic path to adopting federal health insurance. In 1951 Social Security administrators announced a plan to insure retirees for hospital stays, financed by payroll taxes.[2]

The plan rested on the politics of incrementalism. By limiting coverage to elderly beneficiaries of Social Security, reformers hoped to capitalize on the political appeal of the aged as a sympathetic group deserving of government assistance.[3] Truman administration officials presumed that focusing coverage on the elderly would make federal health insurance harder to oppose and dismiss as socialized medicine.

The original 1951 plan, later called Medicare, had extraordinarily limited benefits, calling only for 60 days of hospitalization insurance, another concession to political constraints. By excluding coverage for physician services, Medicare's architects hoped to defuse opposition from the AMA, which had earlier spearheaded resistance to Truman's national health insurance proposal.[4]

Finally, by linking Medicare to Social Security, reformers sought to leverage the popularity of old-age social insurance to propel the enactment of federal health insurance. The connection was programmatic—hospital coverage, like Social Security, would be financed by payroll taxes earmarked for a trust fund and linked to eligibility for Old-Age and Survivors Insurance. It was also political. Medicare proponents' slogan, "health insurance through Social Security," and their references to the "tried-and-true method of Social Security" reinforced the idea that federal health insurance would build on a familiar program with effective financing arrangements.[5] Medicare advocates further assumed that by copying Social Security's social insurance financing and principles—payroll taxes earmarked for a trust fund, universal eligibility for all Americans regardless of income, avoidance of any means test that would stigmatize seniors and limit eligibility to the poor—Medicare would emulate Social Security's popularity, political success, and expansionary trajectory.[6]

But insuring the elderly for hospital stays only was never the end goal of Medicare's designers, either in the 1950s or the 1960s. Over time, the program would expand, its advocates presumed, to cover additional services and new populations. Medicare for All was what the reform leaders of 1965 assumed would be the incremental result of their first step. Medicare's incrementalism was a means to an end, a political strategy designed to secure the passage of a federal health insurance program that would expand substantially in coming years. That presumption was never made public during the Medicare debate, but it was strongly held by the program's architects. As Robert Ball, a key participant in crafting the Medicare strategy and head of the Social Security Administration from 1962 to 1973, later explained, "we all saw insurance for the elderly as a fallback position, which we advocated solely because it seemed to have the best chance politically. . . we expected Medicare to be the first step toward universal national health insurance, perhaps with 'Kiddiecare' as the next step."[7] Despite repeated statements to the contrary during legislative debates in the late 1950s and the early 1960s, Medicare's architects anticipated that after covering the elderly, Medicare would soon expand to insure children, then workers, and eventually all Americans.

The Medicare strategy took an unexpected turn even before the law passed in 1965. After Lyndon Johnson and the Democrats' landslide victory in the 1964 elections made its enactment a certainty, Wilbur Mills, chair of the House Ways and Means Committee and previously a Medicare opponent, maneuvered to alter the legislation. Concerned that Medicare's limited benefits would disappoint beneficiaries and would generate pressure to expand the program to cover physician services via payroll tax funding, and aware that Medicare advocates envisioned it as a first step to a broader federal health insurance program, Mills sought to build a fence around Medicare.[8] With the tacit (and hidden) support of Lyndon Johnson, Mills adapted a Republican alternative plan to Medicare that added voluntary, but subsidized, physicians' insurance to hospitalization coverage.[9] Medicare insurance for physicians (what became Medicare Part B) would be funded by beneficiary premiums and general revenues, not the social insurance financing of hospital coverage (Part A). This enabled Mills, who worried about the consequences of raising payroll taxes too high, to pre-empt the addition of such coverage through Social Security financing.

Mills was also concerned that Medicare would evolve into a broader system of national health insurance. By taking another potential target of federal insurance out of the equation, Mills hoped to weaken the case for later expanding Medicare. He added Medicaid, a plan to cover low-income Americans, to the final Medicare legislation. Mill's initiative built on an AMA proposal and the pre-existing Kerr-Mills program that gave states payments to finance care for low-income residents. The unexpected outcome of Mills's maneuvering was what came to be called a three-layer cake—Medicare Parts A and B, and Medicaid.[10]

The Medicare bill that passed Congress in 1965 thus emerged in a form that was broader than its advocates had expected, but that deviated in key respects from their preferred social insurance model. Nonetheless, even with efforts to constrain Medicare built into the law, program architects believed that federal health insurance would soon expand far past the elderly into national health insurance. The beachhead, they thought, had been established. Now the focus turned to what steps would advance their ultimate goal.

## "Kiddycare" Falls Short

Medicare's designers had good reason to believe in the program's expansionary trajectory. After all, Social Security, built on a similar social insurance model, had expanded greatly since its start in 1935. Moreover, the political conditions at the time of Medicare's enactment seemed auspicious. This was a period of Democratic Party dominance of national politics. From 1933 until 1969, Democrats controlled the White House for all but war hero Dwight Eisenhower's two terms, and enjoyed majorities in the House and Senate for all but four years.

New Deal liberalism had remade American government, securing a much a larger role for the federal government in social welfare policy. Lyndon Johnson's crushing defeat of Barry Goldwater in 1964 and the passage of Great Society legislation appeared to confirm liberalism's ascendance. In that political environment, the step-by-step expansion of Medicare into universal insurance would have seemed not merely quite plausible, but highly likely and perhaps even inevitable.

The initial task was to assure a smooth takeoff for Medicare.[11] Faced with intense resistance from the AMA, including threats of a doctors' boycott, and hoping to avoid the stigma of socialized medicine and to demonstrate that federal health insurance could succeed administratively, program leaders took steps to conciliate the healthcare industry. The Medicare law itself contained an explicit vow that the federal government would not intervene in the practice of medicine.[12] The processing of claims would be handled by private insurers so that hospitals and doctors would not have to deal directly with the federal government. And Medicare adopted permissive payment policies for medical care providers that contained no meaningful cost controls.

In addition to assuring provider participation, Social Security administrators went to great effort to maximize beneficiary enrollment, organizing a nationwide sign-up campaign that relied on mass mailings of Medicare applications and enlisted the postal and forestry services in publicity efforts.[13] Medicare's early success—the program was fully operational just one year after its enactment, and during that first year 93 percent of eligible seniors signed up for Medicare Part B, a voluntary program of physicians' insurance—reflected the administrative skill and preparation of program leaders like Robert Ball, Wilbur Cohen, and Arthur Hess, all of whom had vast experience with Social Security.[14] Medicare's comparatively straightforward programmatic structure also helped to facilitate a successful launch. Enrollment in Part A, for example, was automatic for Social Security beneficiaries, and complex income-based eligibility or subsidy calculations were not necessary since Medicare coverage of the elderly was universal, regardless of income.[15]

With implementation an immense triumph, program leaders turned to plans for expanding Medicare. The question was which step to take next. Medicare leaders had already settled on insuring children. An extension to children would have made Medicare explicitly intergenerational in its beneficiary population, with the program covering both the beginning of life and its end. Children represented another sympathetic group that commanded public support. There were compelling arguments about the moral imperative to provide children with access to medical services. Compared to the elderly, furthermore, children offered a relatively inexpensive population to insure.

Under the leadership of Wilbur Cohen, who was undersecretary and later secretary of Health, Education, and Welfare, "Kiddycare" emerged as the next logical step. The proposal was "to pay for prenatal and postnatal care of all mothers, as well the costs of delivering the baby and the baby's care during the first year of life."[16] As with the rest of Medicare, Kiddycare would be a universal program open to all children, regardless of parental income. Cohen thought enough of Kiddycare's importance that he favored delaying pursuit of expanding Medicare to cover outpatient prescription drugs, another route of programmatic expansion, "until after plans for covering children were launched."[17]

But the plan to add children to Medicare never came to fruition. Opposition from Johnson administration officials to Kiddycare's costs, in the context of concern over the growing costs of the Vietnam War and their implications for domestic fiscal policy, led to its abandonment (plans to add prescription drug coverage to Medicare were also shelved). Johnson's vice president, Hubert Humphrey, reportedly intended to pursue Kiddycare if he won the White House in the 1968 election, but his defeat to Richard Nixon deprived the program of presidential sponsorship.[18] Thus the first step to incremental expansion of Medicare was not taken.

### Dialysis and the Disabled

Despite Kiddycare's fate in the late 1960s, Medicare eligibility did significantly broaden in 1972, with coverage added both for persons with permanent disabilities and patients with end-stage renal disease (ESRD). (Keith Wailoo discusses these expansions in greater detail in Chapter 12 of this volume.) Program leaders viewed an extension of Medicare to beneficiaries of Social Security Disability Insurance, which had been enacted in 1956, as a natural, almost automatic step. Such an extension had been recommended by the 1965 Social Security Advisory Council, proposed by the Johnson administration in 1967, and was passed by both the House and Senate in 1970, only to be held up as part of negotiations over broader Medicare legislation in conference committee.[19] In practice, then, the incremental strategy was alive, but not widely advertised.

In contrast, the expansion of Medicare to kidney disease patients was unanticipated and peculiar, inasmuch as ESRD represented the extension of Medicare to a specific disease category rather than a population group. Indeed, the addition of ESRD coverage was a product of "serendipity... rather than the result of a grand design."[20] The medical procedure for dialysis had been invented in 1960, and thereafter both dialysis advocates and congressional allies sought to secure federal funding that would enable all ESRD patients to access the vital service. Medicare eventually emerged as the programmatic destination for covering dialysis, partly because the addition of disability as a criterion for Medicare eligibility enabled kidney disease to be folded into Medicare's social insurance protection. Put simply, Medicare was the convenient programmatic post to which dialysis could be hitched, so that is where it wound up.

## MEDICARE AS A FISCAL PROBLEM

Medicare's 1972 expansion to persons with disabilities and end-stage renal disease significantly broadened Medicare's reach across American society, diversifying its beneficiary population to persons under age 65. Yet the same 1972 legislation that extended Medicare eligibility also contained warning signs about the difficulties that lay ahead for further program expansion.

The implementation of Medicare was a great success, enrolling virtually all eligible beneficiaries within the first year of operation. But Medicare costs, fueled by the permissive payment policies adopted in 1965, rapidly outpaced the actuarial estimates made at the time of its enactment. The program quickly acquired a reputation among some influential policymakers in Congress and the executive branch as an uncontrollable burden on the federal budget. By 1969, for example, Russell Long, chairman of the Senate Finance Committee, was warning that Medicare had become a "runaway" program; in 1970 his committee issued a landmark report detailing problems with Medicare's payment policies and offering recommendations for its reform.[21]

The report became a foundation of the 1972 Social Security Amendments, which contained the first significant policies aimed at controlling the rate of growth in Medicare spending. The measures included the establishment of organizations to review hospital care provided to Medicare patients, limits on hospital payments, and the authorization of demonstration projects in alternative payment methods.[22] The focus of Medicare policy was shifting.[23] The question of how to contain program spending would come to dominate Medicare politics in ensuing decades, as will be discussed further in later chapters in this volume. Furthermore, intermittent trust fund "crises"—with politicians raising alarm over Medicare's impending "bankruptcy"—would shape program politics and create another barrier to expansion.[24] In retrospect, the extension of Medicare eligibility to the disabled and to kidney disease patients represented not a step toward universal health insurance, but rather both the beginning and the end of Medicare's expansion to new populations beyond the elderly.

## THE SEPARATION

The enactment of Medicare and Medicaid transformed American health politics. Previously, it was widely presumed that spending more on medical care would improve Americans' health. Now, as federal and state governments confronted the rising costs of public insurance programs, health spending became a public policy problem. Spending more on medical care was no longer seen as an unmitigated good. It instead loomed as a serious threat to public budgets and the national economy. Rising costs also threatened Americans' access to medical care. In 1971, President Richard Nixon warned that "medical care costs have gone up twice as fast as the cost of living.... for growing numbers of Americans the cost of care is becoming prohibitive."[25]

Here was America's first healthcare cost crisis, and with it came an extraordinary opportunity to remake American medical care.[26] By fueling medical inflation, Medicare and Medicaid's implementation unexpectedly reopened the debate about overhauling American health care and enacting national health insurance. Reform proposals proliferated in Congress. Meanwhile, the Nixon administration offered its own universal insurance plan, built around requiring employers to provide private coverage (an important development that presaged a fundamental change in the character of health reform plans).[27]

For our story, what is crucial is that this period marks a key disjunction between the Medicare expansion strategy and health reform. Democratic Party reformers offered no shortage of proposals to remake health care during the early to mid-1970s. But these plans did not envision achieving universal coverage incrementally by expanding Medicare group by group, as program architects had during the 1960s. Nor did more ambitious proposals build on the Medicare platform or even invoke its name as its inspiration.

The most influential Democratic voice in Congress on health reform, Massachusetts Senator Edward (Ted) Kennedy, proposed a national health insurance plan, with the federal government providing "identical insurance to all Americans for all essential health care."[28] In terms of both philosophy and policy, Kennedy's plan embraced the aspiration of universalizing

Medicare. It was, in effect, Medicare for All. Yet Kennedy did not explicitly call for Medicare for All, choosing instead to label his plan the Health Security Program.

Why didn't Kennedy simply frame his proposal as Medicare for All? Alternatively, why didn't Democrats seize the opportunity to embrace the Medicare strategy and propose incremental expansions of the program to new groups? The answers are not entirely clear. Medicare's rising costs and its emerging reputation as a fiscal problem likely led Democratic reformers to shift their focus. Some liberal Democrats saw Medicare as overly solicitous of the medical care industry, symbolizing government's failure to stand up to powerful interests. For many moderate and conservative Democrats, in contrast, Medicare had become a budget buster, symbolizing government's fiscal profligacy. Neither group had reason to formulate health reform plans with Medicare as the centerpiece. Nor did the Republicans.

Kennedy imagined his national health insurance program as much broader than Medicare.[29] He argued that, under the Health Security Program, "fragmentation of insurance plans...will cease. Medicare, Medicaid, and other programs will be absorbed in this more comprehensive plan, and thousands of private insurance plans will cease to exist."[30] The problems of American medical care required enacting an entirely new health insurance program, one that would subsume, rather than build on, Medicare. In fact, all of the major health reform proposals considered by Congress in the early to mid-1970s—including Kennedy's national health insurance plan, as well as Nixon's employer mandate proposal and a catastrophic insurance bill sponsored by Senators Russell Long and Abe Ribicoff—had one feature in common: not one of them embraced the strategy of Medicare incrementalism.[31]

Regardless of why Democrats moved away from the Medicare strategy, what is clear is that the 1970s were a pivotal moment for health politics. None of the proposals for universal coverage passed Congress. The advent of stagflation—simultaneous high rates of unemployment and inflation—shook the American economy. Federal budget deficits emerged as a political issue. Liberalism receded as public distrust of government eroded in the wake of Vietnam, Watergate, and economic strains. Deregulation, harnessing market incentives, and reforms that emphasized "public use of the private interest" came into vogue, with some Democratic intellectuals and policymakers embracing a philosophy of neoliberalism that expressed both considerable faith in markets and serious concern about the limits of government.[32]

The changes in the political winds were sufficiently strong that Republican Richard Nixon, who resigned the presidency in 1974, was arguably more liberal on health reform than Democrat Jimmy Carter, who was elected to the White House in 1976. By the end of the 1970s, cost control had become the dominant issue in health policy, supplanting universal coverage and concerns over access to medical services. Medicare policy debates more frequently focused not on expanding the program—either in terms of new populations or covered services—but rather on restraining its growth. Many Democrats abandoned the original Medicare strategy of demographic incrementalism. And some began to embrace models of health reform organized around private insurance, rather than a single system operated by the federal government according to social insurance principles. This shift accorded with the rise of neoliberalism and reflected an adaptation to a more conservative political environment. Even liberal Democrats who had supported single-payer national health insurance accommodated to the new political reality. Kennedy himself, for reasons of legislative pragmatism rather than ideology, came in the late 1970s to favor health reform models that relied extensively on private insurance.[33]

These dynamics—liberalism's political decline, a preoccupation with budget deficits, a focus on controlling federal spending on health care, and a turn to market solutions—would continue to shape American health politics for the next three decades. Medicare for All slipped further away.

DEFICITS AND DEFENSE

The election of Ronald Reagan to the presidency in 1980 furthered the ascendance of conservatism in national politics. The Reagan administration sought to cut taxes, privatize the welfare state, and constrain federal expenditures on domestic programs, all while increasing military spending. Even as the number of uninsured Americans climbed significantly, the administration had no interest in proposals for universal health insurance. It looked at Medicare, as many in Congress did, primarily as a budgetary problem and a potential source of fiscal savings. Nor was the primary concern with system-wide medical spending. That broader focus gave way to a narrower emphasis on how to contain federal spending on Medicare and Medicaid in the context of rising budget deficits. Meanwhile, conservatives promoted pro-competitive healthcare policies that relied on market incentives, consumer choice, and competition between private plans to restrain spending on medical care.[34]

These developments produced two consequences for Medicare. First, driven by budget deficit politics, the 1980s saw the adoption of major new cost containment policies for Medicare payments to doctors and hospitals.[35] Those policies had bipartisan support from Republican presidents (first Reagan and later George H. W. Bush) and Democratic Congresses seeking budgetary savings. Second, the posture of Medicare advocates—both inside and outside Congress—became understandably defensive.[36] Their goal was to protect Medicare against excessive cuts and efforts to privatize Medicare insurance. In 1988, the Reagan administration and Congress did agree on bipartisan legislation that produced the largest expansion in Medicare benefits since the program's enactment (though the Medicare Catastrophic Coverage Act was repealed in 1989).[37] Yet at no time during the 1980s did proposals to expand Medicare substantially to new populations—let alone to create national health insurance—have any chance of becoming law.

MISSING IN ACTION

Universal health insurance returned to the agenda in the early 1990s. Rising health insurance premiums, felt acutely by businesses and their workers, a deep recession that underscored the vulnerabilities of relying on employer-sponsored health insurance, and the surprise emergence of health care as a pivotal issue in Harris Wofford's unexpected victory in a 1991 US Senate special election in Pennsylvania helped bring the issue back to the forefront of American politics.[38] Proposals for overhauling medical care again proliferated in Congress.[39] Health care became a prominent issue in the 1992 elections, and when Bill Clinton defeated George H. W. Bush, giving Democrats their first victory in a presidential contest since 1976, health reform's moment appeared, once again, to have arrived.[40]

Clinton had promised during the campaign to prioritize health reform and, in 1993, his administration developed an ambitious plan for universal health coverage. The plan, which bore the same name as Kennedy's Health Security Act two decades before, illustrated both the changing politics of health care and the shifting of Democratic Party positions. It relied on an employer mandate and private insurance to achieve universal coverage. Moreover, the Clinton plan reflected a version of managed competition, with choice of health plan and competition as its central features (though it also contained robust health spending caps). Neoliberal ideas were now central to the Democratic Party's conceptions of health reform; those ideas did not feature Medicare.[41]

In Congress, a significant—albeit minority—faction of Democrats did back single-payer national health insurance. Some Democrats and liberal policy analysts returned to the idea of using Medicare as a platform for expanding coverage. Congressman Pete Stark, for example, proposed a Medicare Part C to cover the uninsured.[42] But the Clinton administration itself did not embrace such ideas, and Medicare's primary role in the Clinton plan was to serve as a piggy bank to help fund the costs of expanded coverage for the uninsured. A major funding source for Clinton's proposal came from projected cuts in the rate of growth in Medicare payments to medical providers.[43]

Following the 1994 demise of the Clinton plan, the national political agenda turned away from universal health insurance. After winning majority control of both houses of Congress for the first time in 40 years, in 1995 Republicans proposed substantial overhauls to Medicare and Medicaid. Medicare advocates returned to a defensive stance, with the Clinton administration and congressional Democrats resisting GOP proposals to impose a cap on program spending and to expand the role of private insurers within the program. After Clinton vetoed GOP legislation, however, the politics of deficit reduction brought Medicare reform back onto the table, and a bipartisan agreement in 1997 reduced the rate of growth in provider payments while adopting policies to promote private insurer participation in Medicare (or so it was thought at the time; the 1997 law actually had the opposite impact). Medicare politics had again become budget politics.

The Clinton administration and Congress did pursue incremental measures to regulate the health insurance market and expand coverage, including enacting the State Children's Health Insurance Program (SCHIP) in 1996. SCHIP built on similar expansions through Medicaid to low-income children as well as to pregnant women during the mid- to late 1980s. Medicaid, with its joint state-federal structure, means-tested benefits limited to low-income Americans, and general revenue financing—rather than Medicare—emerged as the primary programmatic platform to cover the uninsured.[44] Tellingly, while the Medicaid model gained traction, a 1998 Clinton administration proposal to permit Americans aged 55 to 64 to buy into Medicare went nowhere.[45]

*Reform Rises Again*

In a familiar pattern, the election of a Republican president in 2000, George W. Bush, consigned universal health insurance to the realm of aspiration. The Bush administration's "compassionate conservatism" did not include a place for expanding health insurance coverage.

The administration did support a significant expansion of Medicare benefits to cover the costs of outpatient prescription drugs. Yet the new benefit, enacted in 2003 as part of the Medicare Modernization Act, was to be provided exclusively through private insurance plans, marking a major development in Medicare policy.[46] It represented a programmatic marriage of sorts between the Democratic Party's commitment to universalism and the Republican Party's belief, shared by some Democrats, in the virtues of private insurance and competition—the new prescription drug benefit would be available to all program enrollees, with coverage offered by competing private insurers. The Bush administration and Congress pursued additional policies to ramp up private plan enrollment in Medicare, which the 1997 Balanced Budget Amendments had tried but failed to do. This time those policies worked, helping to boost the percentage of Medicare enrollees in such plans to 24 percent by 2010.[47]

In 1994, Congressman Pete Stark had envisioned a Medicare Part C that would cover the uninsured. Instead, Medicare Part C became a bastion of private insurance within Medicare. Medicare's structure has changed and has become a hybrid of private and public insurance, so that even expanding Medicare to all Americans means something different today than it did half a century ago.[48]

Barack Obama's election in 2008 opened another window for health reform. This time, Medicare played a more prominent role than in earlier reform debates, with liberal policy analysts, politicians, and advocates calling for the uninsured to be given access to a "public option" that would be modeled on Medicare and, depending on the proposal, connected to the original program in terms of cost control measures and other policies. The public option became a rallying cry and central aspiration of many Democrats who wanted the uninsured to have alternatives to private insurance and hoped to challenge the virtual monopoly that insurers had in some states' individual insurance markets.[49]

Democrats included a version of the public option in the health reform bill that passed the House in 2009. But the proposal could not win sufficient support in the Senate, and it was eventually dropped from the legislation that became the 2010 Affordable Care Act (ACA; popularly known as "Obamacare"). Nor did a backup plan to make Medicare available to uninsured Americans aged 55 to 64 make the cut.

Instead, the ACA's health reform model resembled what was previously advanced by the Nixon and Clinton administrations, with a reliance on private plans, consumer choice, means-tested subsidies, and employer financing. (Obamacare, notably, did call for a substantial expansion of Medicaid eligibility.) Medicare cost controls also served as a source of projected savings to help fund the ACA's insurance expansion and as a platform to test a range of new initiatives to reform the delivery of medical care and to control its spending.[50] Additionally, the ACA expanded Medicare's limited prescription drug coverage and enhanced other Medicare benefits.

Democrats, then, had passed the first major overhaul of American health insurance since 1965. Obamacare, however, rested less on the Medicare for All strategy and the concept of social insurance than it did on conservative and neoliberal conceptions of the appropriate shape for healthcare reform.[51] The Obama administration's aim was to patch the existing patchwork of American health insurance, relying on subsidized private insurance and Medicaid expansion to cover the uninsured.[52] "Near" universal insurance had finally arrived in the United States, but when it did, Medicare had been marginalized, playing no role in the ACA's expansion of health insurance.

## LESSONS AND LEGACIES

How did we get to the point where Democrats enacted a major expansion of health coverage without relying on Medicare? Why did the original strategy of incremental expansion of Medicare into universal insurance fail? And what consequences has that failure had for American health policy?

Decisions made at Medicare's start made its subsequent expansion difficult. The permissive payment policies adopted to assure Medicare's smooth implementation helped fuel substantial increases in program spending in its early years. Medicare's reputation as a fiscal problem became a political impediment to program expansion and shifted the agenda to cost containment. This impediment helps to explain both why Medicare did not expand more broadly to new population categories and why Congress rarely expanded program benefits, despite serious limits in its coverage, in the half-century after Medicare's enactment. Put another way, in an effort to secure Medicare's smooth takeoff in 1966, program administrators pursued policies that unintentionally ended up reducing Medicare's political capital, thereby making further population expansions much more difficult. That reputation, in fact, outlived the reality. Since the 1980s, Medicare reforms have succeeded in slowing program spending growth, but Medicare in still seen in some quarters as "unaffordable" and "uncontrollable."[53]

Yet the failure of Medicare for All is certainly not solely—and arguably not even mostly—attributable to decisions made by Medicare's architects. The changing features of American politics and major shifts in socioeconomic conditions had a crucial impact on Medicare's trajectory. The end of Democratic Party dominance over national politics, the ascendance of conservatism, economic stagflation and strain, conflicts over the Vietnam War, Watergate, urban unrest, the rise of pro-market ideology, and welfare state retrenchment—all of these radically altered Medicare's environment. These external developments beyond Medicare's programmatic boundaries would have been impossible to anticipate in 1965, but they made universal coverage via incremental expansion of Medicare a much harder task. Indeed, it is not just Medicare for All that failed, but all efforts at comprehensive health reform from 1966 to 2009.

But building on Medicare was not impossible, and the role of contingency looms large. What if, for example, Robert Kennedy had not been assassinated and instead had won the 1968 presidential elections? It is quite possible that under a second Kennedy administration, the United States could have adopted national health insurance. Additionally, if Hubert Humphrey had defeated Richard Nixon in 1968, that victory might well have empowered Democrats to embrace Medicare expansion. A persistent move forward with Kiddycare could have substantially altered Medicare's course.[54]

It is also worth wondering what would have happened if, after the failure of health reform in the mid-1970s, Democrats had returned to the Medicare strategy. Had Democrats coalesced around a strategy for Medicare expansion in the late 1970s and during the 1980s, and stuck to it despite short-term setbacks (as Medicare's architects did in the late 1950s and early 1960s), then perhaps the Clinton administration's Health Security plan would have looked quite different. Of course, fissures in the Democratic Party and the political and socioeconomic transformations noted above would have made such agreement extraordinarily difficult. Still, strategic choices (and what arguably seem like errors in retrospect) help to explain why Medicare did not occupy a more prominent place in reform models from the 1970s onward.

The failure of Medicare to expand as its designers anticipated has had important consequences for health reform. Kiddycare's demise meant that Medicaid, rather than Medicare, became the primary platform to extend insurance coverage to children and other demographic categories of the uninsured. That legacy was embodied in the Affordable Care Act, which showed that Democrats could pass a health reform law that contained a substantial expansion of Medicaid eligibility, but could not enact legislation that called for even a modest expansion of Medicare or the creation of a Medicare-like federal insurance plan for the uninsured.

Meanwhile, as more Democrats turned away, first from incremental Medicare expansion and then from national health insurance and social insurance, they came to embrace reform models that relied on private insurance and that celebrated consumer choice and competition. Over time, prevailing conceptions of health reform became narrower in their coverage aspirations and more conservative in character—dynamics readily visible in Obamacare, with all of its limitations and complex administration.[55] The troubled rollout of Obamacare's health insurance marketplaces in 2013 underscored the costs of moving away from Medicare's administratively simpler social insurance model.[56]

The irony is acute. Nearly half a century after Medicare's enactment, a Democratic president and Democratic majorities in Congress took additional steps toward universal health insurance, but those steps did not include Medicare. Nothing could better illustrate just how different Medicare's trajectory has been from the path its architects imagined in 1965.

NOTES

1. President Lyndon B. Johnson, "Remarks with President Truman at the Signing in Independence of the Medicare Bill," July 30, 1965, http://www.lbjlib.utexas.edu/johnson/archives.hom/speeches.hom/650730.asp.

2. Theodore R. Marmor, *The Politics of Medicare* (Chicago: Aldine, 1973).
3. Lawrence R. Jacobs, *The Health of Nations: Public Opinion and the Making of American and British Health Policy* (Ithaca, NY: Cornell University Press, 1993).
4. Marmor, *The Politics of Medicare.*
5. Robert Ball, "Perspectives on Medicare: What Medicare's Architects Had in Mind," *Health Affairs* 14 (1995): 62–72.
6. Theodore R. Marmor, Jerry L. Mashaw, and John Pakutka, *Social Insurance: America's Neglected Heritage and Contested Future* (Los Angeles: Sage/CQ Press, 2014).
7. Ball, "Perspectives on Medicare," 62–63.
8. Marmor, *The Politics of Medicare,* 61–81.
9. David Blumenthal and James A. Morone, *The Heart of Power: Health and Politics in the Oval Office* (Berkeley: University of California Press, 2009).
10. Marmor, *The Politics of Medicare,* 64.
11. Judith M. Feder, *Medicare: The Politics of Federal Hospital Insurance* (Lexington, MA: D. C. Heath, 1977).
12. James A. Morone, *The Democratic Wish: Popular Participation and the Limits of American Government* (New York: Basic Books, 1990), 263–264.
13. Michael G. Gluck and Virginia Reno, eds., *Reflections on Implementing Medicare* (Washington, DC: National Academy of Social Insurance, 2001).
14. Marmor, *The Politics of Medicare.*
15. Gluck and Reno, *Reflections on Implementing Medicare.*
16. Edward D. Berkowitz, *Robert Ball and the Politics of Social Security* (Madison: University of Wisconsin Press, 2005), 161.
17. Lawrence R. Jacobs, "The Medicare Approach: Political Choice and American Institutions," *Journal of Health Politics, Policy and Law* 32 (2007): 172.
18. See Berkowitz, *Robert Ball,* 160–163, and Jacobs, "The Medicare Approach," 169–178.
19. Jonathan Oberlander, *The Political Life of Medicare* (Chicago: University of Chicago Press, 2003), 41.
20. Charles L. Plante, "Reflections on the Passage of the End-Stage Renal Disease Medicare Program," *American Journal of Kidney Disease* 35 (2000): S45.
21. Oberlander, *The Political Life of Medicare,* 47–48.
22. Karen Davis, Gerard E. Anderson, Diane Rowland, and Earl P. Steinberg, *Health Care Cost Containment* (Baltimore, MD: Johns Hopkins University Press, 1990).
23. Lawrence D. Brown, "Technocratic Corporatism and Administrative Reform in American Medicine," *Journal of Health Politics, Policy and Law* 10 (1985): 579–599; Theodore R. Marmor, "Coping with a Creeping Crisis: Medicare at Twenty," in *Social Security: Beyond the Rhetoric of Crisis,* ed. Theodore R. Marmor and Jerry L. Mashaw (Princeton, NJ: Princeton University Press, 1988).
24. Oberlander, *The Political Life of Medicare,* 74–106.
25. Richard Nixon, "Special Message to the Congress Proposing a National Health Insurance Strategy," February 18, 1971, *Public Papers of the Presidents of the United States, Richard Nixon, 1971* (Washington, DC: Government Printing Office, 1999), 171.

26. Paul Starr, *The Social Transformation of American Medicine* (New York: Basic Books, 1982).
27. Stuart Altman and David Shactman, *Power, Politics, and Universal Health Care: The Inside Story of a Century-long Battle* (Amherst, NY: Prometheus Books, 2011).
28. Edward M. Kennedy, *In Critical Condition: The Crisis in America's Health Care* (New York: Simon and Schuster, 1972), 239.
29. Telephone interview with Stan Jones, April 2014.
30. Kennedy, *In Critical Condition*, 248.
31. Judith Feder, John Holahan, and Theodore Marmor, eds., *National Health Insurance: Conflicting Goals and Policy Choices* (Washington, DC: Urban Institute, 1980).
32. Charles L. Schultze, *The Public Use of the Private Interest* (Washington, DC: Brookings Institution Press, 1977).
33. Paul Starr, *Remedy and Reaction: The Peculiar American Struggle over Health Care Reform* (New Haven, CT: Yale University Press, 2011); Barry R. Furrow, "Health Reform and Ted Kennedy: The Art of Politics and Persistence," *New York University Journal of Legislation and Public Policy* 14 (2011): 445–476.
34. Theodore R. Marmor, *Understanding Health Care Reform* (New Haven, CT: Yale University Press, 1994).
35. David G. Smith, *Paying for Medicare: The Politics of Reform* (New York: Aldine de Gruyter, 1992); Oberlander, *Political Life of Medicare*; Rick Mayes and Robert A. Berenson, *Medicare Prospective Payment and the Shaping of U.S. Health Care* (Baltimore, MD: Johns Hopkins University Press, 2006).
36. Theodore R. Marmor, *The Politics of Medicare*, 2nd ed. (New York: Aldine de Gruyter, 2000).
37. Oberlander, *Political Life of Medicare*, 53–73; Richard Himmelfarb, *Catastrophic Politics: The Rise and Fall of the Medicare Catastrophic Coverage Act* (University Park, PA: Pennsylvania State University Press, 1995).
38. Haynes Johnson and David S. Broder, *The System: The American Way of Politics at the Breaking Point* (Boston: Little, Brown, 1996).
39. Theda Skocpol, *Boomerang: Clinton's Health Security Act and the Turn Against Government in U.S. Politics* (New York: W. W. Norton, 1996).
40. Jacob S. Hacker, *The Road to Nowhere: The Genesis of President Clinton's Plan for Health Security* (Princeton, NJ: Princeton University Press, 1997).
41. Theodore R. Marmor and Gary J. McKissick, "Medicare's Future: Fact, Fiction, and Folly," *American Journal of Law and Medicine* 26 (2000): 225–253.
42. Robert Pear, "New Health Plan Stresses Medicare," *New York Times*, March 1, 1994.
43. Congressional Budget Office, *An Analysis of the Administration's Health Proposal* (Washington, DC: U.S. Government Printing Office, 1994).
44. Lawrence D. Brown and Michael S. Sparer, "Poor Program's Progress: The Unanticipated Politics of Medicaid Policy," *Health Affairs* 22 (2003): 31–44.
45. John M. Broder, "Clinton Proposes Opening Medicare to Those 55 to 65," *New York Times*, January 7, 1998.
46. Thomas R. Oliver, Philip R. Lee, and Helene Lipton, "A Political History of Medicare and Prescription Drug Coverage," *Milbank Quarterly* 82

(2004): 283–354; Bruce C. Vladeck, "The Struggle for the Soul of Medicare," *Journal of Law, Medicine and Ethics* 32 (2004): 410–415; Douglas Jaenicke and Alex Waddan, "President Bush and Social Policy: The Strange Case of the Medicare Prescription Drug Benefit," *Political Science Quarterly* 121 (2006): 217–240; Jonathan Oberlander, "Through the Looking Glass: The Politics of the Medicare Prescription Drug, Improvement, and Modernization Act," *Journal of Health Politics, Policy and Law* 32 (2007): 187–219; Kimberly J. Morgan and Andrea Louise Campbell, *The Delegated Welfare State: Medicare, Markets, and the Governance of Social Policy* (New York: Oxford University Press, 2011).

47. Jonathan Oberlander, "Voucherizing Medicare," *Journal of Health Politics, Policy and Law* 39 (2014): 470–484.

48. Mark Schlesinger and Jacob S. Hacker, "Secret Weapon: The 'New' Medicare as a Route to Health Security," *Journal of Health Politics, Policy and Law* 32 (2007): 247–291.

49. Jacob S. Hacker, "Healthy Competition: The Whys and How of Public Plan Choice," *New England Journal of Medicine* 360 (2009): 2269–2271.

50. Jonathan Oberlander, "Medicare," in *Health Politics and Policy*, 5th ed., ed. James A. Morone and Daniel C. Ehlke (Stamford, CT: Cengage Learning, 2013): 126–141.

51. Theodore Marmor and Jonathan Oberlander, "The Patchwork: Health Reform, American Style," *Social Science and Medicine* 72 (2011): 125–128.

52. Ibid.

53. Joseph R. Antos, "Premium Support Proposals for Medicare Reform," Statement to the House Committee on Ways and Means, Subcommittee on Health, April 27, 2012; Theodore Marmor, Jonathan Oberlander, and Joseph White, "Medicare and the Federal Budget: Misdiagnosed Problems, Inadequate Solutions," *Journal of Policy Analysis and Management* 30 (2011): 928–934.

54. Jacobs, "The Medicare Approach."

55. Marmor and Oberlander, "The Patchwork."

56. Jonathan Oberlander, "Between Liberal Aspirations and Market Forces: Obamacare's Precarious Balancing Act," *Journal of Law, Medicine & Ethics* 42 (4): 31–41.

# PART II

# THE REMAKING OF VALUES, RELATIONSHIPS, AND SOCIETY

The expanding breadth of Medicare and Medicaid between 1965 and the 1980s highlights how many issues reshaped these programs. The programs became an integral part of the nation's political fabric and medical industry. The aging of the population continued to shape Medicare; ups and downs in the economy and poverty levels influenced Medicaid; the changing politics of entitlements and welfare affected both; and shifting political control of federal and state government continued to define the fate of both programs. In 1982 (17 years after Medicaid's passage), the last holdout state in the union, Arizona, finally signed on to the program. Beneath the story of implementation, however, these programs were slowly remaking values, relationships, and American society in fundamental ways.

As Jill Quadagno argues in Chapter 5, Medicaid has retained much of its poor law legacy; but, as more states adopted the program and as coverage expanded to those above the poverty level, the program also slowly transformed into a middle-class healthcare entitlement. Sara Rosenbaum, in Chapter 6, examines the crucial role played by the courts in rulings that interpreted Medicaid law not merely as a federal grant-in-aid program but also as one that gave beneficiaries legally enforceable rights; in short, the courts of the late 1960s created a Medicaid entitlement that has persisted, even as later courts subsequently eroded those rights. In Chapter 7, Mark Schlesinger turns to how such public programs altered the lives and identities of those they served. Critics saw Medicare as producing dangerously greedy and burdensome elders; advocates saw it as giving rise to healthier and more politically and socially empowered seniors.

# 5

# THE TRANSFORMATION OF MEDICAID FROM POOR LAW LEGACY TO MIDDLE-CLASS ENTITLEMENT?

JILL QUADAGNO

Medicaid, the fourth-largest program in the federal budget, provides the primary public health insurance benefit for over 63 million low-income Americans, or about 20 percent of the population.[1] Medicaid beneficiaries include pregnant women, children and families, individuals with disabilities, and people in poverty.[2] Without Medicaid, most enrollees would be uninsured or would lack coverage for services they need. Medicaid also plays a critical role in long-term care for the frail elderly. As the primary payer for nearly two-thirds of nursing facility residents, Medicaid pays for 40 percent of nursing home care at a cost of about one-fourth of its budget.[3] Medicaid regulations additionally determine the form of long-term care that individuals receive, which historically has been mainly in nursing homes but in more recent years has involved experiments with less institutional types of care. And Medicaid will only become more important in the future, as the Affordable Care Act uses it as the key mechanism to move toward universal coverage.

Given Medicaid's key role in the healthcare system, it is not surprising that a debate has emerged about its quality and value. On one side are critics who consider Medicaid a means-tested program that institutionalizes the legacy of the poor law, stigmatizes beneficiaries, and provides poor quality of care compared to private health insurance.[4] As legal scholar Timothy Jost notes, "a program for the poor will always be politically vulnerable, under-funded, and generally inadequate."[5] On the other side of the debate are advocates who argue that Medicaid has gradually been transformed from a residual benefit for the poor into a middle-class entitlement. As health policy analyst Colleen Grogan puts it, "By the end of the Clinton admin-istration, (Medicaid) looked like a broad entitlement more than a welfare program."[6] This chapter traces the historical evolution of Medicaid, while weighing the merits of each position.

## MEDICAID'S HEALTH INSURANCE BENEFIT

As the chapters in Part I have discussed at greater length, Medicaid origi-nated in a 1950s-era federal grant program that provided funding for states to pay the medical expenses of individuals receiving cash assistance.[7] The Kerr-Mills Act of 1960 expanded this concept by allowing states to cover the impoverished elderly who incurred high medical bills.[8] The 1965 amendments to the Social Security Act that created Medicare also included Medicaid, a slightly expanded version of Kerr-Mills. Medicaid provided health insurance for people who were categorically eligible for the joint federal-state cash assistance programs, Old Age Assistance, Aid to the Blind, and Aid to Families with Dependent Children (AFDC).[9] States could also choose to cover the "medically needy," people whose income was too high to qualify for cash assistance but was insufficient to pay their medical expenses, most of whom were nursing home residents.

Although Medicaid increased funds to the states over what they had been receiving under Kerr-Mills, it allowed states to decide how generous ben-efits would be, or even whether there would be a state program. According to federal regulations, state Medicaid programs had to provide hospital care, physician services, and skilled nursing home services, but the statutes did not specify the amount of services required. States also had to designate a single agency to administer their programs. In some states Blue Cross plans won contracts to implement Medicaid, while in others Medicaid was administered through state health or welfare departments. States with smoothly operating Kerr-Mills programs, such as Pennsylvania and California, had plans ready immediately and ran them efficiently. In other states, however, the agencies responsible for administering Medicaid failed to establish acceptable charges for services, audit hospital books, or assist hospitals in setting up utilization review programs.[10] Thus, the quality of Medicaid programs varied widely.

Within two years Medicaid was absorbing an increasing share of state revenues in the more generous states, crowding out spending for other social services. In New York, for example, the definition of "medically needy" was so generous that nearly half of the state's residents were eligible for benefits. Medicaid's budgetary strains grew after 1972, when Congress converted the joint federal-state Old Age Assistance program, which provided modest benefits to the aged, blind, and disabled poor, into a means-tested federal program, Supplemental Security Income (SSI). All SSI recipients automatically gained entitlement to Medicaid. As state Medicaid budgets rose, cost containment became a pressing concern, and in 1976 Congress severely restricted the definition of "medically needy" to those with an income of 133.5 percent of the AFDC eligibility level. States had the option of continuing to offer benefits to higher income individuals, but they would receive no federal match above the cutoff.[11]

State Medicaid programs changed in numerous ways in the 1970s, in part because of the changing funding structure and in part because of new federal regulations. In the 1980s, federal regulations decoupled Medicaid from AFDC and gave states the option of expanding coverage for children, regardless of parental status or employment. Gradually, the federal government converted optional state expansions into a mandate. In 1988 the federal government mandated coverage of pregnant women and infants with income of up to 100 percent of the federal poverty level (FPL); the following year coverage was added for children age one to five at 133 percent of the FPL.

The availability of Section 1115 waivers also transformed Medicaid. Section 1115 of the Social Security Act allows states to apply for waivers to conduct research and demonstration projects that bypass federal rules and regulations.[12] Although the states had conducted several such experiments throughout the 1980s, most of these were small in scope and were driven mainly by state rather than federal interests. In 1993, however, the Clinton administration began to actively promote states' use of Section 1115 waivers to expand coverage for low-income families, and states responded quickly.[13] By 1997, 16 states had obtained federal approval to launch comprehensive research and demonstration projects to extend Medicaid eligibility either by using higher income levels to cover low-income individuals not eligible under existing programs, through more generous asset tests to determine eligibility, or by incorporating groups not categorically eligible.

As Medicaid expanded to new beneficiary groups and to the near poor and working class, public perceptions of the program were transformed. During the 1995–1996 budget showdown between President Clinton and Republicans, Clinton sought to rally support by arguing that the GOP budget would involve huge cuts to popular entitlement programs—Social Security, Medicare, and Medicaid. No longer was Medicaid solely a "welfare" benefit. The 1996 Democratic Party platform also defined Medicaid as an entitlement and promised to protect the program from "devastating cuts."[14]

The State Children's Health Insurance Program (CHIP) of 1997 increased federal funds to the states to cover low-income children and moved Medicaid even further beyond its poor law legacy.[15] CHIP encouraged states to cover more children by increasing the federal match from 50 percent under Medicaid to 65 percent under CHIP. Equally notable, the Clinton administration allowed states to use CHIP funds to cover uninsured parents.[16]

In 2001 the Bush administration initiated the 2001 Health Insurance Flexibility and Accountability (HIFA) demonstration initiative. HIFA allowed states to increase coverage for adults with income of up to twice the federal poverty levels so long as existing resources were used. Although the HIFA waiver targeted populations with incomes below 200 percent of federal poverty guidelines, it had no upper income threshold. Using available Medicaid and CHIP resources, states could expend unused federal funds to expand coverage to ineligible populations, including parents, single adults, and married couples.[17]

For two decades Section 1115 allowed states to achieve broad program changes outside the legislative process. By 2001, more than 20 percent of federal Medicaid spending was governed by Section 1115 demonstrations. There were limits, however, to what states could achieve through waivers. TennCare provides an example of some of the challenges. Originally TennCare expanded subsidized coverage to all uninsured residents and allowed those ineligible for the subsidy to buy in. In its first year of operation, TennCare enrollment quickly grew close to the federal cap of 1.5 million people (meaning that the federal government would not share in the cost of the number above that). However, the growth in enrollment strained the state budget, and in 1995 Tennessee closed eligibility to uninsured adults. In 2005, faced with spiraling costs, TennCare cut approximately 160,000 people who were not eligible for Medicaid from the rolls; the program's benefits were trimmed.[18] In Oregon, cuts to the program caused some beneficiaries to lose coverage, and those who remained had fewer services and higher cost sharing.[19]

Other waiver experiments were quite successful. MassHealth, which was approved in 1995 and extended in 2001, combined Medicaid and CHIP into one public program that became the core of the Massachusetts Health Care Reform Plan of 2006.[20] Although some observers feared that the Massachusetts plan would falter like other ambitious state-level reforms and, more worrisome, perhaps detract from efforts for federal reform, such dire predictions proved unfounded.[21] Before the law took effect in 2006, about 94 percent of state residents were insured. By 2010 more than 98 percent were insured, including 99.8 percent of all children, making Massachusetts's rate of uninsured the lowest in the nation.[22]

The enactment of the Affordable Care Act has inaugurated a new era for Medicaid. For the first time in more than a century, the federal government has made a commitment to provide universal coverage through a complex mix of private incentives and public support. Its main features include state insurance exchanges, stringent regulations on insurance companies, fines on employers who do not offer coverage, a mandate that individuals purchase health insurance, subsidies to help low-income people purchase such insurance, and a substantial expansion of Medicaid.

The day that President Obama signed the ACA, the state of Florida filed a lawsuit in federal district court challenging the constitutionality of the individual mandate and the Medicaid expansion. Twenty-five other states joined the suit, while 13 states and the District of Columbia filed *amicus* briefs in the Supreme Court supporting the individual mandate and the Medicaid expansion. Two states were on both sides of the case, as their governors and attorneys general took opposite positions.

On June 28, 2012, the Supreme Court held that the individual mandate is a constitutional exercise of Congress's power to levy taxes. The same decision also held the Medicaid expansion to be unconstitutional on the grounds that states did not have adequate notice to voluntarily consent, and because all existing Medicaid funds could be withheld for state noncompliance. Consequently, a five-justice majority ruled that the federal government could not withhold all Medicaid funds for states that refused to comply with the expansion. The practical effect of the Court's decision made the Medicaid expansion optional for states because, if states do not comply, the federal government may withhold only ACA Medicaid expansion funds, not other funds for the rest of the Medicaid program.[23]

One of the federal requirements under the ACA concerns the groups of people who must be covered by a state's Medicaid program. Prior to the ACA, federal law excluded non-disabled, non-pregnant adults without dependent children from Medicaid unless a state obtained a waiver to cover them. Beginning in 2014, the ACA expands Medicaid's mandatory coverage groups by requiring that participating states cover nearly all people under age 65 with household incomes at or below 138 percent of the FPL ($14,856 per year for an individual and $30,657 per year for a family of four in 2012).[24] Some states have already expanded coverage to adults beyond the pre-ACA required income thresholds, but others do not currently cover adults without dependent children at all, or cover parents only at much lower income levels than the ACA's Medicaid expansion minimum. The ACA also provides that the benefit package for the newly eligible Medicaid population must include 10 categories of essential health benefits, ranging from preventive care to mental healthcare services.

Although by 2013 many states had refused to expand Medicaid, federal matching funds have provided incentives to states throughout Medicaid's history, and states have been adept at designing strategies to maximize federal dollars. The federal share of the Medicaid match is significantly more generous for the ACA expansion than for the states' existing Medicaid programs and CHIP. Under the ACA, the federal government will cover 100 percent of the states' costs from 2014 through 2016, gradually decreasing to 90 percent in 2020 and thereafter. Further, the federal government will assume responsibility for some of the costs and segments of the uninsured population that previously came out of state budgets. The effect will be to reduce both state and local government costs for uncompensated care.[25] The political gamble is that these financial incentives will be difficult for states to resist.[26]

Many of the recalcitrant states have already received federal support behind the scenes. State receipt of federal support suggests "a substantial level of seriousness about reform."[27] By 2013, all but four states had received infrastructure planning grants. This includes all 21 states party to the lawsuits. In this respect, the states are behaving in the long-standing tradition of public resistance with backstage cooperation. But does the ACA put "Medicaid at par with Medicare and Social Security—America's middle class entitlements," as at least one policy analyst has claimed?[28]

## MEDICAID'S POOR LAW LEGACY

Although Medicaid has been transformed from a program for the very poor into a benefit that reaches into the middle class, it is important not to overstate the case. Before the ACA, the majority of states maintained such strict eligibility criteria that most low-income adults did not qualify for Medicaid. Further, complex enrollment procedures prevent many individuals from actually claiming their benefits. Every state requires participates to re-enroll at least every 12 months, but some require more frequent assessments of eligibility. This process contrasts with Social Security and Medicare, both of which provide automatic entitlement to benefits on a permanent basis to all qualified individuals. As a result, nearly half of all Medicaid and CHIP recipients have had some interruption in coverage.[29]

Another problem is that eligibility criteria differ for adults and children within families and even for children of different ages. In 2014 the income eligibility standards in Iowa were 375 percent of FPL for children aged 0–1, 167 percent of FPL for children aged 1–18, 375 percent of FPL for pregnant women, and 133 percent of FPL for parents and other adults. In Mississippi, the standards varied even more: 194 percent of FPL for infants aged 0–1, 143 percent of FPL for children aged 1–5, 133 percent of FPL for children aged 6–18, 194 percent of FPL for pregnant women, and 24 percent of FPL for parents. Thus, some members of a family may be Medicaid-eligible while others are not, and children—who are the best-protected Medicaid recipients overall—may "age out" of coverage.[30]

The patchwork network of state agencies administering Medicaid claims additionally complicates the question of whether or not Medicaid has truly become an entitlement. States typically house the agencies that administer Medicaid within either health or welfare departments. These agencies are responsible for enrolling and credentialing providers, evaluating claims, monitoring the quality of services, and policing fraudulent providers. Each state has its own rules and procedures; prior to the ACA, there were few national requirements. Although states are required to enter basic information about recipients into the central Medicaid Management Information System, few states actually fully abide by this requirement. State agencies have been lax in fulfilling these duties in part because Medicaid's lower payments, compared to those of private insurers, has created a shortage of providers. As a result, the overall performance of states is uneven.[31]

The shortage of providers stems from a variety of factors. Many low-income persons—not only those enrolled in Medicaid but also individuals who have no insurance—often have difficulty finding physicians who are willing to accept them as patients. One study found a gradual decline in physicians who accept Medicaid patients, from 87.1 percent in 1997 to 85.4 percent in 2001. The number of physicians who have closed their practices to new Medicaid patients has also increased, especially in higher-income areas.[32] Among office-based physicians, 30 percent do not accept new Medicaid patients, and in some specialties, the rate of non-acceptance is much higher: 40 percent in orthopedics, 44 percent in general internal medicine, 45 percent in dermatology, and 56 percent in psychiatry. Payment reductions from managed care have also made it more difficult for physicians to cross-subsidize the care they provide to uninsured or Medicaid patients, adding to administrative complexity and creating problems obtaining specialist care. Relatively low payment rates and high administrative costs are particularly contributing to decreased involvement with Medicaid among physicians in solo and small-group practices.[33] Nor are these entirely financial decisions: physicians also may be reluctant to see Medicaid patients because they often have complicated behavioral health, transportation, and social service needs that require physician and staff time.[34] Thus, the care of Medicaid patients has become increasingly concentrated among a smaller proportion of physicians: those who practice in large groups, hospitals, academic medical centers, and community health centers.

The ACA will increase the number of Medicaid-insured patients, but it may have other unintended consequences. Because of the flexibility allowed under the ACA, Medicaid may be in a process of fundamental transformation. In September 2013, Arkansas was granted a waiver to pursue a so-called "private option," which will allow state residents to use Medicaid dollars to subsidize coverage obtained through private insurance. Up to six other states may pursue some form of Arkansas's plan. Two, Iowa and Pennsylvania, had already filed waiver requests in 2013. The Arkansas, Iowa, and Pennsylvania plans all feature free-market aspects in the expansion of coverage—a unique "hybrid" strategy that could be palatable to Republicans and conservative Democrats who object on principle to expanding any government program.[35]

Critics who see Medicaid as an entitlement on par with Medicare and Social Security are likely to oppose the private insurance option. Yet there are also potential advantages to this strategy. One possible advantage is that Medicaid patients with private plans will no longer be stigmatized in physician practices, because they will no longer be identifiable. Further, it is possible that these plans will be no more difficult for health systems to administer than any private insurance plan, solving the administrative headaches associated with Medicaid. This option, moreover, provides political cover for Republicans who campaigned on a promise to rescind Obamacare. Thus, ironically, the route that may allow Medicaid to move beyond its poor law legacy and become truly a middle-class entitlement is through the private insurance industry.

## MEDICAID AND LONG-TERM CARE

In 2011 Medicaid was the primary payer for over 63 percent of skilled nursing facility (SNF) residents, dwarfing the 4.5 percent of these residents supported by Medicare.[36] Medicaid has become the default source of long-term care funding, because Medicare mainly covers acute care services. The exception is when a Medicare beneficiary is released to an SNF directly from an inpatient hospital stay of at least three days, not including the day of discharge. Even then, only the first 20 days are fully covered, with a portion of the cost covered up to a hundred days.

Health policy analysts vehemently disagree over the quality of Medicaid's long-term care benefit, both to those who use it and to the public at large.

Critics such as political scientist Laura Katz Olson have charged that Medicaid's long-term care benefit results in a "bifurcated structure" for long-term care that separates those with substantial resources from those without.[37] By contrast, Colleen Grogan and Eric Patashnik have argued that Medicaid has increasingly been cast as "a core entitlement for the mainstream aged" that protects people with a long history of employment and tax payment.[38] Both perspectives contain an element of truth.

It is certainly the case that Medicaid has become a de facto nursing home benefit for the middle class. A core provision of Medicaid is the "medically needy" category, which allows individuals who have large medical expenses relative to their income to receive coverage for long-term care.[39] Though not universal, this benefit has expanded over time, and by 2009, 34 states had medically needy programs. States also extend eligibility through a special income rule called the "300 percent rule," which allows frail individuals with incomes up to 300 percent of the SSI level to qualify for Medicaid for nursing home care.[40]

There is, however, a catch: in addition to the income eligibility rules, Medicaid applicants must also satisfy an asset test. Individuals who have assets over the federal limit are not eligible for Medicaid until they have "spent down" their resources below the limit. Given the high cost of nursing home care, which in 2011 ranged from $60,986 annually in South Dakota to $114,975 in New York (for a semiprivate room), few individuals can afford to pay for more than a few months in most cases. As a result, about 60 percent of nursing home residents enter as private payers and then become Medicaid eligible when they deplete their resources. Another one-third are eligible at admission.[41]

During the spend-down process, Medicaid applicants are allowed to spend their money on anything, not just on their care. They cannot, however, give resources away for less than fair market value. Medicaid has a "look-back" period of five years to see whether assets were improperly transferred. The look-back period was instituted by Congress in 1993 because of suspicion that middle-class elderly persons were sheltering their assets to qualify for Medicaid; the original rule stipulated that assets had to be transferred prior to three years before an individual could apply for Medicaid. The Deficit Reduction Act of 2005 increased the look-back period for asset transfers to five years, with the penalty period beginning when the individual applied for Medicaid, not when funds or assets were transferred. While the value of a primary residence (up to $750,000) is excluded from the eligibility calculations, federal law includes a "clawback" clause that requires states to recover the amount Medicaid spent on an individual's long-term care services from his or her estate after death. Although state probate laws vary, they generally include as part of an estate all real and personal property, such as a home and other assets. In addition, individuals must name the state as the sole beneficiary for any annuities they hold equal to the amount of the Medicaid-funded assistance.[42] Some states do allow Medicaid recipients to put excess income above the Medicaid limit into a trust to help them to qualify for Medicaid. At death the trust proceeds then go first to repay the state for long-term care provided.

In limiting the transfer of generational wealth, these rules place Medicaid squarely in the category of care for the indigent. The exceptions for spousal transfers of wealth make this clear: if one spouse requires long-term care services, Medicaid does not require the other spouse to give up all assets and income so that the spouse needing care can qualify. Every state has its own "spousal protection" rules to allow the healthy spouse to remain in the community, but the rules allow the healthy spouse to keep anywhere from $22,000 to $110,000 in assets. The estate of the Medicaid beneficiary is exempt from recovery if the community-dwelling spouse is still alive, but the states may recover from the spouse's estate after his or her death.

The Medicaid long-term care recovery rule clearly distinguishes the program from Social Security and Medicare. The latter programs are funded by payroll taxes and are viewed as an earned right. This is the case even though the link between Medicare benefits vis-à-vis taxes paid is tenuous at best. People also pay taxes at both the state and federal level that fund Medicaid, yet these taxes are not viewed as constituting an earned right to benefits. Thus, the government does not expect any recovery of benefits paid to Social Security and Medicare recipients, but does demand recovery from Medicaid nursing home recipients.

Because income and asset tests vary from state to state, Medicaid applicants face a bewildering array of rules and regulations. Most people have no idea how the Medicaid rules in their state operate until a health crisis forces them to apply for benefits. Then they are ill-prepared to deal with the consequences.[43]

Despite the byzantine rules, Medicaid has had a significant impact on the type of care that frail older people receive, with the bulk of resources being spent on institutional care, as Judith Feder explains in Chapter 13 of this volume. Congress has gradually allowed states to apply for waivers to experiment with alternative methods of providing services, given concerns that Medicaid was encouraging unnecessary institutionalization. The Home and Community-Based Services Waiver program (HCBS) lets states provide low-income and disabled individuals with a variety of services to help them avoid institutional care. These include personal care, homemaker services, day care, and case management. By 2005, all 50 states had HCBS waivers.[44] In 2006, Congress created the Money Follows the Person (MFP) program, which provides states funds to move Medicaid beneficiaries who reside in nursing homes back to their own homes or to alternative community housing. States have nevertheless faced major challenges in implementing the program, including a lack of appropriate housing, a paucity of well-trained workers to provide services to individuals leaving nursing facilities, and an inadequate network of home-and-community-based services. The ACA expanded the MFP program. As of 2014, 44 states and the District of Columbia were participating in the demonstration.[45]

Another effort to reduce unnecessary institutionalization is the Program of All-Inclusive Care for the Elderly (PACE). PACE is an optional benefit under both Medicare and Medicaid for older people who meet their state's standards for nursing home care. It features comprehensive medical and social services that can be provided at an adult day care center, private home, nursing home, or assisted living facility. Most recipients of PACE services are able to remain in their own homes while receiving services, rather than be forced to move into a nursing home. Currently, however, PACE is available only in states that have taken the option of offering the program through Medicaid. Thirty-one states had PACE enabling legislation in 2014, but not all states had programs operating, and never on a statewide basis.[46]

Although there have been efforts to reverse course and decrease funding for institutional care, these efforts have been piecemeal, as Judith Feder explains in Chapter 13 of this volume. Individuals seeking HCBS as an alternative to nursing home care are also discouraged by variations in eligibility rules. Some states apply more restrictive income eligibility criteria to waiver recipients compared to nursing home residents; some states only provide the medically needy and spend-down options to nursing home residents; and many states do not provide the same level of income and spousal asset protection to waiver recipients compared to nursing home residents.[47] Thus, although the percentage of funding for HCBS relative to nursing home care has steadily increased, institutional care still predominates.

A final question is quality. Individuals who are Medicaid-eligible might find their options limited, compared to patients with the ability to pay from private funds. In part, access is limited because Medicare pays almost three times as much as Medicaid, so in many states nursing homes have attempted to maximize revenues by saving fewer beds for Medicaid patients.[48] As a result, Medicaid patients have longer waits to gain admission and end up in less desirable homes. Low reimbursement rates can also affect access. For example, in Illinois, state officials concerned about the rising cost of Medicaid halted nursing home reimbursement rate increases for three years in the 1990s. In response, many nursing homes began to limit the number of Medicaid patients they would accept, and some stopped taking Medicaid patients altogether.[49]

There is also evidence that facilities with high Medicaid occupancy are of poor quality compared to those with a different patient mix.[50] This issue is especially a problem for African Americans, who are much more likely than white patients to be concentrated in nursing homes that have serious deficiencies, lower staffing ratios, and financial vulnerabilities.[51]

Has Medicaid reached the status of an entitlement, or does it remain mired in its poor law legacy? Formally, Medicaid is an "entitlement" program, because "it features an open-ended funding commitment by the federal government, which matches at varying rates whatever the states spend."[52] Thus, states have guaranteed federal financial support for a portion of their Medicaid programs. Further, the states are legally required to offer the basic package of services to all beneficiaries who meet the eligibility requirements. Medicaid might also be considered an entitlement because its benefits extend well beyond the poor to reach into the middle class, both in terms of health insurance coverage and long-term care in nursing homes.

Medicaid also provides significant value to beneficiaries. It improves access to care and reduces unmet health needs. Compared to the uninsured, the majority of children and adults covered by Medicaid have a usual source of care, and few children and relatively few adults with Medicaid postpone or go without needed care due to cost. This is in sharp contrast to the uninsured, who report significant cost barriers that prevent them from receiving care.[53]

Other aspects of Medicaid, however, cast doubt on its status as an entitlement in the broader sense of the word. In this definition, an entitlement is equivalent to social insurance: "The central image of social insurance is the earned entitlement, publicly administered benefits for which all similarly situated persons are eligible by virtue of their financial contributions to the system or the taxes they pay.... Equitable treatment... is the controlling standard."[54] The core social insurance programs are Social Security and Medicare, which are granted to individuals as an earned right on a permanent basis once eligibility has been determined. By contrast, Medicaid is much more unstable. Beneficiaries may move on and off coverage as income changes. Coverage can vary not only over time but also among individuals in the same family, because eligibility standards differ for children on the basis of age and for adults of different statuses.

Medicaid also has limits on access. Some providers refuse to accept Medicaid beneficiaries for various reasons, while others set quotas on the number they will accept. The quality of the Medicaid benefit also varies according to place of residence. Some states have quite generous Medicaid programs with income limits well above the federal standard, while others are quite stingy. Although the ACA will even out some of the disparities in coverage, states will still differ in regard to eligibility rules and how Medicaid programs operate. Thus, the quality of health insurance will remain uneven across states. Overall, then, the Medicaid benefit is not fully an entitlement because of instability in coverage, limits on access, and variation in quality across regions and providers.

The Medicaid long-term care benefit funds many middle-class people through its medically needy and spend-down provisions, which is why this part of the program is often described as an entitlement. Yet there are many aspects to this benefit that negate this argument. Unlike Social Security and Medicare, the Medicaid long-term care benefit forces applicants to prove their eligibility in ways that some see as demeaning. It is not given as a right. Even after individuals have qualified, they are forced to turn over all their income except for a small personal care allowance. And because of the recovery rule, Medicaid long-term care beneficiaries must reimburse the state for the cost of their care after death. Access to care can also be a problem, even for fully qualified beneficiaries. Many nursing homes discriminate against

Medicaid-eligible elderly, preferring Medicare and private pay patients. Those that do accept a high percentage of Medicaid-eligible patients often provide poorer quality of care.

Surveys show that the vast majority of older people would prefer to remain in their own homes and community, and efforts have been made to reverse the course of institutionalized care set a half-century ago. There are now a variety of experiments with HCBS to service the frail elderly in the community. However, these services are only available to some individuals and are never universally offered on a statewide basis. In part, this is due to fears that the costs would be exorbitant, and in part because of a shortage of service providers. As a result, Medicaid still contains incentives to provide care in institutional, rather than less restrictive, settings. In the long-term care benefit, too, then, Medicaid is not equivalent to Social Security and Medicare, because of uneven eligibility requirements, harsh estate recovery rules, discrimination by facility operators, and lack of choice regarding type of care for many beneficiaries.

## Notes

1. Laura Katz Olson, *The Politics of Medicaid* (New York: Columbia University Press, 2010).
2. Frank Thompson, *Medicaid Politics* (Washington, DC: Georgetown University Press, 2012).
3. Henry J. Kaiser Family Foundation, "The Medicaid Program at a Glance," March 4, 2013, http://kff.org/medicaid/fact-sheet/the-medicaid-program-at-a-glance-update/.
4. Laura Katz Olson, *The Not-So-Golden Years: Caregiving, the Frail Elderly and the Long Term Care Establishment* (Lanham, MD: Rowman and Littlefield, 2003).
5. Timothy Jost, *Disentitlement?* (New York: Oxford University Press, 2003), 178.
6. Colleen Grogan, "Medicaid: Designed to Grow," in *Health Politics and Policy*, ed. James Morone, Theodor Litman, and Leonard Robins (Independence, KY: Engage Learning, 2014), 142–163.
7. David G. Smith, *Entitlement Politics* (Hawthorne, NY: Aldine De Gruyter, 2002).
8. Colleen Grogan and Christian Andrews, "Medicaid," in *The Oxford Handbook of U.S. Social Policy*, ed. Daniel Beland and Kimberly Morgan (New York: Oxford University Press, 2014), 337–354.
9. Jill Quadagno, *One Nation, Uninsured: Why the US Has No National Health Insurance* (New York: Oxford University Press, 2005).
10. Olson, *The Not-So-Golden Years*.
11. Quadagno, *One Nation, Uninsured*.

12. Ben Kail, Jill Quadagno, and Marc Dixon, "Can States Lead the Way to Universal Coverage? The Effect of Health Care Reform on the Uninsured." *Social Science Quarterly* 90 (2009): 1–20.

13. Leighton Ku and Bowen Garrett, "How Welfare Reform and Economic Factors Affected Medicaid Participation: 1984–1996," Urban Institute Discussion Paper (Washington, DC: The Urban Institute, 2000).

14. Colleen Grogan and Eric Patashnik, "Universalism within Targeting: Nursing Home Care, the Middle Class and the Politics of the Medicaid Program," *Social Service Review* 7 (2003): 45.

15. Peter Cunningham, "SCHIP Making Progress: Increased Take-Up Contributes to Coverage Gains," *Health Affairs* 22 (2003): 163–172.

16. Kaiser Commission on Medicaid and the Uninsured, *Medicaid Section 1115 Waivers: Current Issues*, Key Facts (Washington, DC: The Kaiser Family Foundation, 2005).

17. Gretchen Engquist and Peter Burns, "Health Insurance Flexibility and Accountability Initiative: Opportunities and Issues for States," *State Coverage Initiatives, Robert Wood Johnson Foundation.* Issue Brief 3 (August 2002): 1–6.

18. Kaiser Commission on Medicaid and the Uninsured, *Medicaid Section 1115 Waivers.*

19. Jonathan Oberlander, "Health Reform Interrupted: The Unraveling of the Oregon Health Plan," *Health Affairs* 26 (2007): 96–105.

20. Michael Cooper, "Conservatives Sowed Idea of Health Care Mandate, Only to Spurn It Later," *New York Times*, February 14, 2012.

21. Peter Jacobson and Rebecca Braun, "Let 1000 Flowers Wilt: The Futility of State Health Care Reform," *University of Kansas Law Review* 55 (2006–2007): 1173–1202.

22. Huma Kahn, "Has Mitt Romney's Massachusetts Health Care Law Worked?" *The Note*, May 12, 2011, http://abcnews.go.com/blogs/politics/2011/05/has-mitt-romneys-massachusetts-health-care-law-worked.

23. Henry J. Kaiser Family Foundation, "The Medicaid Medically Needy Program: Spending and Enrollment Update," December 12, 2012, http://kaiser-familyfoundation.files.wordpress.com/2013/01/4096.pdf.

24. Grogan, "Medicaid."

25. Henry J. Kaiser Family Foundation, "The Medicaid Medically Needy Program."

26. Ae-sook Kim and Edward Jennings, "The Evolution of an Innovation: Variations in Medicaid Managed Care Program Extensiveness," *Journal of Health Politics, Policy, and Law* 37 (2012): 815–849.

27. Lawrence R. Jacobs and Timothy Callaghan, "Why States Expand Medicaid: Party, Resources, and History," *Journal of Health Politics, Policy and Law* 38 (2013): 1025.

28. Grogan, "Medicaid."

29. Olson, *The Politics of Medicaid.*

30. Quadagno, *One Nation, Uninsured.*

31. Olson, *The Not-So-Golden Years.*

32. Peter J. Cunningham, "Mounting Pressures: Physicians Serving Medicaid Patients and the Uninsured, 1997–2001," *Center for Studying Health System Change* 6 (December 2002): 104.

33. Peter Cunningham and Jessica May, "Medicaid Patients Increasingly Concentrated among Physicians," *Center for Studying Health System Change* 16 (2006): 1–4.

34. Lawrence Casalino, "Professionalism and Caring for Medicaid Patients—The 5 percent Commitment?" *New England Journal of Medicine* 369 (2013): 1775–1777.

35. Henry J. Kaiser Family Foundation, "Medicaid Expansion Through Premium Assistance: Arkansas, Iowa, and Pennsylvania's Proposals Compared," April 14, 2014, http://kff.org/health-reform/fact-sheet/medicaid-expansion-through-premium-assistance-arkansas-and-iowas-section-1115-demonstration-waiver-applications-compared/.

36. Henry J. Kaiser Family Foundation, "Overview of Nursing Facility Capacity, Financing, and Ownership in the United States in 2011," June 28, 2013, http://kff.org/medicaid/fact-sheet/overview-of-nursing-facility-capacity-financing-and-ownership-in-the-united-states-in-2011/.

37. Olson, *The Not-So-Golden Years*, 17–18.

38. Grogan and Patashnik, "Universalism within Targeting," 58.

39. Henry J. Kaiser Family Foundation, "The Medicaid Medically Needy Program."

40. Henry J. Kaiser Family Foundation, "The Medicaid Program at a Glance."

41. Olson, *The Politics of Medicaid*, 137.

42. Olson, *The Politics of Medicaid*.

43. Quadagno, *One Nation, Uninsured*.

44. Centers for Medicare and Medicaid Services, *State Waiver and Demonstration Programs* (Baltimore, MD: CMS, 2003).

45. "Money Follows the Person," http://www.medicaid.gov/Medicaid-CHIP-Program-Information/By-Topics/Long-Term-Services-and-Supports/Balancing/Money-Follows-the-Person.html.

46. "PACE Benefits," http://www.medicaid.gov/Medicaid-CHIP-Program-Information/By-Topics/Long-Term-Services-and-Supports/Integrating-Care/Program-of-All-Inclusive-Care-for-the-Elderly-PACE/PACE-Benefits.html.

47. Enid Kassner and Lee Shirey, "Medicaid Financial Eligibility for Older People: State Variations in Access to Home and Community-Based Waiver and Nursing Home Services," AARP Public Policy Institute, April 2000, http://assets.aarp.org/rgcenter/health/2000_06_medicaid.pdf.

48. Debra Street, Jill Quadagno, Lori Parham and Steve McDonald, "Reinventing Long-Term Care: The Effect of Policy Changes on Trends in Nursing Home Reimbursement and Resident Characteristics: Florida, 1989–1997," *The Gerontologist* 43 (2003): 118–131.

49. Madonna Harrington-Meyer and Michelle Kesterke-Storbakken, "Shifting the Burden Back to Families." in *Care Work*, ed. Madonna Harrington Meyer (New York: Routledge, 2000), 217–228.

50. David Grabowski, Joseph Angelelli, and Vincent Mor, "The Relationship of Medicaid Payment Rates, Bed Constraint Policies, and Risk-Adjusted Pressure Ulcers," *Health Services Research* 39 (2004): 793–812.
51. David B. Smith, Zhanlian Feng, Mary Fennel, Jacqueline Zinn, and Vincent Mor, "Separate and Unequal: Racial Segregation and Disparities in Quality Across U.S. Nursing Homes," *Health Affairs* 26 (2007): 1448–1458.
52. Thompson, *Medicaid Politics*, 18.
53. Henry J. Kaiser Family Foundation, "The Medicaid Program at a Glance."
54. Theodore Marmor, Jerry Mashaw, and Philip Harvey, *America's Misunderstood Welfare State* (New York: Basic Books, 1990), 27.

# 6

# HOW THE COURTS CREATED
# THE MEDICAID ENTITLEMENT

SARA ROSENBAUM

We speak of entitlement in political and moral terms. Ultimately, however, the question of entitlement is a legal one that focuses on whether an individual has a legal claim to some form of right, property, or benefit.[1] In a privatized healthcare system, the question of legal entitlement to healthcare financing looms large, given the consequences of being without an enforceable right to health insurance and the benefits and services it pays for.

Unlike Medicare, the Medicaid statute both lacks explicit rights-creating language and fails to address the separate question of whether private individuals have the right to seek judicial redress against state agencies for violation of federal law. Despite its incredible complexity, the federal Medicaid statute is silent on both counts, leaving it to the courts to sort out matters of fundamental importance to the program's purpose, structure, operation, and future.

Medicaid's historical trajectory as a rights-creating law that grants individuals access to the courts mirrors the philosophical and political trajectory of the courts themselves, as shaped by the US Supreme Court, which has the final word on the meaning of federal laws. Under the Court's increasingly restrictive standards applicable to the question of when government programs create individual rights, key portions of the Medicaid statute continue to be treated as privately enforceable rights. But beneficiaries and providers increasingly meet with judicial skepticism over whether they can turn to the courts when they claim governmental violations of pivotal portions of the statute that are essential to its success but whose terms do not pass the modern Court's high bar for determining when grant programs that aid the poor can be said to create "rights."

Thus, as a law, Medicaid raises two central questions: First, does its legal framework create "rights," and if so, to what? Second, are private individuals and entities able to seek judicial review of state actions that allegedly violate federal law? These questions are integral to understanding what Medicaid guarantees to the tens of millions of people who depend on the program for affordable medical care.

Where Medicare is concerned, Congress answered both questions at the time of initial enactment. Medicare rested—and continues to rest—on a statutory architecture that establishes a legal claim of entitlement to a defined set of benefits. Over the decades, the Medicare legal entitlement has survived a deluge of amendments, but the fundamental concept—an entitlement to coverage for specified benefits—remains intact. Medicare makes repeated references to "individuals entitled to benefits under this title."[2] Nor does Medicare leave any doubt regarding its legal relationship with participating providers; providers and suppliers that furnish covered and medically necessary care to patients are legally entitled to payment in accordance with Medicare payment methodologies. In recognition of legal entitlement, the Medicare statute explicitly establishes a federal legal enforcement process that provides a detailed process of administrative and judicial review of claims of coverage.[3] Even alternative coverage approaches that would eliminate Medicare's defined benefit structure in favor of a premium support model that eliminates defined-benefit government insurance in favor of subsidized private coverage (much like the approach to subsidized coverage under the Affordable Care Act) do not purport to eliminate the entitlement; rather, they would downgrade it.

Medicaid presents a vastly different situation. Unlike Medicare, the legal architecture of Medicaid was—and is—that of a classic grant-in-aid program enacted pursuant to the Constitution's Spending Clause, which empowers

Congress to spend funds to promote the general welfare. The essence of grant-in-aid laws is a detailed description of the relationship between the two governments—federal and state—that engage in joint administration. Of course, Medicaid's ultimate beneficiaries are the children and adults who fall within its eligibility parameters and thus are qualified to receive covered benefits. Nonetheless, the chief focus of Medicaid's legal framework is the rights and obligations of two sovereigns: their terms of engagement, as it were.[4] Participating states operating approved state plans are entitled to federal payments, calculated in accordance with the law's open-ended funding formula.[5] Furthermore, states have an express right to pursue their legal entitlement to payment through federal administrative and judicial proceedings. In exchange for this guarantee, the law gives the secretary of Health and Human Services (HHS) (previously the Department of Health, Education, and Welfare [HEW]) the power to enforce the terms of the bargain.[6] Even so, the federal enforcement process, which in its most extreme form can involve the withdrawal of federal funding, is used sparingly (to put it mildly).

Nowhere does the Medicaid statute specify a legal entitlement to medical assistance on the part of eligible individuals. Indeed, the original Act began (and still begins today) with the statement that federal funding is to be provided "for the purpose of enabling each State, as far as practical under the conditions within such state, to furnish medical assistance. . . . "[7]—a distinctly inauspicious opening clause in a statute in the context of legal entitlement. Nor did—or does—the statute establish a process of federal administrative and judicial review by which program beneficiaries or providers can challenge state actions that they believe conflict with federal rights or legal safeguards.[8]

How Medicaid was transformed from a Spending Clause grant-in-aid program into a law that vests program beneficiaries with certain legally enforceable rights and a right of access to the courts is the subject of this chapter. Simply put, the Medicaid legal entitlement is the product of a remarkable judicial gloss overlaid on the statute, the result of a fundamental doctrinal shift in how the courts viewed governmental benefits. In recent decades, an increasingly conservative judiciary has sought to reverse course, tightening up considerably on its earlier rulings, while making it more difficult for beneficiaries and providers to seek judicial intervention.

The twin questions of whether Medicaid is a rights-creating statute, and whether and when the courts can intervene to protect private interests, now stand at the forefront of a profound philosophical battle over the proper role of the courts in enforcing the terms of Spending Clause programs. Medicaid exists as a legal entitlement, and its beneficiaries can secure access to the courts, not because Congress said so, but because the courts said so. And courts can and do change their minds.

That an older Supreme Court initially characterized Medicaid as a legal entitlement, or that the modern Supreme Court has backtracked on earlier positions, should come as no surprise to those familiar with the extent to which social and political context shape judicial philosophy.[9] The arc of Medicaid as an enforceable legal right parallels the arc of social justice as an American concept over the past half century. Lawrence Friedman, a leading scholar of the role of courts in society, has observed that the law made by legislatures, agencies, and courts is both a product and a reflection of society.[10] As American culture has shifted in its attitudes toward the poor and disenfranchised, so have the courts. Furthermore, given Medicaid's size as the largest of all means-tested entitlements, it is perhaps inevitable that Medicaid should have emerged as the biggest prize for those who favor retrenchment and the main event in the federalism battle, in which states test the power of the federal government.[11]

There may come a time when federal lawmakers will resolve this battle by simply block-granting Medicaid to the states, thereby eliminating all vestiges of individual legal entitlement.[12] In fact, this is exactly what lawmakers did in 1996 when they replaced Aid to Families with Dependent Children (AFDC) with the Temporary Assistance to Needy Families (TANF) program. As with the Children's Health Insurance Program (CHIP), enacted in 1997, Congress could restructure Medicaid to expressly disavow the existence of legal rights.[13] For now, Medicaid perseveres intact, even if its future remains tentative. Then again, where Medicaid is concerned, this somewhat precarious legal state of affairs has existed for decades.

The body of judicial case law interpreting Medicaid's provisions and meanings is almost as vast as the Medicaid program itself. Attempting to discuss all of the Medicaid cases ever litigated would be like counting the stars in the sky. By necessity, this chapter is selective, focusing on the milestone cases that have spelled out the relationship between states and providers and individuals. Some of the cases discussed here directly arose under Medicaid, while others—especially the early cases—involved efforts by lawyers representing the poor to clarify the legal status of the AFDC program, the original proving ground for welfare rights litigation. (The degree to which AFDC similarly came to be understood as a privately enforceable legal entitlement helps explain the fact that Congress did not merely amend AFDC in 1996 but repealed it altogether, in order to stamp out all vestiges of judicial precedent over the meaning of cash welfare assistance).

My intent throughout this chapter is to illustrate the great building blocks of judicial entitlement policy: whether a law creates a legal entitlement that cannot be denied, reduced, or terminated without due process; when a law can be said to set minimum legal standards governing the nature, size, and scope of an entitlement; and when the courts will permit individuals who are the intended beneficiaries of Spending Clause programs to seek the protection of the courts when vital interests are at stake, rather than having to rely exclusively on the political process or the discretionary powers of a federal enforcement agency.

## The Threshold Question: Does Medicaid Create a Legal Entitlement to Benefits?

Medicaid's judicial recognition as a legal entitlement required a profound shift in how society understood the status of government benefits more generally. Nineteenth-century law produced an important step forward in recognizing government as an actor in the lives of the poor, primarily through the enactment of English and American laws that empowered state and local governments to provide relief to the poor.[14] At the same time, these laws vested governments with broad discretion in terms of who would be helped, what form that help would take, and how much help would be provided. In this worldview, the poor had no legal right to assistance. Government had the power to help, but it also had the power to draw distinctions, often arbitrary, between the worthy and "unworthy" poor.

Under the old political regime, aid could be furnished in humiliating ways. People could be forced to appear before county boards to beg for assistance, and they could leave empty-handed for no particular reason. Those who were deemed deserving received help. Those who were not (e.g., adults deemed "able-bodied,"[15] women who bore children out of wedlock, the unemployed, those deemed social pariahs) received nothing.

This general societal attitude regarding the relationship between government and those who depended on it for survival was codified in the original Aid to Dependent Children provisions of the Social Security Act of 1935, whose purpose was to encourage the care of children in their own homes (later expanded to encompass the encouragement of family self-support and a strengthening of family life).[16] The federal government provided open-ended financing to states that chose to participate, while conferring on state governments the power to determine what constituted dependency, the standard of aid to be furnished, and the conditions under which aid would be given.[17] Assistance could be abruptly terminated. Aid was a means of softening the harshest edges of a free market economy, but only on conditions deemed politically acceptable to appointed or elected leaders, whose political outlook varied from state to state and community to community.

From the outset, AFDC was understood to encompass health care within the "standard of need" that established family eligibility for assistance. Of course, payments were so low ($3,800 over a year for a single parent with children in 1970) that using AFDC benefits to buy health care was impossible.[18]

The advent of discrete federal healthcare financing programs in 1950 continued in this tradition: entitlement funding to states would be coupled with broad powers to define what would constitute medical assistance. The arrival of federal healthcare financing in the form of the Kerr-Mills Act in 1960 had an incalculable effect on later court decisions, because it established an obligation on the part of participating states to aid certain groups of eligible individuals and to pay private providers of health care.

Medicaid emerged from these earlier laws as a system of federally supported third-party financing on behalf of eligible individuals who, as long as they met the program's eligibility criteria, were qualified to receive covered services from participating providers, including private providers.[19] The original statute was specific: it defined the categories of people for whom coverage was mandated, as well as those for whom coverage was optional. The statute also defined the "medical assistance" for which federal funding was available as a series of distinct categories of healthcare items and services, some of which were required; others were optional.[20]

Such was the governmental state of play in 1965, a year after publication of perhaps the most seminal law review article ever to address the relationship between individuals and government. In 1964, several years after the

US Supreme Court's decision in *Flemming v. Nestor*,[21] the *Yale Law Journal* published an article by Charles Reich, entitled "The New Property."[22] The article took its cue from the Court's decision in *Flemming*, which held that Barbara Nestor's Social Security spousal benefits could be lawfully terminated following the deportation of her husband, Ephram Nestor, for anti-American activities as a member of the Communist Party.[23] Nestor had worked a sufficient number of quarters in a Social Security–covered job to qualify for payments as vested benefits, but a five-member majority for the Court nevertheless concluded that termination was lawful, because Social Security retirement benefits did not amount to the type of property interest protected from arbitrary government action under law. In the majority's view, Social Security was fundamentally different from, say, funds held in a bank account or—tellingly—the contractual interest created through commercial insurance coverage. The Court recognized that individuals earned a right to Social Security benefits, but concluded that to treat such benefits as an accrued property right would deprive the government "of the flexibility and boldness in adjustment to ever-changing conditions which it demands."[24]

Taking its cue from *Flemming*, Reich "articulated a vision of individual liberty and government largesse that aimed to push the welfare state under the protective umbrella of the Constitution."[25] Reich essentially argued that benefits conferred by government, whether in the form of licenses or income and in-kind assistance, were "steadily taking the place of traditional forms of wealth,"[26] and that, as such, merited recognition as property and the extension of constitutional protection. Reich's arguments—precisely the opposite of the position taken by the *Flemming v. Nestor* majority—would dramatically alter how later courts viewed legal provisions such as those found in Medicaid and other means-tested government programs, for decades to come.

Reflecting Reich's enormous influence, as well as at least an implicit rejection of the Court's reasoning in *Flemming v. Nestor*, the 1965 Medicaid statute—even as it spoke primarily of the legal relationship between governments and eschewed the express legal guarantees accorded Medicare beneficiaries—contained exceedingly important provisions where subsequent judicial interpretation would be concerned. First, the law defined groups of individuals whom states would be mandated to assist.[27] Second, the statute obligated participating states to provide "fair hearings" (i.e., an impartial administrative review under state law) to any individual whose claim to medical assistance was denied, reduced, or terminated.[28] Third, the statute directed states to allow all people who wanted to apply for Medicaid to be allowed to do so; should an individual be found eligible, the statute further obligated states to provide medical assistance with "reasonable promptness."[29] Significantly, in its Handbook of Public Assistance (Supplement D), a foundational document interpreting and explaining the original Medicaid statute, the US Department of Health, Education, and Welfare (HEW, the predecessor to HHS) clarified that it considered Medicaid to amount to a form of public insurance that operated alongside the newly created Medicare program.[30]

Taken together, these statutory provisions, supplemented by HEW's interpretation of the law as a form of insurance, appeared to confer upon Medicaid the type of government-created benefit envisioned by Reich under his "new property" theory, meaning that the program was more than simple government largesse that could be denied or taken away without due process. But although the early Medicaid statute picked up on Reich's thinking, it did so in an ambiguous fashion, never using Medicare's clear language of legal entitlement. For this reason, it ultimately fell to the courts to give Medicaid its legal meaning.

Medicaid's early years as a law coincided with a time in the life of the American judiciary when courts took an expansive view of what constituted protectable property interests and essentially flung open the courthouse doors, inviting those who depended on this "new property" to seek judicial protection against arbitrary government conduct. The decade following Medicaid's enactment thus coincided with an explosion of judicial decisions exploring the relationship between government and people. Eighteen US Supreme Court decisions, including a trilogy of three landmark cases discussed below, created the judicial context for Medicaid's emergence as a legal entitlement.[31] These three cases, each of which dealt with the nature of entitlements and their enforcement, arrived in the nation's highest court as part of a systemic effort by welfare rights advocates to enshrine Reich's "new property" concept into law for the poorest Americans.

The first of these cases, *King v. Smith*, involved an Alabama mother of four whose AFDC benefits had been revoked.[32] The state treated her boyfriend, who was occasionally a presence in her home, as a "substitute father" for her children, thereby disqualifying her and her children from financial assistance because they were not "deprived" of the support of both parents. (By the time lawyers brought *King*, states were engaged in widespread efforts to adopt "man in the house" or "man assuming the role of spouse" barriers to cash welfare assistance, including midnight raids on homes.) In *King*, the Court held that states that participated in a federally funded welfare program were obligated to conform to legally binding federal requirements and, furthermore, that private individuals who were the intended beneficiaries of a Spending Clause program had the right to seek the aid of the courts in challenging state conduct that allegedly violated federal standards.[33]

In *Rosado v. Wyman,* the second case, the Court addressed the enforcement process itself.[34] *Rosado* concerned the question of whether New York's method for calculating welfare benefits satisfied federal requirements or violated the law's welfare assistance formula. In *Rosado*, the Court moved the *King* principles a step further, holding that welfare recipients could turn directly to the courts to seek protection from unlawful state action and did not have to wait to see if a federal enforcement agency would provide relief. Indeed, as the Court pointed out, the federal AFDC statute (like Medicaid) gave private individuals no right to federal agency assistance against state violators. (In 1970, this silence on Congress's part was understood as clearing the way for beneficiaries' access to the courts; 40 years later, as discussed below, a near-majority of the Court would take the position that such silence was evidence that Congress intended that the two sovereigns work matters out with each other, cutting beneficiaries out of the action entirely.)

The final case in the trilogy, *Goldberg v. Kelly,*[35] concerned the procedures that governments are constitutionally required to follow when reducing or terminating public assistance, in this case, again, cash welfare benefits. The Court's decision in *Goldberg* effectively sounded the death knell to the proposition that means-tested welfare programs amounted to no more than government largesse that can be denied, reduced, or terminated at will and without constitutional due process. *Goldberg* set a particularly high standard for the termination of programs that, like AFDC or Medicaid, are means-tested and thus respond to "brutal need." In such situations, assistance cannot be terminated until a state's preliminary decision to end assistance becomes final following full procedural due process.[36]

The Court's central holdings in these cases were immediately understood by the lower courts to extend to Medicaid, a welfare program closely tied to AFDC (indeed, Medicaid's mandatory eligibility groups included AFDC recipients). The courts viewed Medicaid, with its open-ended financing, its ties to welfare, and its description of state coverage obligations, as a program that conferred legally enforceable expectations on the part of those for whom benefits were intended while protecting recipients of aid from the arbitrary denial, termination, or reduction of assistance without due process of law.

Medicaid's structure, with its clearly defined eligibility groups, a clearly defined set of benefits, and open-ended federal financing, served to create a potential crucial bulwark against the loss of these protections as an increasingly conservative US Supreme Court began retrenching on its earlier positions. Perhaps the most important signal of judicial retrenchment came in *Pennhurst State School v. Halderman*,[37] decided in 1981, in which the Court held that the Mental Health and Mental Retardation Act of 1966, which provided grants to states to aid in the treatment of persons with mental disabilities, created no federal right to treatment in the least restrictive alternative. It was in *Pennhurst* that the Court first signaled the existence of clear limits on the extent to which Spending Clause programs that were intended to assist states address the needs of vulnerable populations would be interpreted as creating legally enforceable rights in the intended beneficiaries of such programs. For conservative theorists, *Pennhurst* has become a sort of legal touchstone going forward, with its vivid imagery (the majority decision was written by then-Justice Rehnquist, who later would become the Court's Chief Justice) of public welfare programs as a "contract" between sovereigns, rather than a means of vesting rights in the poor.[38]

## THE SCOPE QUESTION: WHAT IS THE EXTENT OF THE RIGHT TO MEDICAID?

Even as the Court was showing signs of retrenchment in *Pennhurst*, Medicaid and welfare enforcement litigation proceeded in the lower courts, with beneficiaries often winning sweeping holdings barring various types of state efforts aimed at curbing eligibility, reducing benefits, or effectuating change in the scope and nature of coverage without procedural due process. Yet despite the breadth of these decisions, many of which favored beneficiaries, courts also showed their willingness to find limits in the extent of states' legal obligations under the law.[39] At the same time, beneficiaries won many cases. While no official scorecard of Medicaid wins and losses exists, legal scholar Tim Jost has estimated that in 1999 and 2000, respectively, plaintiffs prevailed in 53 and 48 percent of cases, with stronger win records for beneficiaries than providers.[40]

The Medicaid statute sets forth a series of standards that govern the amount, duration, and scope of coverage. Certain categories of eligible individuals must be given benefits, while other eligibility groups are optional.[41] Certain classes of services are required, while others are optional.[42] The statute also imposes a test of reasonableness to which states must adhere in setting limits on the amount, duration, and scope of covered benefits (that is, the extent of medical assistance they will cover).[43] Early HEW policies interpreted certain tests of reasonableness to apply to both required and optional services,[44] while other regulations prohibit arbitrary discrimination based on condition, only in the case of coverage of required services.[45] This prohibition would bar a state, for example, from placing limits on physician care for mental illness while permitting all medically necessary care for physical health problems. (In this regard, Medicaid's nondiscrimination rules effectively created mental health parity long before the concept of mental health parity first was introduced by Congress into the private health insurance market in 1996 and then considerably broadened in 2008.)[46]

The list of benefits contained in the statute, coupled with the law's reasonableness of coverage standard and early and relatively expansive interpretive rules, led to extensive litigation against states that attempted to limit or reduce the scope of coverage.[47] In some cases, states tried simply to reduce the scope of coverage (e.g., permitting eyeglasses for adults following glaucoma surgery but denying coverage for refractive conditions, a move held to violate the regulatory purpose of eyeglasses, defined as to improve vision).[48] In other cases, states attempted to exclude required treatment for certain specified conditions (such as banning gender reassignment surgery for transgendered persons).[49] Cases also challenged states' refusal to cover drug therapies for AIDS patients;[50] the refusal to fund nontherapeutic abortions;[51] the refusal to fund certain types of medically necessary treatment in the absence of federal funding; and the imposition of flat normative limits (e.g., three physician visits per month for non-emergency care) on coverage for adults or flat limits on adult hospitalization to 14 days per year).[52]

Taken together, these cases demonstrated that the courts were willing to hear not only challenges that denied eligibility for coverage entirely, but also cases in which the extent and scope of coverage were the focus of state conduct. In these cases, plaintiffs were typically not individual beneficiaries who had been denied a particular treatment as medically unnecessary, but classes of beneficiaries attempting to halt an across-the-board reduction in the scope of a state's Medicaid plan as unlawful under controlling federal standards. Beneficiaries won many of these cases, but they also lost legal battles, especially disputes involving across-the-board limits applicable to all people, not just those with certain conditions. Supreme Court prec-edents have established a tolerance for normative limits in Medicaid, even when such limits have the effect of reducing coverage below levels needed by people with disabilities, because under the Court's rulings, federal dis-ability law does not affect the *design* of coverage.[53] At the same time, the courts remained vigilant over public coverage limits that seemed to select out certain conditions for more restrictive coverage (e.g., transgenderism, HIV/AIDS, mental illness), while allowing commercial insurance plans considerably more discretion over benefit design.[54] Furthermore, in evaluat-ing Medicaid's reach, the courts also have been willing to exclude treatments that lacked a medical basis (e.g., elective abortions).[55]

In *Harris v. McCrea*,[56] which involved a federal constitutional challenge to Congress's decision to bar federal funding for abortions not connected with rape, incest, or the life of the mother (a policy codified in the so-called Hyde Amendment, an annual rider on federal appropriations laws), the Supreme Court articulated another limitation on Medicaid's scope, one with echoes of *Flemming v. Nestor.* In *Harris*, the Court established the proposition that Congress can itself limit the scope of the Medicaid entitlement without vio-lating beneficiaries' equal protection and due process rights, simply by with-drawing federal funding for certain procedures and treatments. Congress can do so even when access to the underlying treatment is considered a fun-damental right. While the right to abortion may be fundamental, the federal government has no obligation to finance the exercise of such rights, even when the absence of funding acts as a de facto deprivation of those rights.

The one exception to the courts' willingness to grant states a fair degree of flexibility on the amount, duration, and scope of coverage has been Medicaid's Early and Periodic Screening, Diagnosis, and Treatment (EPSDT) benefit, which establishes a special and uniquely broad level of coverage for Medicaid-enrolled children and adolescents up to age 21.[57] Added to the statute in 1967 as a required Medicaid benefit and dramatically expanded by Congress in 1989, EPSDT is extraordinarily comprehensive and encompasses literally all treatments, items, and services, that, when medically necessary, fall within the federal definition of "medical assistance."[58] Given this sweeping and definitive language regarding what must be covered for children, the courts have been unusually vigilant in denying state efforts to limit medically necessary care to children and adolescents. Not only have courts overturned discriminatory coverage rules, but they have virtually always rejected the use of fixed coverage norms that are applied across the board. Thus, while a state might limit inpatient hospital care to 14 days per year in the case of adults, a similar limitation, if applied to children, would be considered unlawful. Not surprisingly, perhaps, states and federal lawmakers opposed to such a sweeping entitlement in children have argued for revisions to federal law that would scale back the scope of EPSDT, but such efforts have been rejected. (The CHIP program is not only a non-entitlement program, it requires benefits far more limited in scope than EPSDT.)

## Does Medicaid Create Rights for Providers?

A second aspect of Medicaid's history as an enforceable legal entitlement concerns participation and payment. Medicaid provider participation tends to be intertwined with participation in Medicare, since Medicaid participation frequently is derivative of Medicare participation status. In general, the courts have treated participation in a government insurance program as a "new property" interest, with an attendant emphasis on due process in the denial or revocation of that right. At the same time, the courts have been less than uniform on this matter, with some having determined that participation does not rise to the level of a right protected by the Constitution.[59]

States do retain a certain amount of discretion over provider participation; for example, they have the power to limit participation to providers that are deemed "qualified" to participate in the program.[60] At the same time, however, beneficiaries' right to free choice among qualified providers means that, in the absence of special federal waivers that permit states to limit beneficiary choice to only certain providers,[61] states cannot screen out providers other than for health and safety concerns (at which point they undoubtedly would no longer be "qualified").

The beneficiary entitlement to free choice of qualified provider has been most memorably used, perhaps, in cases in which politically motivated state lawmakers attempted to use Medicaid (the biggest source of public financing for family planning services) to punish Planned Parenthood by excluding it from Medicaid participation because of its involvement in both family planning and abortion. Two separate federal appellate courts have ruled that beneficiaries' right to choose the qualified provider of their choice bars an arbitrary state exclusion based solely on the fact that Planned Parenthood also provides treatment that Medicaid does not cover.[62]

Medicaid vests considerable discretion in states over provider payment. But certain classes of providers do have payment protections that have been recognized in the federal courts as enforceable rights. Nowhere is recognition of payment rights clearer than in the case of community health centers (federally funded clinics providing comprehensive primary health care in low-income and medically underserved communities). Because of the large proportion of completely uninsured patients served by health centers, Congress amended federal law in 1990 to grant health centers the right to reasonable payment levels in order to shield their grant funds (intended for care of the uninsured) from the impact of cost-shifting by state Medicaid programs, whose payment rates typically are very low. Efforts by health centers to enforce their payment rights tend to succeed.[63]

## When Can Medicaid Beneficiaries Seek the Protection of the Courts?

It is not enough to have a legal interest to protect; one must have the right to go to court to protect that interest, rather than relying on the political process or federal enforcement agencies, when one's interests are threatened. Access to the courts is not automatic. Not only must courts have the official power to hear a case (a power referred to as "jurisdiction"), but individuals must also have the right to seek judicial redress (the "right of action") to be able to turn to a court rather than an administration agency, or more simply, the political process. This is why Congress was so careful to spell out a right of action in the Medicare statute, in addition to detailing the terms of the individual legal entitlement.

In Medicaid, when and how private actors (beneficiaries and providers) can go to court is a question fraught with tension. In fact, it was hospitals' attempt to enforce their legal entitlement to payment under a now-repealed provision of the Medicaid program that led to the Supreme Court's most far-reaching decision regarding Medicaid as a judicially enforceable legal entitlement. Ten years after its 1981 *Pennhurst* decision, the Court held in *Wilder v. Virginia Hospital Association* that the federal Medicaid statute entitled hospitals to a reasonable level of payment.[64] The case involved a suit brought by Virginia's hospitals over the state's low Medicaid payment rates; the Court held that the Boren Amendment, which would be repealed six years later as part of the 1997 Balanced Budget Act, entitled the hospitals to "reasonable and adequate" payment levels.[65] But the Court's decision, which remains controlling despite the demise of Boren, underscored that even in the wake of *Pennhurst*, the Justices in fact regarded Medicaid as a statute that created judicially enforceable rights.

*Wilder* also clarified that, when an enforceable right under Medicaid is involved, claimants have a right to bring suit under a special (and ancient) post–Civil War statute, 42 U.S.C. §1983. Section 1983 was enacted by Congress to ensure private individuals' access to the courts in cases of alleged deprivation by states of their "rights" secured by the Constitution or federal law. The Court's willingness to consider the hospitals' claims in *Wilder* meant that it regarded Medicaid as the type of "rights"-creating law for which §1983 provided a pathway to judicial review. A decade previously, the Court had, in fact, laid the basis for this decision in a case involving AFDC benefits, which were also considered a right that could be enforced under §1983.[66]

Even as *Wilder* seemed to settle the question of Medicaid's status as a legal entitlement whose terms could be interpreted by the courts under §1983, the question for an increasingly conservative Court in the wake of *Wilder* became *which* portions of public welfare programs generally can be said to create "rights." After all, Congress does not label pieces of statutes as rights-creating or otherwise. Laws such as Medicaid are extremely complex statutory schemes with countless moving parts. Some portions of the law speak to entitlement, while others speak to the program's extensive operational requirements, which of course, are integral to the proper working of the entitlement itself. In the judicial philosophy period that produced *King* and *Rosado,* it was sufficient that claimants seeking the help of the courts be the intended beneficiaries of a program. The Court treated program beneficiaries as having an "implied right of action" under the Constitution's Supremacy Clause, which allowed them to come to court when the threat of injury was the result of a possible state violation of federal law. But as the

Court became more conservative, it moved toward rejecting the concept of an implied right of action, at least in Spending Clause cases. For the courts to be involved in such cases, plaintiffs had to be able to point to an *express* right of action.

Where a legal entitlement was on the line, *Wilder*, of course, meant that §1983 was available. But under what circumstances would a legal entitlement be said to exist? And what about other cases, where critical state duties were on the line, but the Medicaid entitlement itself (i.e., eligibility for coverage) was not directly implicated? In a succession of cases spanning the decade between 1992 and 2002, the Court took an increasingly narrow view of when it would consider a federal Spending Clause statute as creating legal "rights" for purposes of §1983.[67] This line of cases culminated with *Gonzaga University v. Doe*.[68] Writing for a seven-member majority in a case involving the Federal Educational Rights and Privacy Act (FERPA), Chief Justice Rehnquist held that in the absence of clear congressional intent to confer a right, the Court would not deem the existence of one. In other words, general language describing how a social welfare program should work was not enough to create a right conferred by federal law for purposes of §1983. Instead, courts were expected to find hard evidence, in the terms of the statutes themselves, of congressional intent to confer a right, that is, a measurable benefit, on specific individuals.

This strategy of narrowing access to §1983 was accompanied by other cases in which the Court sought to stamp out the notion of an implied right of action. A key decision in this regard was *Alexander v. Sandoval*,[69] in which the plaintiffs sought to enjoin Alabama officials from allegedly engaging in de facto (i.e., discriminatory in effect) discrimination on the basis of race in administering a federally funded program through the use of language restrictions on who could participate in the program. Holding that Title VI of the 1964 Civil Rights Act sanctioned only cases of *intentional* discrimination, the Court effectively dismissed the case, since Title VI created no right of action for de facto discrimination claims, and plaintiffs could not rely on an implied right of action under the Supremacy Clause. Following *Sandoval*, the entire question of when, if ever, the Court will allow plaintiffs to enter court on an implied right of action theory moved to the forefront.

This question is crucial to Medicaid, whose hundreds of pages describe not only the legal entitlement to coverage but also the many duties of states that make coverage real and accessible for people. For example, the statute provides that states must allow people who want to do so to apply for Medicaid, and additionally assigns states the duty to determine eligibility with reasonable promptness and to actually provide medical assistance with reasonable promptness.[70] These duties clearly are integral to the program's operations, but does the language create a "right"? Some lower courts have said "yes," while others have said "no." Similarly, Medicaid obligates states to set provider payment levels that are sufficient to ensure that Medicaid patients have access to care comparable to that enjoyed by privately insured patients.[71] Is this directive (known informally as the "equal access" provision) a general obligation of the state, or is it a right? Courts similarly have split on this question.[72]

Shortly after *Sandoval* was decided, the Court appeared to soften its draconian position on when injured parties asserting Medicaid claims could—or could not—get into court. In 2003, the Court decided *Pharmaceutical Research and Manufacturers Association v. Walsh*,[73] which involved a lawsuit brought by pharmaceutical manufacturers against the state of Maine over how it was administering its prescription drug coverage program. The companies lost, but that was not the point. The point, in fact, was that the Court heard the claim *at all*, since the case did not involve any entitlement provision of the statute but instead challenged a state's general operation of its program. (Only Justice Thomas, in his concurrence, pointed out the oddity of hearing the case.)[74]

Despite the fact that it seemed to sanction continuing litigation over non-entitlement provisions of Medicaid in *Walsh*, in 2012 the Court agreed to hear a case that once again squarely considered the question of whether providers and beneficiaries have the right to obtain judicial review of state agency conduct under Medicaid, even when a right was not on the line.

*Douglas v. Independent Living Center of Southern California* regarded a series of Medicaid provider payment reductions made by the state of California in the wake of the 2008 financial crisis.[75] Several groups of providers and beneficiaries sued to enjoin the reductions, basing their claim on Medicaid's equal access provision. The Court of Appeals for the Ninth Circuit (whose region includes California), in an earlier case, already had determined that the equal access provision was *not* a rights-creating statute; hence, plaintiffs could not invoke §1983. As was the case with the pharmaceutical companies who brought *Walsh*, however, the *Douglas* plaintiffs argued that because the state was violating federal law in how it was administering Medicaid, they had the ability—under the Supremacy Clause of the US Constitution—to go to court.

In *Douglas*, moreover, the stakes were especially high because the states—somewhat surprisingly—had the Obama administration on their side. Along with the states, the solicitor general argued that, in the absence of a legal right that meets the *Gonzaga* test, claimants have no ability to obtain judicial review of state Medicaid agency actions, even when they face direct injury, because these non-entitlement portions of the statute are left to the exclusive enforcement powers of the federal executive branch.

At the time the Court heard the arguments in *Douglas*, the Centers for Medicare and Medicaid Services (CMS), which administer the federal Medicaid program, were still reviewing California's rate reduction proposals. (In fact, CMS takes years to resolve these types of matters, meaning that in the absence of a court injunction barring the state action on legal grounds, the plaintiffs could face extensive injury.) Shortly after the arguments concluded, however, CMS finally reached its decision, permitting some of California's cuts and rejecting others. To understand just how practically and politically impossible it is for providers and beneficiaries to turn to CMS when faced with injury, an amicus brief filed in *Douglas* by former HHS officials on their behalf argued that Medicaid's many protections were "logistically, practically, legally, and politically" unenforceable by the federal government.[76]

In the end, because of the CMS action, the Court sent *Douglas* back to the lower courts with the pivotal issue unresolved. The Court's four-member liberal wing effectively persuaded Justice Anthony Kennedy to essentially kick a potential blockbuster away on the ground that since the federal agency with enforcement authority finally had sorted matters out, the case was now sufficiently resolved to punt it without deciding the ultimate question. By ducking matters (over the angry dissent of Chief Justice Roberts, who argued that the time had come for an unequivocal ruling that closed the courthouse doors to Spending Clause cases in which rights are not involved), the Court left for another day the question of whether the courts are available when a federal duty, but not a federal right, is on the line.

Ironically perhaps, after the high drama of *Douglas*, the Court has continued to hear additional Medicaid cases that, like *Douglas*, raise questions regarding state violations of federal duties, not the violation of a right. In 2013 the Court decided *Wos v. E.M.A. ex rel Johnson*,[77] which involved a challenge to the legality of North Carolina's process for imposing liens on beneficiary proceeds arising from injury awards. The plaintiff in *Wos* did not claim that a right had been violated; instead, the claim was that the state had allegedly violated federal Medicaid law regulating the imposition of liens on beneficiary property. In reaching the merits of the claim (and holding for the beneficiary), Justice Kennedy stressed in his ruling that the Court was acting in the absence of *any* federal agency action. Unlike *Douglas,* not only had CMS not reviewed the lawfulness of North Carolina's conduct, but the agency had never even articulated federal standards for states to follow. Putting *Douglas* and *Wos* together, one can infer that as long as the federal agency has not stepped in to manage the problem, the Supreme Court will continue to permit claims of general statutory violations that rest on Supremacy Clause right-of-action theory, even where no federal rights are involved.

However, in 2014 the Supreme Court once again agreed to hear a replay of *Douglas,* this time in a case involving Idaho legislature's refusal to appropriate funds sufficient to pay a federally-approved payment rate to providers of health care services for children with disabilities. In this case, *Exceptional Child Center Inc. v Armstrong,*[78] the Court will once again consider whether providers and beneficiaries can seek the help of the courts when states refuse to comply with federal Medicaid requirements governing the accessibility of health care.

This overview of the role played by the courts in breathing life into the Medicaid statute underscores the extent to which the courts have shaped the fundamental policy concepts on which the entire program rests. Unlike Medicare, Medicaid lacked both explicit rights-creating language as well as a statutory right of action to privately enforce legal rights. Had they been enacted in another era, it is possible that the courts might have left Medicaid's benefits and protections to federal and state discretion. But Medicaid's enactment coincided with a profound shift in judicial philosophy regarding the fundamental meaning of government programs intended to benefit individuals. As the courts moved decisively to develop a framework of entitlement and enforcement, Medicaid became the beneficiary of this seismic shift in judicial philosophy.

This early flowering of rights theory began to erode by the 1970s. Over the past 40 years, the erosion has been significant. Medicaid litigation has become a series of staged battles in which a rights theory of government benefits is on the line. Courts move from provision to provision, determining which are rights-creating, and which are not. Section 1983 offers a secure pathway to the enforcement of rights (secure is, of course, a relative term; Congress always could repeal §1983). But the pathway to private enforcement of Medicaid's many important provisions that do not create individual rights is far from a solid certainty. For the time being, the US Supreme Court appears to have found a means of reconciling Spending Clause statutory provisions with the reach of the Supremacy clause. This could, however, change, and the Court could at some point order a full-scale retrenchment from judicial review of Medicaid claims that do not involve one of the handful of designated "rights." This possibility looms large, especially if Medicaid litigation intensifies in the wake of the sweeping eligibility, coverage, and enrollment reforms contained in the Affordable Care Act—reforms that all are designed to make the program work better for millions of the nation's most disadvantaged residents.

What would happen to Medicaid if these private enforcement underpinnings were to be removed—that is, if the Supreme Court were to close the door to most forms of private legal actions, proclaiming that Medicaid is no more than a contract between sovereigns? We don't know the answer to this; hopefully, we never will. Most federal and state officials at least privately acknowledge the importance of the courts in shaping the policy and politics of programs for the poor. A few are even thankful.

## Notes

1. Timothy Stoltzfus Jost, *Disentitlement: The Threats Facing Our Public Health Care Programs and a Rights-Based Response* (New York: Oxford University Press, 2003).
2. See, e.g., Social Security Act §1802, 42 U.S.C. §1395a(a).
3. Social Security Act §§405(g) and 1395ff(b). For the relationship between the Social Security appeals system and the system used in Medicare, as well as the scope of appeals rights, see *Heckler v. Ringer*, 466 U.S. 602 (1984).
4. In its statutory provisions, Medicaid is the stuff of legend. The law is said to boast the single longest sentence among all federal statutory enactments. Moreover, courts have taken notice of Medicaid's intricacies, most famously perhaps in *Friedman v. Berger*, 547 F.2d 724, 724 n.7 (2d Cir, 1976), in which, as he struggled through a complex Medicaid eligibility case, Judge Henry Friendly, one of the most eminent legal jurists of the twentieth century, concluded that Medicaid was "almost unintelligible to the uninitiated." This observation was made almost 40 years ago, when Medicaid was still relatively simple.

5. See 42 U.S.C. §1396b(a), which states clearly that the secretary "shall pay" amounts owed under variable federal payment formulas to states.
6. See Sara Rosenbaum, "Suing States over Threatened Access to Care: The Douglas Decision," *New England Journal of Medicine* 366 (April 12, 2012): e22.
7. 42 U.S.C. §1396-1 (2014).
8. States must provide fair hearings to individuals whose claims to assistance are denied or not acted upon with reasonable promptness; Social Security Act §1902(a)(3), 42 U.S.C. §1396a(a)(23). A state fair hearing, at which a state's actions are examined against the state's plan for medical assistance, typically lacks a legal basis for considering whether the state's actions violate federal law.
9. For an excellent discussion of the degree to which politics and culture lead courts to remake the relationship between individuals and government, see John T. Noonan, Jr., *Narrowing the Nation's Power: The Supreme Court Sides with the States* (Berkeley: University of California Press, 2002).
10. Lawrence M. Friedman, *Law in America* (New York: Modern Library, 2002), Ch. 1.
11. For the dissenters in *NFIB v. Sebelius* (132 S. Ct. 2566 [2012]), Medicaid's size alone was sufficient to render the program an unconstitutional coercion on the states, despite the fact that participation remains voluntary as a legal matter.
12. For a review of Medicaid's block grant history, see Jeanne M. Lambrew, "Making Medicaid a Block Grant Program: An Analysis of the Implications of Past Proposals," *Milbank Quarterly* 83 (2005): 41–63.
13. Even in the case of governmental benefits conferred as non-entitlements, basic constitutional due process principles would bar governments from arbitrarily terminating assistance. But the insertion of rights-extinguishing language into the law would have the effect of enabling government to freely (at least from a legal perspective) deny assistance to eligible persons (e.g., through the creation of waiting lists) or to vary the scope or duration of coverage.
14. See the historical discussion in Robert Stevens and Rosemary Stevens, *Welfare Medicine in America: A Case Study of Medicaid* (New York: Free Press, 1974).
15. This phrase continues to haunt welfare reform, as evidenced by how opponents of the Affordable Care Act describe the Act's Medicaid adult expansion, made optional for states in *NFIB v. Sebelius* 132 S. Ct. 2566 (2012). See, e.g., Josh Archambault and Jonathan Ingram, "Will Governor Pence Walk Away from His Medicaid Expansion? 5 Things to Watch," *Forbes*, July 30, 2014, http://www.forbes.com/sites/theapothecary/2014/07/30/will-governor-pence-walk-away-from-his-medicaid-expansion-5-things-to-watch/, describing the "Obamacare" plan to create a "new entitlement for able-bodied adults."
16. Committee on Ways and Means, US House of Representatives, *The Green Book* (Washington, DC: Government Printing Office, 1997).
17. Stevens and Stevens, *Welfare Medicine*; Edward Sparer, "The Right to Welfare," in *The Rights of Americans*, ed. Norman Dorsen (New York: Pantheon, 1971), 77–96; Frances Fox Piven and Richard Cloward, *Regulating the Poor: The Functions of Public Welfare* (New York: Vintage Books, 1971).
18. Committee on Ways and Means, *The Green Book* (GPO, 1998) Table 7-5.
19. 42 U.S.C. §1396a(a)(10).
20. 42 U.S.C. §1396d.

21. *Flemming v. Nestor*, 363 U.S. 603 (1960).
22. Charles Reich, "The New Property," *Yale Law Journal* 73 (1964): 733–787.
23. Karen M. Tani, "Flemming v. Nestor: Anticommunism, the Welfare State, and the Making of the New Property," *Law and History Review* 26 (2008): 379–414.
24. *Flemming*, 363 U.S. at 610.
25. *Flemming*, 363 U.S. at 622.
26. Reich, "New Property," 768.
27. 42 U.S.C. §1396a(a)(10)(A)(i).
28. 42 U.S.C. §1396a(a)(3).
29. 42 U.S.C. §1396a(a)(8).
30. Department of Health, Education, and Welfare, *Handbook of Public Assistance, Supplement D* (1966) §1000.
31. Jost, *Disentitlement*, 91.
32. *King v. Smith*, 392 U.S. 309 (1968).
33. *King* 309 U.S. at 332. This assertion, contained in a footnote in *King*, was later made a direct part of the Court's legal doctrine in *Townsend v. Swank*, 404 U.S. 282 (1971). See Jost, *Disentitlement*, 92.
34. *Rosado v. Wyman*, 397 U.S. 397 (1970).
35. *Goldberg v. Kelly*, 397 U.S. 254 (1970).
36. *Goldberg*, 397 U.S. at 269. The decision explicitly cited "The New Property" as part of the conceptual basis for its central holding that welfare was a right, not a privilege, and therefore had to be accorded due process protections.
37. 451 U.S. 1 (1981).
38. *Pennhurst v. Halderman*, 451 U.S. at 17. Writing for the court, Justice Rehnquist stated, memorably: "[L]egislation enacted pursuant to the spending power is much in the nature of a contract: in return for federal funds, the States agree to comply with federally imposed conditions. The legitimacy of Congress's power to legislate under the spending power thus rests on whether the State voluntarily and knowingly accepts the terms of the 'contract.'"
39. For a comprehensive overview of Medicaid litigation, see National Health Law Program, *The Advocate's Guide to the Medicaid Program*, http://www.medicaid-guide.org/.
40. Jost, *Disentitlement*, 36.
41. See, 42 U.S.C. §1396a(a)(10)(A) (i) and (ii).
42. 42 U.S.C. §§1396a(a)(10)(A) and 1396d(a). For example, physician services and hospital care are required, while other key services, such as prescribed drugs, are optional.
43. 42 U.S.C. §1396a(a)(17).
44. 42 C.F.R. §440.30(b)(1).
45. 42 C.F.R. §440.230(b)(2).
46. At the same time, Medicaid suspends coverage for beneficiaries who become residents of "institutions for mental diseases," a holdover from Congress's early desire not to federalize the cost of state mental institutions, especially at a time when the pressure for deinstitutionalization was increasing. In this regard, Medicaid is more limited than private insurance plans sold in the individual and small group markets, which post-ACA must cover mental health rehabilitative services

regardless of the location of the service as an "essential health benefit"; 42 U.S.C. §18031(b).

47. See discussion in Sara Rosenbaum, David M. Frankford, Sylvia A. Law, and Rand E. Rosenblatt, *Law and the American Health Care System*, 2nd ed. (St. Paul, MN: Foundation Press, 2012), Ch. 11.

48. *White v. Beal*, 413 F. Supp. 1141 (E. D. Pa. 1976). Under such circumstances, a state's only option would be to eliminate coverage of eyeglasses entirely, since eyeglasses are an optional benefit. Some states took such draconian steps in the face of losses, not exactly the result intended by litigants.

49. *Pinneke v. Preisser*, 623 F.2d 546 (8th Cir. 1980); *Rush v. Parham*, 625 F.2d 1150 (5th Cir. 1980).

50. *Reagan v. Weaver*, 842 F.2d 194 (8th Cir. 1989).

51. *Beal v. Doe*, 432 U.S. 438 (1977).

52. *Curtis v. Taylor*, 625 F.2d 645 (5th Cir. 1980); *Alexander v. Choate*, 469 U.S. 287 (1985).

53. *Alexander v Choate*, 469 U.S. 287.

54. *Law and the American Health Care System*, Ch. 8.

55. *Beal*, 432 U.S. at 444: "Nothing in the language of Title XIX requires a participating State to fund every medical procedure falling within the delineated categories of medical care. Each State is given broad discretion to determine the extent of medical assistance that is 'reasonable' and 'consistent with the objectives' of Title XIX."

56. 448 U.S. 297 (1980).

57. 42 U.S.C. §1395d(a)(4)(B) and 1396(r).

58. Sara Rosenbaum and Paul Wise, "Crossing the Medicaid/Private Insurance Divide: The Case of EPSDT," *Health Affairs* 26, no. 2 (2007): 382–393.

59. Jost, *Disentitlement*, 42–43.

60. 42 U.S.C. 1396a(a)(23).

61. 42 U.S.C. §§1396a(a)(23), 1396n(b).

62. *Planned Parenthood of Indiana v. Commissioner of Indiana State Department of Health*, 699 F. 3d 962 (7th Cir., 2012). See also *Planned Parenthood of Arizona Inc. v. Betlach*, 727 F. 3d 960 (9th Cir., 2013). For an excellent article discussing the Indiana case as well as the struggle over whether Medicaid creates privately enforceable rights, see Nicole Huberfeld, "Where There Is a Right, There Must Be a Remedy (Even in Medicaid)," *Kentucky Law Journal* 102 (2013–2014): 327–355.

63. See e.g., *California Association of Rural Health Clinics v. Douglas*, 783 F. 3d 1007 (9th Cir., 2013).

64. *Wilder v. Virginia Hospital Association*, 496 U.S. 498 (1990).

65. Pub. L. 105-33, §4711. Readers now should begin to pick up on the fact that as Congress and the states have grown more conservative, and as Medicaid costs have exploded, lawmakers have been receptive to changes in the statute that eliminate key entitlements.

66. *Maine v. Thiboutot*, 448 U.S. 1 (1980).

67. *Law and the American Health Care System*, Ch. 11.

68. 536 U.S. 273 (2002).

69. 532 U.S. 275 (2001).

70. 42 U.S.C. §1396a(a)(8).
71. 42 U.S.C. §1396a(a)(30(A).
72. Sara Rosenbaum, "Medicaid Payment Rate Lawsuits: Evolving Court Views Mean Uncertain Future for Medi-Cal" (California Health Care Foundation, 2011), http://www.chcf.org/publications/2009/10/medicaid-payment-rate-lawsuits-evolving-court-views-mean-uncertain-future-for-medical.
73. *Pharmaceutical Research and Manufacturers of America v. Walsh*, 123 S. Ct. 1855 (2003).
74. *Pharmaceutical Research and Manufacturers of America*, 123 S. Ct. at 1874 (Justice Thomas concurrence).
75. 132 S. Ct. 1204 (2012).
76. *Douglas v. Independent Living Center of Southern California*, Brief for Former HHS Officials as Amici in Support of Respondents (2011 Westlaw 3706105).
77. *Wos v. E.M.A. ex rel Johnson*, 133 S. Ct. 1391 (2013).
78. 567 Fed. App. 496; cert. granted 135 S. Ct. 44, U.S (Oct. 2, 2014).

# 7

# MEDICARE AND THE SOCIAL TRANSFORMATIONS OF AMERICAN ELDERS

## MARK SCHLESINGER

Every public program alters the lives of its beneficiaries. Financial transfer programs augment financial resources, social insurance programs enhance financial security, and programs delivering services address specific functional needs. How effectively they do so is, of course, a matter of considerable debate and ideological discord. Their intended impacts, however, are not the only—nor always the most consequential—ways that public programs affect the lives of those they serve.

Participating in a program can also alter beneficiaries' social roles and identities. For programs serving groups deemed worthy, and addressing needs considered legitimate, these broader effects can be quite positive. Veterans programs, for example, are frequently celebrated as a social reciprocation for past contributions; receiving such benefits honors those contributions and those who have made them.[1] In other cases, receiving benefits from association with a public program can be deeply pejorative. Programs laden with the specter of undue dependency carry a penumbra of stigma that can both delegitimize the program in the eyes of the public and deter participation among eligible individuals.[2]

How public programs alter the lives and identifies of those they serve is particularly consequential for understanding Medicare's relationship with its beneficiaries, transforming them into a new political constituency, shifting their image from passive and dependent to active and engaged. These are potentially long-lasting effects. Once someone enrolls in Medicare, he or she remains a beneficiary for life. But unlike Social Security, which has equally long connections with beneficiaries, Medicare does not just deliver checks: it shapes the nature of services and clinical relationships that profoundly affect its beneficiaries' well-being and life course.[3]

These extended exposures and life-changing influences matter. They matter for how deep a stake beneficiaries have developed in the program over the past five decades, as well as how much they depend upon its future viability. They amplify the ways in which public attitudes toward the Medicare program diffuse into public perceptions of the beneficiaries whom it serves. Though inarguably powerful, these transformations have had a rather mixed impact. On the positive side, they have given rise to new social roles through which the elderly and disabled can contribute to the public good. On the negative side, they have cast beneficiaries, especially elders, as dangerously greedy and burdensome. Exploring how these conflicting images interact with each other and intersect with the program's legitimacy reveals some useful insights into the distinctive political dynamics of Medicare. It also illuminates ways in which the program might, in the future, constructively transform beneficiaries' social identity yet again.

## Shaping Beneficiary Identity: A History in Three Acts

Medicare has dramatically enhanced the well-being and altered the healthcare experiences of its beneficiaries over the past 50 years.[4] The program moved groups previously without reliable access to medical care—the elderly, the disabled, and the chronically ill—from the fringes of the American medical enterprise to its center. Along the way, it has also reshaped the infrastructure of health care through its payment policies, altering medical education, service delivery, and the organization of medical practices.[5] These are singular accomplishments. But they're also old news—all these consequences were evident by the program's twenty-fifth anniversary.[6]

Medicare's influence over the social identity of its beneficiaries has emerged more gradually. Nonetheless, the five decades after the program's enactment have provided sufficient perspective to clearly demarcate three eras of identity change. In the first, American elders were transformed from passive recipients of public benefits into engaged (and, for a brief period, seemingly powerful) political actors. The second era recast the elderly from worthy beneficiaries to "greedy geezers" who were overly demanding of scarce public resources for their health benefits, to the neglect of other vital societal needs. In the third era, beneficiaries' roles within the healthcare system became the target for change, as they were encouraged to become active consumers of medical care rather than passive patients.

The best-documented illustration of Medicare's impact on its beneficiaries' identity involves the growing political stature and engagement of the elderly, starting in the 1960s.[7] To be sure, elders' empowerment was not due to Medicare alone. The program's enactment in 1965 coincided with expanding Social Security benefits as well as the initiation of other public policies—for example, the Older Americans Act (OAA), also established in 1965—that reduced elders' anxiety about economic deprivation, freeing their attention for events in the political realm. Nevertheless, there are good reasons to attribute much of the political mobilization that followed to Medicare itself.

It is difficult to imagine today just how politically disconnected American elders were in the mid-twentieth century. Beset by economic hardship and limited education, those over the age of 65 voted far less often than did younger adults; age disparities were even larger for other forms of political participation. These gaps in participation were both caused by and a cause of very limited interest group representation for the elderly in national politics. The American Association of Retired Persons (now known solely by its acronym, AARP), though founded in 1958, had little political voice in its early years.[8] And, as Julian Zelizer discusses in Chapter 1 of this volume, the National Council of Senior Citizens (NCSC), an organization formed largely by retired union members, had only limited influence on the debate over Medicare.[9]

By contrast, the flurry of legislation that accompanied Medicare's initial enactment (as well as the amendments that followed soon after, in

1967) induced the formation of numerous interest groups within the Beltway that held representation of the elderly as part of their core mission.[10] The number of organizations focused in this manner roughly doubled. Moreover, the program galvanized such existing membership organizations as the AARP and NCSC into action, both as representatives of their constituents' interests and as an infrastructure for mobilizing their membership's political involvement.[11]

Political participation among older Americans began to steadily increase—a trend that persisted for the next four decades in the face of declining political engagement among Americans generally.[12] With the bedrock of support for elders' basic needs coming from national policies, public affairs were simply far more salient for this age group than for most of the populace. The contested passage of Medicare signaled the need to safeguard the program to its beneficiaries, most of whom had quickly come to recognize it as vital to their well-being.[13] Motivated to protective action, attentive to affairs within the Beltway, and alert to political threats, the elderly were gradually transformed into "über-citizens."[14]

During the 1970s and through the late 1980s, the perceived political influence of the elderly and groups representing them grew steadily, to the extent that political scientists came to view them as among the "advantaged" interests in American politics.[15] Even as the economic circumstances of the average older American improved, public and elected officials continued to see the elderly as worthy of collective support, their status legitimated by their past contributions to society.[16] Elders' increasing rates of political participation also made politicians cautious about taking stands that might alienate their older constituents. The political posturing of elder membership organizations, which claimed to represent (and potentially mobilize) millions of elder votes, heightened their concerns.[17] As a consequence, many elected officials began to view Medicare as the "third rail" of American politics—dangerous to touch, even lightly (see Chapter 8 by Mark Peterson in this volume).

All this made the political events of the late 1980s quite unexpected. At mid-decade, Congress had begun considering reforms to limit the substantial out-of-pocket expenses that seriously ill beneficiaries accumulated under Medicare's cost-sharing provisions.[18] In 1988, Congress finally enacted reforms that expanded coverage for prescription drugs and capped copayment obligations, most extensively for lower-income beneficiaries. Passage of the Medicare Catastrophic Coverage Act (MCCA), however, depended on a political compromise between Democrats in Congress and officials from the Reagan administration who attempted to limit the impact on the federal budget. The costs of improved benefits were to be supported entirely by an income tax surcharge on Medicare beneficiaries, in effect representing a form of income-adjusted premium for the program.[19]

Officials from AARP had worked closely with congressional staff in crafting the amendments, with the promise that their members would rally around the legislation.[20] These assurances in hand, Congress enacted the MCCA with broad bipartisan support. Celebration ensued, with elected officials convinced they had done right by the elderly—particularly those in limited financial circumstances. Yet within 12 months, a million elders had written angry protests to Congress, and the majority of age-related membership organizations had broken ranks with the AARP to oppose the legislation.[21] Within 18 months, Congress repealed most of the MCCA's provisions, with an equally large bipartisanship majority, over the AARP's plaintive objections.

This dramatic reversal of fortune was historically unprecedented—not just for Medicare, but for *any* social policy. It left a lasting imprint on elders' political image. Because elders split in their reaction to the MCCA, the AARP lost credibility as a peak interest group that could represent—and mobilize—its membership behind a cohesive vision of older Americans' collective interests.[22] Elders' political renaissance after 1965 had given the AARP considerable credibility as a political force. Yet by the late 1980s it was merely one node in an entire ecology of age-related membership groups, each capable of activating a subset of Medicare's older beneficiaries, each with its own distinct (and sometimes conflicting) political agenda.[23]

The late 1980s thus shattered the illusion of a univocal political presence for American elders. The MCCA debacle, moreover, shifted politicians' stereotypes about their older constituents. Although the MCCA's tax surcharge fell largely on the upper end of the income distribution, misleading campaigns by some interest groups evoked the specter of extensive tax burdens for middle-class elders.[24] As a result, Congress faced a barrage of letters from both middle- and upper-income beneficiaries. That experience left many members of Congress with the broad impression of elders as selfish and self-oriented actors who were unwilling to sacrifice anything financially on behalf of the economically disadvantaged within their own age cohort.[25]

Many politicians felt personally betrayed by this turn of events. In part, they were responding to a few particularly dramatic incidents, including a televised episode of older Americans beating on the car of the chairman of the House Ways and Means Committee with protest placards. But politicians had also been "primed"—predisposed to notice particular aspects of complex social phenomena—by a newly emerging discourse within the Beltway, one that recast age-related social policies, and Medicare in particular, in the context of an emerging lexicon of "intergenerational equity."

As political commentators bemoaned Americans' persisting inattention to public affairs, one might expect that the growing political engagement of older American would have been greeted with some enthusiasm, as a role model for younger citizens. So it was—to a point. However, the combination of elders' disproportionate political participation, combined with politicians' perception of their self-interested behavior, also evoked concerns about an imbalanced political playing field, with elders' needs trumping those of other age groups. This change marked the beginning of a second era in the transformation of elders' image in American society, an act in which their political engagement led them to be increasingly characterized as "greedy geezers"—and to be so perceived within the Beltway.

The rubric of "intergenerational equity" emerged in the late 1980s in two flavors.[26] The stronger version portrayed the burgeoning political influence of older Americans as an active threat to other vital interests, as the "gray lobby" strategically garnered an expanding share of tax dollars to serve elders' interests. The milder version focused more on comparisons across generational cohorts. This alternative framing suggested that elders' political voice could lock in place social policies that would break the fiscal bank for later generations, even if elders were not overly acquisitive and sought only to defend existing entitlements.[27]

These warnings came from varied sources, reflecting a variety of motives. Yet it was hard to overlook the implicit ideological agenda permeating many of these claims. Despite the best efforts of conservative pundits, social insurance and other age-targeted programs had previously remained free from the stigma associated with means-tested initiatives, even for those who became long-term "dependents," relying on public benefits for decades. But here was a fresh take on the ways in which public benefits corroded the values of their recipients: in this case, by making them more selfish. Thus the term "greedy geezer" found its way into the social policy lexicon and media coverage of the day, extolled with greatest fervor by conservative pundits.

Medicare played a starring role in these scenarios.[28] Absent an aggregate budget, its rapidly growing costs and financing from general federal revenues made it an apparent threat to resources for other federal programs. Medicare's incomplete insurance coverage—at that time omitting outpatient prescription drugs, long-term care, and preventive screenings—left advocacy groups constantly asking for better coverage (and thus additional federal spending), as they sought to enhance elders' access to care and financial security. At the same time, media reports conveyed unnerving projections of Medicare's future solvency (the program operates under its own trust fund) creating flashpoints for repeated political controversy.[29] This combination of catalysts caused the intergenerational equity motif in healthcare to capture far more media attention in the United States than in Canada, where elders' medical expenses were growing equally quickly, but were incorporated into a health care program shared by all Canadians.[30]

The intergenerational equity paradigm identified some valid concerns regarding the sustainability of a welfare state reliant on age-targeted programs. Yet these useful insights were interspersed with other assertions that were almost entirely divorced from reality, serving largely to fan anxieties and prejudice against older Americans. Nor was this muddle much clarified by contemporary media coverage or the flurry of academic conclaves devoted to these concerns, which for the most part simply restated the erroneous fears, rather than carefully assessing them. To better understand the implications of this debate—and Medicare's role—for Americans' persisting impressions of the elderly, it's helpful to clarify a few key points.

- *A false presumption of self-interest*: Those raising intergenerational equity concerns anticipated that elders' magnified political voice, relative to younger Americans, would inevitably lead to greater demands for age-related public benefits.[31] But that assumption was inaccurate. Compared to younger Americans, elders have always been *less* supportive of expanded benefits for their age group and more concerned about the burden those benefits might place on younger taxpayers.[32]
- *A real divergence in life-course experiences*: There are, nonetheless, well-documented age gradients in support for various service-benefit programs for the obvious reason that needs vary over the life course.

For example, Americans over the age of 65 are more aware of the prevalence and costs of home care for the elderly than are younger adults, but less familiar with the costs and burdens associated with child care or education.[33] Familiarity breeds concern, and concern fuels support for policies to help with these burdens.[34]

- *A trumped-up tension from artificial priorities*: If one wants to find them, apparent intergenerational tensions are easy to induce simply by imposing an artificial choice among policy options. Consider a 1999 national survey that asked in two ways about helping the uninsured. The first query presented expanding insurance coverage as one option among eight, with a single top choice allowed; the second asked about possible priorities for spending down the federal surplus, with multiple answers permitted. The apparent differences between policy support among the old and the young are striking, if illusory (Figure 7.1). When asked to choose a single preferred policy, elders seemed to forsake the uninsured in favor of improved drug coverage under Medicare: they are half as likely to rate the former as their top priority. Yet when the same respondents were asked about the uninsured as a spending priority on the very same survey, elders were actually *more* supportive of additional public funding than were younger Americans.

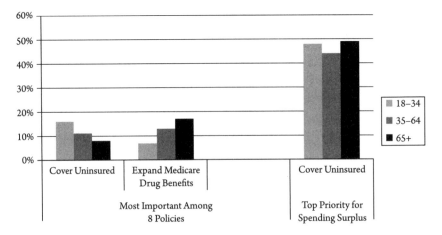

FIGURE 7.1 Perceived Importance of Insurance Expansions, 1999.

Source: Roper Center for Public Opinion Research: Survey by Henry J. Kaiser Family Foundation: December 3–13, 1999. Dataset: USPSRA1999-HNI021.

• *A real growth in sensitivity to fiscal burdens*: The economic shocks of the 1970s weakened Americans' optimism about future prosperity. This, in turn, heightened the public's concerns about the fiscal burdens associated with long-term commitments to particular age groups and their willingness to compare fairness across age cohorts. Under these circumstances, concerns about the solvency of Medicare's trust fund grew more politically salient.[35]

The muddling of valid concerns with inaccurate fears made for a potent mix, leading even sophisticated pundits to some alarming conclusions concerning intergenerational equity. For example, one nationally syndicated columnist steeped in the debate warned, "the AARP has become America's most dangerous lobby. If left unchecked, its agenda will plunder our children and grandchildren." The prospect of massive future outlays for programs like Medicare and Social Security, he ominously forewarned, threatened to rend to tatters both "the economy and the social fabric."[36]

Despite the media furor over "greedy geezers," the trope had only a mixed and modest effect on public opinion. Characterizing elders as an active political threat never really caught on, or at least it never materialized in public opinion data. Consider, for example, the response to a survey question fielded over three different decades: "on the whole, how much influence do you think retired older Americans have in this country today—too much influence, just about the right amount, or too little influence?" In 1981, well before concerns about intergenerational equity had garnered any media attention, almost two-thirds of the public (64 percent) felt that elders had too little influence; hardly anyone (3 percent) felt that their influence was excessive (Figure 7.2, left bar). By 1994, coverage of intergenerational equity in the mass media had been fairly extensive in the United States,[37] but Americans' attitudes had barely changed (Figure 7.2, middle bar). Though fewer Americans felt that elders had too little influence (down to 53 percent), only a tiny minority (6 percent) believed that they had too much. The 2004 survey yielded nearly identical results (Figure 7.2, right bar).

Public opinion polls did, however, demonstrate growing caution about the fiscal burdens associated with age-targeted programs like Medicare.[38] Between the mid-1980s (the initiation of the intergenerational equity debate) and the late 1990s, public support for more generous age-targeted benefits fell, and doubts about the role of entitlement programs more

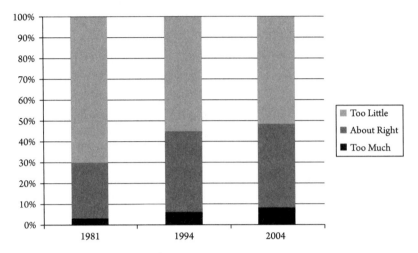

FIGURE 7.2 Perceived Influence of Older Americans.

Sources: Roper Center for Public Opinion Research.

(1) 1981: Survey by Louis Harris and Associates June 15–31, 1981. Dataset: USHARRIS.81AGE.RO9A.

(2) 1994: Survey by FGI Research September 6–29, 1994. Dataset: USFGI.94AGE.RC11.

(3) 2004: Survey by FGI Research March 11–April 25, 2004. Dataset: USAARP.06AGING.RNH11.

generally rose.[39] These changes were not trivial: over about a decade, the proportion of the public favoring benefit expansions fell from 57 percent to 47 percent. While doubts about the sustainability of federal entitlement programs were largely limited to young adults, reduced support for benefit expansions was most pronounced among elder respondents—six times as large a drop as among young adults. These shifts in popular attitudes were clearly more cautious than punitive—the proportion of the public that favored cutting age-targeted benefits did grow, but remained minuscule (up from 3 percent to 6 percent over this time period).[40]

Though more difficult to track or quantify, the intergenerational equity paradigm also left its imprint on policy elites. Policymakers embraced evaluating public policies in terms of generational cohorts, a practice previously relegated to a handful of academic publications.[41] By the end of the 1990s, this approach had become an accepted lens for thinking about Medicare's performance and prospects in policymaking circles.[42] Policymakers similarly expressed a growing caution about long-term cost commitments and burdens associated with age-targeted programs, mirroring the concerns evident in public opinion.[43]

Elderly advocates responded by establishing coalitions of interest groups (sporting proclaimed intergenerational compacts) addressing needs all along the life course. They also called attention to a growing presence of elders as volunteers and catalysts for civic engagement, hoping that this enhanced social contribution might at least partly offset the perceived burdens of age-targeted programs.[44] These varied forms at strategic positioning clearly had their impact within the Beltway, including assessments of the intergenerational impact of the Medicare program.[45] They did not, however, entirely mollify the concerns of elected officials, who were increasingly intent on revising expectations for older Americans along rather different lines.

Beginning in the 1990s, a growing number of policymakers emphasized the need for older Americans to act like medical consumers rather than patients, to help stem the rising tide of Medicare spending. This emphasis ushered in a third era of social identity effects for Medicare recipients. Bringing elder Americans back into the mainstream of American medicine had been a major impetus behind the passage of Medicare. Modeling Medicare's benefits on existing Blue Cross/Blue Shield plans and having private insurers act as fiscal intermediaries for the program were more than just administrative conveniences. These measures also reflected a strong presumption that insurance arrangements and access to care for beneficiaries should be consistent with those available to working-age Americans.[46]

And so it was, for much of the program's first quarter-century.[47] Yet by the late 1980s, it was clear that health insurance for working-age Americans was undergoing some profound changes, with conventional fee-for-service coverage increasingly displaced by various forms of managed-care plans. Employers, moreover, placed a growing emphasis on their employees' choice among health plans to encourage insurers (and their affiliated providers) to be more responsive to consumer needs. Americans' experience with these emergent insurance arrangements was decidedly mixed.[48] Nonetheless, they held considerable appeal for a coalition of liberal and conservative elected officials: the former saw in them the potential to reshape American health care in some pro-social ways; the latter hoped to use market discipline to constrain rising medical costs.[49]

In this context, conventional Medicare benefits seemed increasingly anachronistic—and increasingly divergent from the insurance available to working-age Americans. To be sure, some private health plans had enrolled Medicare beneficiaries since the early 1980s as demonstration projects. But most older Americans had limited access to these alternatives and little interest in insurance choices: through the early 1990s, less than 5 percent enrolled in a private plan alternative to conventional Medicare.[50]

That prompted Congressional action. In a series of amendments to the Medicare program enacted in 1992, 1997, and 2003, Congress incorporated a far larger role for private insurers as a complement to conventional Medicare. These legislative initiatives created Medicare Part C to give beneficiaries more private insurance alternatives to conventional Medicare enrollment and Medicare Part D to supplement conventional Medicare coverage with prescription drug benefits available *only* through private insurers.

A consistent aspiration connected these program amendments: encouraging beneficiaries to choose among health insurance alternatives.[51] Proponents envisioned a variety of possible advantages with enhanced choice, ranging from greater innovation in service delivery, to market pressures to add benefits historically omitted from conventional Medicare, and (less realistically) to cost-constraining competition. Less explicitly, policymakers also sought to transform beneficiaries themselves, from passive patients to active consumers.

Policymakers presented this new expectation for Medicare beneficiaries as both an opportunity and an obligation. The opportunity came from offering an abundance of choices regarding coverage, provider networks, and cost-sharing provisions, each of which would allow elders to select plans that best matched their health needs. The sense of obligation emerged from the intergenerational equity debate playing itself out at the same time: given the rising costs and burdens imposed by Medicare, beneficiaries should shoulder their share by making more carefully informed, cost-conscious choices in healthcare settings.[52]

Expecting elders to become active consumers was no small ask. Through the late 1980s, those over 65 were the age group least engaged as active medical consumers. To be sure, they came to the doctor's office well prepared in certain ways. Because chronic illness rises with age, older people tend to be more knowledgeable about health matters than are younger adults. Given this greater salience, elders have always been more attentive to health-related issues in the media and generally have a more sophisticated understanding of treatment options.[53]

But other crucial attributes of medical consumerism were missing through the 1980s. Compared to younger adults, elders were far less willing to question authority in healthcare contexts. They were also less prepared to think about making trade-offs among valued aspects of health plans.[54] When researchers assessed consumer attitudes in health care in 1987, those over the age of 65 were less than half as likely (17 percent vs. 38 percent) to be identified as having the crucial attributes of active medical consumers.[55]

Ready or not, Medicare beneficiaries were exposed to abundant opportunities for insurance choice over the next quarter-century. Although the number of participating private insurers fluctuated from year to year and varied by geographic region, elders never faced a dearth of options: in 2013, the average beneficiary could choose among 18 Part C plans and 31 Part D plans.[56] That left virtually every beneficiary either considering or making choices among plans: enrollment in Part D, though voluntary, was close to universal. By 2014, 30 percent of beneficiaries were enrolled in a Part C plan; in the state with the highest Part C penetration rate (Minnesota), the majority of beneficiaries were enrolled in a plan other than conventional Medicare.

Many elders responded by embracing consumerism. By 2006, the prevalence of an active consumer orientation was as common among those 65 and older as among younger adults, a dramatic change from two decades earlier.[57] This did not mean that elders necessarily made wise choices. Quite the contrary: many elders enroll (and stay enrolled) in Part D plans that are more expensive for the particular drugs they have been prescribed than would be the case with other plans available to them.[58] Most enrollees in Part C stay with the private plan they first selected, even if their health needs subsequently change or more highly rated plan options have emerged in their local market.[59]

This transformation of beneficiaries into empowered but inept consumers may not, in the long term, prove the most consequential outcome of Medicare privatization, because program changes also resonate in beneficiaries' political identity and engagement. Adding Parts C and D to the program meant that beneficiaries typically contacted private insurers as they accessed care and sought to understand their benefits. These changing patterns of day-to-day interaction have the potential to alter beneficiaries' relationship to the Medicare program itself in several potentially important ways.

First, privatization may weaken beneficiaries' political identification with the program. Enrollment in conventional Medicare implied that the choices being made in Washington, D.C., had direct consequences for beneficiaries' benefits, their access to medical care, and their financial security. That

personal salience led elders to pay attention to public affairs.[60] But enrollment in a private plan creates an organizational buffer, a distancing between
the politics of Medicare and the practices that shape their own insurance
coverage and health care. To be sure, this distancing may hold some benefits—both for the individual and the program—but may come at the price
of reducing elders' engagement as political actors.

Second, privatization can weaken beneficiaries' collective identity. When
every elder in America was enrolled in a single national program, they could
share information, compare experiences, and learn from one another about
how the program operates and how they could best relate to it. With beneficiaries enrolled in a thousand different private plans, this sense of shared
fate and common purpose will almost certainly be adulterated; over time, it
could evaporate entirely.[61]

Finally, an expanded role for private insurers will likely undermine beneficiaries' willingness to speak up when they experience problems with their
insurance benefits. Historically, Medicare has relied on a variety of ombudsman programs to identify systematic patterns of problems.[62] But a larger role
for private insurers may make it harder for beneficiaries to discern how best
to respond to problematic experiences. Is the problem in question the fault
of the health plan—or the ways in which Medicare regulates Parts C and D?
To avoid facing the same problem again, would it be more efficacious
to voice a grievance or to switch to a different plan? In those cases where
exit supplants voice, individual beneficiaries may find themselves in a better plan, but the Centers for Medicare and Medicaid Services (CMS) will
have no ability to identify repeated problems in their original plan. In other
cases, beneficiaries may be so uncertain about whether to exit or file a grievance that in the end they do neither, leaving them still vulnerable and CMS
ill-informed.[63]

In all these ways, privatizing Medicare can erode the program's political
base and its beneficiaries' collective identification with it. These processes
are likely mutually reinforcing: if beneficiaries feel less collective identification, they will also be less likely to file grievances about problematic
practices, because one of the primary motivations for grievances in health
settings is to reduce the odds of the same problem befalling someone else. If
beneficiaries care less about one another, that motivation is weakened.

Because these political side effects are likely to emerge only gradually
over time, it remains too early to fully detect the impact of Parts C and D.

Nonetheless, a few warning signs have already appeared. Beneficiaries who live in the regions of the country in which Part C enrollment is highest report lower levels of identification with both the program and with other Medicare beneficiaries.[64] The addition of Medicare Part D in 2003, although a substantial expansion of program benefits, did not generate the same pattern of subsequent political activation among the elderly that was evident after Medicare's enactment in 1965.[65] These fragments of evidence are certainly consistent with the anticipated impact of privatization depicted above. Only time will tell how persistent and substantial their effects will be.

## A Layering of Altered Social Identities

So far, we have explored three different eras in which older Americans' interactions and connections with the Medicare program reshaped their social identities. Each of the three followed on those that came before. It is probably more accurate to view these eras as a progressive layering-on of identities, rather than a process of sequential identity displacement. Though activating older Americans as consumers may have weakened their political connectedness to Medicare, it has not (yet) altered in any observable manner the ways in which policymakers and elected officials perceive elders and their advocates as political actors. Nor has older beneficiaries' embrace of a consumer role eliminated the intergenerational tensions around either the Medicare program or elders' role in American society. These transformed identities coexist in contemporary American society to create a complex, often confusing mix.

Consider two examples. The first is drawn from the political realm, the second from Medicare's administrative practices. Amid the contentious and ideologically laden debate over healthcare reform during the first Obama administration, one pattern in public opinion stood out: the elderly were strikingly and consistently less supportive (typically by 8–10 percentage points) of the reform package than were younger adults. This pattern was indisputable. The real question was why these differentials emerged.

Many analysts interpreted elders' opinion of the Affordable Care Act (ACA) through the lens of two decades of scholarship on intergenerational equity. Elders' apparent lack of support for benefits extended to others brought to mind their seemingly selfish orientation in the debate over the MCCA. As political scientist Andrea Campbell has put it,

"Public opinion polls showed repeatedly that seniors were more opposed to the Obama healthcare reform effort than were younger citizens. After all, they already have national health insurance, and many had difficulty imagining how coverage would be expanded to another one-sixth of the population without negatively affecting them.... It is difficult to reform a healthcare system in which those with national health insurance believe they have earned it and resent its extension to those they believe have not earned it...."[66]

To be sure, this sort of interpretation was an easy reach. Poll after poll documented elders' reduced enthusiasm for health insurance reform. In one telling example from mid-2009, only 61 to 65 percent of elders supported extending Medicare enrollment to those aged 55 to 64, while over 80 percent of working-age adults approved.[67] For many pundits, such findings sealed the deal on their impressions of elders as selfish and apparently unwilling to share their precious Medicare (financed by younger Americans' payroll taxes).

But this was clearly an interpretation, not a self-evident conclusion. After all, almost two-thirds of the elderly *did* favor expanding Medicare to the middle-aged—hardly a serious impediment to reform. Moreover, the survey questions that evoked these age-related patterns neglected to inform respondents that younger Medicare enrollees would actually pay a fair premium. Including the premiums in the survey question yielded dramatically different responses. Overall support dropped, and the age-related differential virtually disappeared: 54 percent of those under 65 favored expanding Medicare enrollment in this manner, compared to 50 percent of those over 65 (Figure 7.3, right-hand columns).

But the broader question remains: Did elders express less support for the ACA because they felt working-age Americans were less deserving of coverage (even if they paid fair premiums), or for some other reason? The evidence suggests the latter. Elders were not resisting the expansion of insurance options so much as opposing the ACA as a package of initiatives, as best they understood it.[68] Elders expressed less support than younger Americans for *any* provision in the legislation. For example, 8 percent fewer elders had a positive assessment of the act's regulation of private insurance than was expressed by those younger than 65, though those regulations had no plausible impact on their own coverage or care.[69] They demonstrated a similar distrust for virtually every aspect of the reforms.

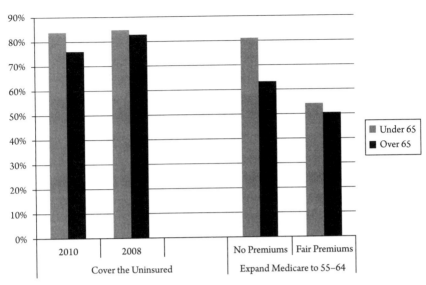

FIGURE 7.3 Age Differences in Support for Insurance Expansion.

Sources: Roper Center for Public Opinion Research and Hacker et al (2013).

(1) 2010: Survey by Research Associates International (RAI), January 3–10, 2010. Dataset: USPSRA.012510.R30QF2.

(2) 2008: Survey by Research Associates International (RAI), January 8–13, 2008. Dataset: USPSRA.012408A.R28QF2.

(3) Medicare for 55–64, No Premiums: Survey by RAI, April 2–8, 2009. Dataset: USPSRA.09HTPAPR.R07C.

(4) Medicare for 55–64: With Premiums: Jacob Hacker, Philip Rehm, Mark Schlesinger, "The Insecure American: Economic Experiences and Policy Attitudes Amidst the Great Recession," *Perspectives on Politics* 11 (2013): 23–49.

Several factors explain this opposition. A third believed (mistakenly) that the ACA included "death panels." A majority were aware (accurately) that the ACA's budget projections relied heavily on promised reductions in the future growth of Medicare spending. This complex mélange of impression and misimpression was not exactly the recipe to endear the initiative to older voters.[70]

These reasons are *not* equivalent to judging younger adults as undeserving of insurance or resenting efforts to extend health insurance to these age groups. Indeed, a poll that asked about expanding insurance to the uninsured in 2008 (before there was an ACA to react against) showed virtually no age-related differential (Figure 7.3, left columns). When coupled with historical evidence of support for insurance expansions from earlier surveys (recall Figure 7.1), these numbers suggest that older Americans are not, in fact, any less supportive of covering the uninsured than younger Americans. The ensuing media debate, in which pundits and scholars insisted that older Americans posed a daunting roadblock to the passage of the ACA, seems to have more to do with the persistence of the intergenerational equity debate than reality.

The second example of how prior identity transformations continue to shape contemporary policy discourse about elders and Medicare involves a set of long-term care reforms associated with "consumer-directed home care." Historically, Medicare has paid for home care largely as an extension of Part A hospital coverage and as a means to facilitate shorter inpatient stays. To this end, it contracts with home care agencies throughout the country to provide a certain number of home care visits to each hospitalized beneficiary. Quality care is thought to be promoted by contracting with accredited home care agencies run by well-trained professionals.

Since the turn of the twenty-first century, financing for home care services outside Medicare have been shifting away from this conventional professional services paradigm. It has been increasingly displaced by a "consumer-directed" model that emerged from the independent-living movement among people with disabilities. This alternative paradigm accords greater autonomy to the recipient of care (or the recipient's family, acting as proxy decision-makers) by providing them to cash to purchase services on their own. A number of European countries and state Medicaid programs have made such consumer-directed (aka "cash and counseling") models the centerpiece of long-term care.[71] As a result, both healthcare advocates and policymakers are now considering to what extent Medicare should also embrace this model.

Inevitably, this assessment will be shaped in part by whether Medicare beneficiaries are seen as willing and capable consumers.[72] To be sure, consumer choice in home care differs in many ways from selecting among health insurers; it involves a more personal set of decisions and fewer skills evaluating comparative performance metrics. Nonetheless, the process of consumer activation may be similar.[73] Certainly, policymakers' impressions of elders as capable consumers will be shaped by their prior efforts to imbue Medicare beneficiaries with consumerist aspirations in selecting among insurers.

Given the popularity of consumer-directed home care among contemporary policymakers, elders' mixed experience with medical consumerism deserves careful attention. Although Americans over the age of 65 are now as likely as younger adults to embrace medical consumerism, those who adopt a strong consumerist orientation for health care remain in the minority for all ages.[74] Roughly 15 percent of older Americans reject consumer autonomy in any medical setting; just over 50 percent favor a shared decision-making model where the extent of their autonomy varies by context. For some in this latter group, home care will be a realm in which they wish to retain considerable control; for others (because this care is often needed in the aftermath of a debilitating hospital stay), consumer autonomy loses much of its appeal.

It is therefore important for advocates and policymakers to guard against simplistic stereotypes. Making greater allowances for consumer-directed home care seems a sensible approach, as long as expectations for greater choice are not imposed on beneficiaries unwilling or unable to take on these responsibilities. Indeed, even in many of the European countries that have most successfully embraced these cash-benefit models for long-term care, a majority of home care recipients still prefer a service benefit over a cash voucher.

## Constructively Harnessing the Potential for Identity Transformation

Given Medicare's ability to alter the social identities of those it serves, might policymakers in the future be able to leverage this influence in constructive ways? Consider a single case in point: an alternative form of consumer empowerment for Medicare beneficiaries. Could the grievance process for Medicare's own Parts C and D be changed to transform older Americans into the "watchdogs" of the healthcare system, thereby enhancing their public image by assuring that health care is made better for all Americans?

Imagine a system in which Medicare beneficiaries were incentivized or otherwise encouraged to voice complaints about their insurance plans, doctors, or hospitals directly to CMS, instead of simply selecting another provider. In that role, they would give voice to their personal experiences and, by so doing, would help to identify what works well and badly. They would be encouraged to provide feedback through several conduits. They could provide periodic assessments of their experiences through responses to open-ended questions appended to existing patient experience surveys, which the typical elder completes on a regular basis. The goal would be for beneficiaries, as both patients and consumers, to provide detailed, thoughtful assessments of their encounters with healthcare providers and insurers—the sort of probing accountings that one might expect from the most insightful book reviewers on Amazon.com. More problematic episodes would be reported as they occur though a newly established grievance or ombudsman program that would investigate and rectify bad practices by either insurers or clinicians, benefiting all Americans but with Medicare beneficiaries as the catalyzing agents.

This alternative approach to medical consumerism seems promising at several levels. For the individual elder, giving voice to consumer experiences is a far more realistic aspiration for empowerment than is exit from unsatisfactory situations, particularly with regard to health plans. Switching plans often requires disrupting established relationships with healthcare professionals: always a dubious ask, but particularly so for older populations with prevalent chronic conditions and long-standing relationships with clinicians.[75] A social role that emphasizes voice as the operative form of empowerment would unify Medicare beneficiaries' political engagement with their activation as consumers a quarter-century later. Finally, at the societal level, an active role for elders as healthcare watchdogs directly addresses concerns related to intergenerational equity by assigning elders a vital, very public role that makes their continued contribution to society clear and concrete.

Is this sort of transformation feasible? Could it be incorporated into Medicare's practices without disrupting other vital aspects of its mission? While this chapter cannot definitely answer that question, the move certainly seems promising, both for the potential it holds as a concrete proposal and for the broader array of ways in which advocates, social scientists, and policymakers might think more constructively about how Medicare shapes the social identities of its beneficiaries.

Medicare has influenced the social identify and expectations of its beneficiaries since the program's inception. These effects persist in current debates and permeate visions of the program's future. To be sure, these interactions have been a bit of a mixed bag. Some of the influences emerged as the deliberate consequences of policymakers' actions, while others were largely unintentional. Some involved Medicare as an active agent, others as a passive symbol. Some affected beneficiaries' engagement with the program itself, others their broader role in society. Some worked primarily by transforming beneficiaries' own expectations, others their public image. But within this diversity there is a common thread—the interaction has always been bidirectional. Medicare has shaped the social identity of its beneficiaries, while also having its own prospects altered by the evolution of that identity.

These influences have deeply transformed how most Americans view the elderly: from passive recipients of benefits to engaged consumers and citizens. Many of these changes have been salubrious, for both elders themselves and their public image. These positive manifestations include both the immediate changes wrought in elders' attitudes and behaviors, as well as the ways in which advocates for the aging responded to incipient intergenerational tensions. These latter, more indirect, consequences include the emergence of (still largely nascent) intergenerational compacts across the life course and various forms of enhanced civic engagement among their members.

But not all of these influences were positive. Elders' growing political voice raised the specter of political threat. Elders' response to the MCCA, which they saw as violating the implicit social contract of Medicare (e.g., a cross-generational financing of benefits), led many elected officials, pundits, and scholars to perceive them as excessively self-oriented. Elders' embrace of consumer empowerment left them with the façade of empowered choice, in settings where their actual choices often yielded quite problematic outcomes.

The full consequences of these identity transformations have yet to fully play out, particularly as they interact with one another to create new hybrid expectations. Social norms, roles, and expectations are, of course, shaped by a variety of factors, with public policy often playing only a minor influence. But in domains where the services provided through those programs are so vital to personal identity and well-being, as is true for the health care of the elderly and disabled, the influences of public programs such as Medicare on identity take on additional force. It behooves us to try to understand them more fully.

In addition to gaining a fuller understanding of these influences, policymakers must be attentive to their implications and mindful of the variegated ways in which they affect Medicare's beneficiaries. It is not enough to know that Medicare galvanized political engagement among older Americans; one must be equally aware that not all subsets of elders were as fully mobilized or as effectively represented in political discourse. It is not enough to understand that the caustic portrayal of the older Americans as greedy and selfish is inaccurate; one must recognize that intergenerational tensions may still arise because different generational cohorts deem some age-related needs as more salient than others, creating a sense of competition for scarce tax dollars. It is not enough to appreciate the extent to which older Americans now strive to be informed medical consumers; one must also recognize that a substantial portion will fail to live up to these aspirations, and a goodly number of others will not even feel capable of trying to meet them. It is only when policymakers, policy advocates, and political pundits are attentive to the true variation that underlies these stereotypes that Medicare policymaking—indeed, health policymaking more generally—will have suitably responded to these lessons from Medicare's first half century.

## NOTES

1. In an era of deep distrust of entitlement programs, the notion of a positive penumbra to program participation may raise some eyebrows. Yet various initiatives that are perceived as benefits earned through past contributions to society, including veterans' benefits and social insurance programs, maintain positive associations. See Fay Lomax Cook and Edith Barrett, *Support for the American Welfare State: The Views of Congress and the Public* (New York: Columbia University Press, 1992); John Williamson, Diane Watts-Roy, and Eric Kingson, eds. *The Generational Equity Debate* (New York: Columbia University Press, 1999).
2. Linda Gordon, *Pitied but Not Entitled: Single Mothers and the History of Welfare* (New York: Free Press, 1994).
3. Cynthia Mathieson and Hendaikns Stam, "Renegotiating Identity: Cancer Narratives," *Sociology of Health & Illness* 17 (1995): 283–306; Kathy Charmaz, "Struggling For a Self: Identity Levels of the Chronically Ill," *Research in The Sociology Of Health Care* 6 (1987): 283–321.
4. Curiously, the program was much less successful at ensuring financial security for its beneficiaries, a disturbing shortcoming for a social insurance program. See Marilyn Moon and Matthew Storeyguard, *One-Third At Risk: The Special Circumstances of Medicare Beneficiaries with Health Problems* (New York: Commonwealth Fund, 2001); Michael Graetz and Jerry Mashaw, *True Security: Rethinking American Social Insurance* (New Haven, CT: Yale University Press, 1999).
5. Rick Mayes and Robert Berenson, *Medicare Prospective Payment and the Shaping of U.S. Health Care* (Baltimore, MD: Johns Hopkins University Press, 2006).
6. David Blumenthal, Mark Schlesinger, and Pamela Brown Drumheller, *Renewing the Promise: Medicare and Its Reform* (New York: Oxford University Press, 1988); Karen Davis and Diane Rowland, *Medicare Policy: New Directions for Health and Long-Term Care* (Baltimore, MD: Johns Hopkins University Press, 1986).
7. Robert Hudson and Judith Gonyea, "Baby Boomers and the Shifting Political Construction of Old Age," *The Gerontologist* 52 (2012): 272–282; Andrea Campbell, *How Policies Make Citizens: Senior Political Activism and the American Welfare State* (Princeton, NJ: Princeton University Press, 2003); Robert Binstock, "Older People and Voting Participation: Past and Future," *The Gerontologist* 40 (2000): 18–31.
8. Hudson and Gonyea, "Baby Boomers."

9. See also Jonathan Oberlander, *The Political Life of Medicare* (Chicago: University of Chicago Press, 2003); Theodore Marmor, *The Politics of Medicare* (Chicago: Aldine, 1971).

10. Jack Walker, "The Origins and Maintenance of Interest Groups in America," *American Political Science Review* 77 (1983): 390–406.

11. Henry Pratt, *The Gray Lobby* (Chicago: University of Chicago Press, 1976).

12. Andrea Campbell and Robert Binstock, "Politics and Aging in the United States," in *Handbook of Aging and the Social Sciences*, 7th ed., ed. Linda George (London: Elsevier, 2011). 265–280.

13. Campbell, *How Policies Make Citizens.*

14. Andrea Campbell, "Participatory Reactions to Policy Threats: Senior Citizens and the Defense of Social Security and Medicare," *Political Behavior* 25, no. 1 (2003): 29–49.

15. Anne Schneider and Helen Ingram, "Social Construction of Target Populations: Implications for Politics and Policy," *American Political Science Review* 87, no. 2 (1993): 334–347.

16. Cook and Barrett, *Support for the American Welfare State.*

17. See also Hudson and Gonyea, "Baby Boomers," 277.

18. Mark Schlesinger and Pamela Brown Drumheller, "Medicare and the Burden of Health Care Costs on Older Americans," in Blumenthal, Schlesinger, and Drumheller, *Renewing the Promise*, 31–57.

19. Christine Day, "Older Americans' Attitudes toward the Medicare Catastrophic Coverage Act of 1988," *The Journal of Politics* 55, no. 1 (1993): 167–177.

20. Richard Himelfarb, *Catastrophic Politics* (University Park: Pennsylvania State University Press, 1995).

21. Debra Street, "Maintaining the Status Quo: The Impact of Old-Age Interest Groups on the Medicare Catastrophic Coverage Act of 1988," *Social Problems* 40, no. 4 (1993): 431–444.

22. Day, "Older Americans' Attitudes."

23. Street, "Maintaining the Status Quo."

24. Street, "Maintaining the Status Quo."

25. Himelfarb, *Catastrophic Politics*; Hudson and Gonyea, "Baby Boomers."

26. Theodore R. Marmor, Timothy M. Smeeding, and Vernon L. Greene, eds., *Economic Security and Intergenerational Justice: A Look at North America* (Washington, DC: The Urban Institute, 1994).

27. Phillip Longman, *Born to Pay: The New Politics of Aging in America* (Boston: Houghton Mifflin, 1987).

28. David Cutler and Louise Sheiner, "Generational Aspects of Medicare," *American Economic Review* 90, no. 2 (2000): 303–307.

29. Oberlander, *Political Life of Medicare.*

30. Victor Marshall, Fay Lomax Cook, and Joanne Gard Marshall, "Conflict over Intergenerational Equity: Rhetoric and Reality in a Comparative Context," in *The Changing Contract across Generations*, ed. W. Andrew Achenbaum and Vern L. Bengston (New York: Aldine de Gruyter, 1993), 119–140.

31. Why they assumed that political motives would be exclusively self-interested remains unclear, but probably had more to do with their broad presumptions

about human nature than with any notions (and certainly not any evidence) specifically related to older citizens.

32. Becca Levy and Mark Schlesinger, "When Self-Interest and Stereotypes Collide: Older Individuals' Opposition to Federal Programs That Benefit Their Age Group," *Journal of Aging and Social Policy* 17 (2005): 25–39; Mark Schlesinger and Karl Kronebusch, "Intergenerational Tensions and Conflict: Attitudes and Perceptions about Social Justice and Age-Related Needs," in *Intergenerational Linkages: Hidden Connections in American Society,* ed. Vern L. Bengston (New York: Springer, 1994), 152–184; Laurie Rhodebeck, "The Politics of Greed? Political Preferences among the Elderly," *The Journal of Politics* 55, no. 2 (1993): 342–364; Michael Ponza, Greg Duncan, Mary Corcoran, and Fred Groskind, "The Guns of Autumn? Age Differences in Support for Income Transfers to the Young and the Old," *Public Opinion Quarterly* 53 (1988): 441–466.
33. Schlesinger and Kronebusch, "Intergenerational Tensions and Conflict."
34. Mark Schlesinger and Karl Kronebusch, "The Sources of Intergenerational Burdens and Tensions," in Bengston, *Intergenerational Linkages,* 184–209.
35. Oberlander, *Political Life of Medicare.*
36. Robert Samuelson, "America's Most Dangerous Lobby," *San Diego Union-Tribune,* November 16, 2005.
37. Marshall, Cook, and Marshall, "Conflict over Intergenerational Equity."
38. Although most Americans recognize that Medicare enrolls people with disabilities, the public still views the program as primarily benefiting its older enrollees. See Schlesinger and Kronebusch, "Sources of Intergenerational Burdens and Tensions."
39. Merril Silverstein, Joseph Angelelli, and Tonya Parrott, "Changing Attitudes Toward Aging Policy in the United States During the 1980s and 1990s: A Cohort Analysis," *Journal of Gerontology* 56B (2001): S36–S43.
40. It seems a rather remarkable coincidence that the proportion of the public wishing to cut entitlement benefits was at exactly the same level and changed at exactly the same extent (from 3 percent to 6 percent) as those who felt that elders had too much influence on American society (Figure 7.2). Of course, that might suggest that it is not coincidental at all. But since no extant survey asked the same respondents both of these questions, their connection cannot, at this point, be conclusively established.
41. Matthew W. Wolfe, "The Shadows of Future Generations," *Duke Law Journal* 57 (2008): 1897–1932; Bayard Catron, "Sustainability and Intergenerational Equity: An Expanded Stewardship Role for Public Administration," *Administrative Theory & Praxis* 18 (1996): 2–12.
42. Victor Fuchs, "Medicare Reform: The Larger Picture," *The Journal of Economic Perspectives* 14, no. 2 (2000): 57–70; Julie Lee, Mark McClellan, and Jonathan Skinner, "The Distributional Effects of Medicare," *Tax Policy and the Economy* 13 (1999): 85–107.
43. Hudson and Gonyea, "Baby Boomers."
44. Fay Lomax Cook, "Social Security and Senior Participation," *The Gerontologist* 45 (2005): 131–133; Robert Harootyan and Robert Vorek, "Volunteering, Helping, and Gift Giving in Families and Communities," in Bengston, *Intergenerational Linkages,* 77–111.

45. Michael Gusmano and Mark Schlesinger, "The Social Roles of Medicare: Assessing Medicare's Collateral Benefits," *Journal of Health Politics, Policy, and Law* 26 (2001): 37–80.
46. Blumenthal, Schlesinger, and Drumheller, *Renewing the Promise.*
47. Karen Davis, Cathy Schoen, Michelle Doty, and Katie Tenney, "Medicare versus Private Insurance: Rhetoric and Reality," *Health Affairs* (web exclusive) 2002: W311–24, doi: 10.1377/hlthaff.w2.311.
48. Robert Blendon et al., "Understanding the Managed Care Backlash," *Health Affairs* 17 (1998): 80–94.
49. Jacob Hacker, *The Road to Nowhere* (Princeton, NJ: Princeton University Press, 1997); Mark Schlesinger, "On Values and Democratic Policymaking: The Fragile Consensus around Market-Oriented Medical Care," *Journal of Health Politics, Policy, and Law* 27, no. 6 (2002): 889–926.
50. Marsha Gold et al., *Monitoring Medicare+Choice: Medicare Beneficiaries and Health Plan Choice, 2000* (Washington, DC: Mathematica Policy Research, 2001).
51. Thomas McGuire, Joseph Newhouse, and Anna Sinaiko, "An Economic History of Medicare Part C," *Milbank Quarterly* 89 (2011): 289–332; Mark Duggan et al., "Providing Prescription Drug Coverage to the Elderly: America's Experiment with Medicare Part D," *The Journal of Economic Perspectives* 22, no. 4 (2008): 69–92.
52. Schlesinger, "On Values."
53. Mohan Dutta-Bergman, "Developing a Profile of Consumer Intention to Seek Out Health Information beyond the Doctor," *Health Marketing Quarterly* 21 (2003): 91–112.
54. Judith Hibbard et al., "Is the Informed-Choice Policy Approach Appropriate for Medicare Beneficiaries?" *Health Affairs* 20 (2001): 199–203.
55. Judith Hibbard and Edward Weeks, "Consumerism in Health Care: Prevalence and Predictors," *Medical Care* 25 (1987): 1019–1032.
56. The number of participating insurers peaked in 2008–2009, when the average beneficiary could select among 48 Part D plans and 32 Part C plans. See Marsha Gold et al., *Medicare Advantage 2013 Spotlight: Enrollment Market Update* (Menlo Park, CA: Kaiser Family Foundation, 2014); Jack Hoadley et al., *Medicare Part D Prescription Drug Plans: The Marketplace in 2014 and Key Trends. 2006–2013* (Menlo Park, CA: Kaiser Family Foundation, 2014).
57. Elizabeth Murray et al., "Clinical Decision-Making: Patients' Preferences and Experiences," *Patient Education and Counseling* 65 (2007): 189–196.
58. Jason Abaluck and Jonathan Gruber, "Choice Inconsistencies among the Elderly: Evidence from Plan Choice in the Medicare Part D Program," *The American Economic Review* 101 (2011): 1180–1210.
59. Marsha Gold et al., *Medicare Advantage 2013*; Gretchen Jacobson et al., *How Are Seniors Choosing and Changing Health Insurance Plans?* (Menlo Park, CA: Kaiser Family Foundation, 2014.
60. Andrea Campbell, "Policy Feedbacks and the Impact of Policy Designs on Public Opinion," *Journal of Health Politics, Policy, and Law* 36, no. 6 (2011): 961–973.
61. John Geyman, *Shredding the Social Contract: The Privatization of Medicare* (Monroe, ME: Common Courage Press, 2006).

62. Charlene Harrington, Susan Merrill, and Jeffrey Newman, "Factors Associated with Medicare Beneficiary Complaints about Quality Of Care," *Journal for Healthcare Quality* 23 (2001): 4–14.
63. The British National Health Service is experiencing similar tensions as it introduces greater consumer choice into its system. See Judith Allsop and Kathryn Jones, "Withering the Citizen, Managing the Consumer: Complaints in Healthcare Settings," *Social Policy & Society* 7 (2007): 233–243.
64. Mark Schlesinger, Kathy King, and the Study Panel on Medicare and Markets, *The Role of Private Plans in Medicare: Lessons from the Past, Looking to the Future* (Washington, DC: National Academy of Social Insurance, 2003).
65. Kimberly Morgan and Andrea Campbell, *The Delegated Welfare State: Medicare, Markets, and the Governance of Social Policy* (New York: Oxford University Press, 2011).
66. Campbell, "Policy Feedbacks," 966.
67. Helen Halpin and Peter Harbage, "The Origins and Demise of the Public Option," *Health Affairs* 29 (2010): 1117–1124.
68. Which was not very well, since the legislation was far too complex and its origins far too politically contested for much of the public to have an accurate understanding of its provisions. Mollyann Brodie et al., "Liking the Pieces, Not the Package: Contradictions in Public Opinion during Health Reform," *Health Affairs* 29 (2010): 1125–1130.
69. Data from Roper Center for Public Opinion Research, survey by Research Associates International (RAI), July 13–18, 2011. Dataset: USPSRA.11HTPJUL. R06F.
70. Daniel Gitterman and John Scott, "Obama Lies, Grandma Dies: The Uncertain Politics of Medicare and the Patient Protection and Affordable Care Act," *Journal of Health Politics, Policy, and Law* 36 (2010): 555–563.
71. Melissa Castora-Binkley et al., "Inclusion of Caregiver Supports and Services in Home- and Community-Based Service Programs," *Journal of Aging & Social Policy* 23 (2011): 19–33; Barbara Da Roit and Blanche Le Bihan, "Similar and Yet So Different: Cash-for-Care in Six European Countries' Long-Term Care Policies," *Milbank Quarterly* 88 (2010): 286–309.
72. Because the disability rights movement has for the past 40 years embraced a consumer-directed model, there is little doubt that this subset of beneficiaries would embrace these sorts of reforms.
73. Kyoungrae Jung, Dennis Shea, and Candy Warner, "Agency Characteristics and Changes in Home Health Quality after Home Health Compare," *Journal of Aging and Health* 22 (2010): 454–476.
74. Murray et al., "Clinical Decision-Making."
75. Brian Elbel and Mark Schlesinger, "A Neglected Aspect of Medical Consumerism: Responsive Consumers in Markets for Health Plans," *Milbank Quarterly* 87 (2009): 633–682.

# PART III

# RETRENCHMENT, REFORM, AND REACTION

In the 1970s and 1980s, two forces threatened the future of Medicare and Medicaid: rising costs and the resulting cost containment efforts, on the one hand, and the rightward turn in American politics, on the other. Out of these uncertain times came political experimentation, economic reform, and innovations that merged Republican market ideas and distrust of the federal government with the old Great Society ideal that still buoyed these programs. In many ways, today's design of both programs owes much to this era of retrenchment and reform and to the political reaction against those reforms.

Looking at this era closely, Mark Peterson, in Chapter 8, examines how Medicare has gone from being labeled as "socialistic" in the 1960s to becoming a bedrock institution of social policy by the 1970s. Yet, as he also observes, the 1980s and 1990s produced a new twist, as the program formerly known as "the third rail of American politics" suddenly became "touchable" by reformers on the right. In Chapter 9, Uwe Reinhardt describes how, out of this drive to limit the rising cost of Medicare, innovation emerged—specifically, the use of DRGs (diagnosis-related groups) and physician fee schedules as the means for limiting hospital and physician payments, respectively. As Frank Thompson observes in Chapter 10, innovation in the embattled Medicaid program brought a new trend toward executive waivers—giving states latitude to experiment while preventing the program's conversion to block-grant funding. And yet, despite the retrenchment, reform, and reaction, American public opinion continued to regard Medicare as one of the nation's most popular government programs. Andrea Campbell's Chapter 11 explores how that public support has allowed Medicare and Medicaid to weather economic and political battles.

# 8

# THIRD RAIL OF POLITICS
## THE RISE AND FALL OF MEDICARE'S UNTOUCHABILITY

MARK A. PETERSON

In 1991 I participated in one of Capitol Hill's annual rituals. President George H. W. Bush was set to transmit his federal budget plan for fiscal year 1992 to Congress. That morning, other legislative aides and I in the Office of Senator Tom Daschle, Co-Chair of the Democratic Policy Committee and a member of the Senate Finance Committee, were allocated assignments on what particular domains of the president's proposed budget we would read and quickly assess. Each of us would prepare memos to inform Senator Daschle on our assigned text and write up pithy rapid responses available to the communications staff. This being well before the launch of the Web, we gathered as a group to await copies of the printed document hot off the presses.

As a legislative assistant for health policy, I was given one of the easier tasks—identifying and characterizing the administration's intentions for the Medicare program. Nothing should be "easy" about evaluating either Medicare or federal budget plans, each of which harbors a level of complexity that could stymie the best of minds, but that was not the point. As we fully anticipated, the president wanted to reduce Medicare spending and also initiate means-testing so that wealthier beneficiaries would pay higher premiums for Part B physician coverage. My memo to Senator Daschle later that day reported that the "budget presents a combination of severe cuts in Medicare coupled with a few modest reforms. Sen. Bentsen [Chair of the Senate Finance Committee] has already gone on record stating that these cuts are unacceptable." To bring home the consequences to the senator's constituents, in boldface I wrote, "No hospital, physician, or Medicare beneficiary in South Dakota will be able to escape the effects of these cuts."

Regarding the Part B means-testing provision, while recognizing that it was not necessarily a "bad idea in principle," I highlighted, again in boldface, that "most senior groups are adamantly opposed to this plan (sounds like Catastrophic all over again)." "Catastrophic" served as a reminder of the political rebellion among seniors that triggered the extraordinary congressional repeal of the Medicare Catastrophic Coverage Act (MCCA) in the year after its 1988 enactment (see Chapter 7 by Mark Schlesinger in this volume). That remarkable episode became the synecdoche for what happens to policies and politicians when they mess with Medicare.

Long before the creation of President Bush's fiscal year 1992 budget and my memo in response, Medicare had been dubbed, along with Social Security, a "third rail of American politics." Like the high-voltage third rail that powers a subway train, "touch it and you die." As with many metaphors, the associated image exaggerated reality, but that theme defined the politics of challenging President Bush's Medicare initiatives—they could be thwarted by fashioning them as too close to the rail's supposed lethal current.

Fifty years after Medicare's enactment, and almost a quarter-century since my personal dabbling in third-rail politics, it is important to examine what gave Medicare such "juice." Given the significant transformations in American politics that have transpired since the elder Bush served in the White House, it is equally important to ask whether the program retains its political shield against major disruptions. While Paul Starr, in Chapter 16 of this volume, explores the ways that government health programs have become "entrenched" in American politics, and Keith Wailoo, in Chapter 12, addresses the drive for expansion, this chapter offers a policy perspective on how the core social insurance idea of Medicare—publicly financed universal health insurance coverage for senior citizens—went from being cast as "socialistic" and well outside the acceptable mainstream sensibilities of American politics, to being a bedrock institution of American social policy, and then to becoming "touchable" by reformers. I explore how the conservative Republican revolution, which wrested control of Congress from long-standing Democratic majorities in the 1994 election, challenged the program's third-rail meme, making Medicare reform possible, even if still politically treacherous. All the while, the fiscal challenges facing Medicare have mounted—driven by baby boomer retirement, a proportionally smaller taxpaying workforce, and rising costs in the healthcare system overall—making the program a fixture of political and policy debate.

In this changed context, during which the Republican Party routinely put transformative plans for Medicare front and center on the healthcare policy agenda, the "touch it and you die" motif, whatever its past credence, seems decidedly outdated. Has the power of the third rail been truly cut? Not entirely, I argue; it still retains its power to cripple politically. Elected officials who *propose* significant revisions to Medicare may not suffer political death or even severe burns, but we cannot yet know what would happen to them if their plans actually became law. Even many right-wing, anti-government activists from the Tea Party movement that populate much of the Republican electoral base warn officials in various versions to "keep your government hands off my Medicare."[1] All that can be said so far is that touching Medicare with bold schemes to outright nix its social insurance principles has produced little in the way of either overt political harm for trying or transformative shifts in policy and law. I close this chapter with a reminder that third-rail politics, even as tempered as they have become, helps ensure not policy stasis, but rather relative stability in Medicare's fundamental architecture. At the same time, it undermines the viability of potentially beneficial policy reforms advocated by either the left or right.

## From "Socialist" Threat to American Bedrock: Powering the Third Rail

As described in Chapter 1 of this volume by Julian Zelizer, Medicare, now covering over 50 million Americans and second only to Social Security in federal expenditures for domestic programs, began contentiously as a feeble stepchild to President Harry Truman's failed effort to enact—or even generate formal congressional debate about—a publicly financed national health insurance program. In the early 1950s, his advisers began to focus on coverage for just the elderly as a possible first step toward universal coverage. And incremental it was. When formally introduced by congressional Democrats in the late 1950s and adopted as a centerpiece of President John F. Kennedy's domestic agenda, the policy ambitions were remarkably timid—just anemic coverage of hospital care, with physician services left out entirely, for recipients of Social Security.[2] That was it. Even this proposed pinky in the water of government involvement in healthcare financing was attacked by opponents as deeply contrary to American liberties and values, a first step on the road to Soviet-style socialism. In 1961, as part of its "Operation Coffee Cup" campaign against Medicare, the American Medical Association (AMA) widely distributed a speech by Ronald Reagan that argued, if people did not get appropriately mobilized,

> this program, I promise you, will pass just as surely as the sun will come up tomorrow. And behind it will come other federal programs that will invade every area of freedom as we have known it in this country. Until one day...we will awake to find that we have socialism. And if you don't do this, one of these days you and I are going to spend our sunset years telling our children and our children's children what it once was like in America when men were free.[3]

The shifting political terrain in the decades after World War II, however, eventually transformed Medicare's prospects from the "politics of legislative impossibility" to the "politics of legislative certainty," as first explained by Theodore Marmor in his classic study of the program's evolution.[4] The 1964 elections—with President Lyndon Johnson's historic landslide and huge gains by Democrats in the House and Senate—finally broke the logjam that had prevented Medicare's enactment, as several of the chapters in this volume have explored. By triggering collaboration between Johnson and House Ways and Means Committee Chair Wilbur Mills, a previous Medicare skeptic, the electoral rout also led to an enacted Medicare program that was far more expansive and comprehensive than originally proposed. The most notable addition included the Medicaid program for certain categories of the non-elderly poor.[5] Some of the usual rhetorical pangs of an overreaching government remained alive in the conservative opposition at the end of debate, but the votes on final passage in 1965 were overwhelming and bipartisan—in the House, 85 percent of the Democrats were joined by 47 percent of the Republicans voting in favor, while in the Senate the figures were 81 percent and 41 percent.

Given the initial socialist trope promoted by opponents to just the original hospital coverage proposal, the political turnaround in the passage of Medicare is quite stunning. At least for those over 64 years old, the 1965 law established a robust and highly popular social insurance program consistent with the parameters of the "international standard" for national healthcare systems.[6] Except for some nuances at the very margin, enrollment is universal for this population (defined by Social Security eligibility); the vast majority of the funding is from federal taxes based on income, not the beneficiary's medical risk or need; and the coverage of services is comprehensive (especially as defined by the health insurance paradigm at the time). Moreover, the federal government, as the sole payer (other than patient cost sharing), has the capacity to adjust payments and impose some cost controls. With beneficiaries inclusive of rich and poor, the program is not just a "safety net" for the disadvantaged.[7] As exhibited by other advanced democracies, these social insurance principles can be fulfilled by myriad distinctive program designs, ranging from tax-financed and government-delivered health services (Britain) to services provided through competing private insurance plans (the Netherlands). As created, Medicare resembles most the "single-payer" Medicare program in Canada, incorporating public financing of privately delivered healthcare services. Since then, however, there has been some subsequent movement that hints at the Dutch model.

A year after enactment, over 19 million senior citizens were enrolled in the program. By the time I was drafting memos to Senator Daschle in 1991, that figure would grow by 60 percent. Senior citizens had, by then, been joined by nearly 3.5 million long-term disabled.[8] As Jonathan Oberlander has described in *The Political Life of Medicare*, soon after Medicare's implementation and for decades hence, American health politics operated under a "Medicare consensus" characterized by bipartisan agreement and relative tranquility. Although policymakers modified the program's provisions, sometimes substantially, none of their modifications disrupted, and some even reinforced, the core social insurance structure of the program—especially from the beneficiaries' perspective. As with Social Security, the third-rail of this unusual form of US social policy soon became bolted into place because of the reinforcing combination of general public enthusiasm for Medicare, among both its beneficiaries and the public at large; escalating stakeholder interests, both institutional and geographic; and the incidence of the program's benefits and costs.

As Jill Bernstein and Rosemary Stevens noted in a 1999 report, "If there is one 'absolute' in polls about Medicare, it is that Americans place a very high value on the program." Three-quarters of the public agrees that the program is a "commitment made a long time ago that cannot be broken."[9] Andrea Campbell, in Chapter 11 of this volume, similarly recounts the strong and enduring public support that the program has received from its early days to the present, even during periods when it has seemed most vulnerable to retreat and redefinition.

As an existing program in which most people have major material stakes, any proposed changes in Medicare benefits run into a general political hurdle in the health policy arena: overcoming the public's basic premise that a reform should " 'do no harm' to them personally."[10] Even imagined perils can thwart programmatic changes. The Medicare Catastrophic Coverage Act (MCCA) of 1988 became law because members of Congress *thought* they were extending *desired* benefits to Medicare enrollees, but it was soon repealed by Congress following an outcry from constituents. Although 91 percent of the elderly supported the proposed law in May 1988 and two-thirds remained favorable at the time of its passage in December 1988, by eight months later, support had collapsed to only 40 percent. During the intervening months, the National Committee to Preserve Social Security and Medicare had conducted a major—and to be sure, entirely misleading—opposition campaign (see Mark Schlesinger's discussion in Chapter 7 of this volume).[11] Few politicians have lost standing in their constituencies by attacking either the explicit cuts in Medicare proposed by others or revisions that have come to be viewed as threatening and harmful to beneficiaries.

Organized interests are a second contributing factor to Medicare's third-rail status. The media, the public, and even social scientists frequently turn first and foremost to the power of "special interests" to explain policy outcomes, including policy stalemate. In surveys of the public and congressional staff that we conducted about a decade ago as part of the Institutions of American Democracy project, roughly three-quarters of each agreed with the proposition that special interests have an adverse effect on policymaking by Congress.[12] Given its size and importance to multiple constituencies,

Medicare politics would seem to be particularly hospitable terrain for organized interests. At the beginning, Medicare's enactment had little to do with interest-group advocacy, and proponents largely failed at obtaining later expansions.[13] Once in place, however, the program has generated a protective sphere of three distinct sets of interests with readily identifiable stakes in the program—beneficiaries, healthcare providers (in the broadest sense of the term), and communities—all of whom have access to Capitol Hill and would presumably seek to block policy options that would impose identifiable costs.

The already enormous Medicare beneficiary population is projected to nearly double as all baby boomers reach eligibility. Medicare and Social Security have together provided the stakes and resources that permit the Medicare population to become particularly well mobilized and engaged with its present and future prospects. Not only do senior citizens in general have the highest voting rates in the electorate, but these programs have given lower-income elderly the incentive and the means (time and money) to engage in political participation at higher rates than younger citizens in comparable economic circumstances.[14] The AARP is the most prominent of the many formally organized interests representing this constituency. Although its influence has waned from its peak a few decades ago, as Mark Schlesinger argues in Chapter 7, with a membership of about 40 million people (52 percent of Americans age 50 or older), the AARP can claim to be the largest voluntary association in the country, reaching the potential to mobilize significant numbers of citizens in every congressional district. It also possesses a sizable professional research staff, a team of lobbyists, and ready access to Congress.[15]

Medicare was enacted despite the vociferous opposition of the American Medical Association, then perhaps the single most influential interest group in America.[16] Organized medicine no longer has that kind of sway in American politics,[17] but, as noted by Bruce Vladeck, former administrator of the agency that manages Medicare (and a Ph.D. in political science), it has become part of the "Medicare-Industrial Complex" spawned by Medicare. As Vladeck has characterized it, the "Medicare-Industrial Complex" is vast, representing not only physicians and hospitals, but also laboratories, home health agencies, producers of medical supplies, pharmaceutical companies, and, perhaps most important, private insurance companies who serve as Medicare contractors.[18] Anyone who has spent time working on health policy issues on Capitol Hill has experienced the constant flow of representatives from this Medicare-Industrial Complex into members' personal offices, hearing rooms, committee markup sessions, breakfast chats, and political action committee (PAC) fundraisers. The barrage of formal correspondence, reports, faxes, e-mails, and briefings provided by individuals or professional and industry coalitions is impossible to miss: in the space of one year I noted meeting with representatives from 84 healthcare associations, think tanks, unions, firms, advocacy centers, and grassroots organizations, most of whom would have included Medicare among their policy interests.

Under the rubric of "distributive politics" (also known more cynically as "pork barrel politics"), Vladeck also identifies a third category of programmatic claimants: communities hoping to secure local spending.[19] One economic study in 2004 estimated that federal health spending accounts for an average of 4.4 percent of "metropolitan gross product," and that health-services jobs accounted for 6.6 percent to 12.0 percent of all employment in sampled communities.[20] Towns, cities, and states are well represented in Washington, and individually are usually accorded unfettered contact with the members of Congress who represent them.

Taken at face value, these features of the Medicare interest-group domain suggest an arena of well-positioned and resource-rich organizations likely to be antagonistic, in whole or in part, to Medicare reforms that alter the central premises and commitments of the program.[21] And in some cases, as Sara Rosenbaum has discussed in Chapter 6 of this volume, healthcare providers may even be able to argue that such cuts represent a denial of their constitutional rights.

The barriers to change may be greatest for those elements of a plan that would impose explicit losses on beneficiaries. This constituency is well mobilized politically and pays close attention to policy debate on these issues.[22] Public opinion polls repeatedly reveal both public and senior citizen opposition to many of the specific proposals to limit benefits, from raising the age of eligibility to increasing cost-sharing (except for the more affluent) or subjecting beneficiaries to increased financial risk.

A third aspect of Medicare's staying power comes from the political effects of trying to change features of the program. Political scientists have long recognized that not only does the political setting shape policy outcomes, but that the attributes of policies themselves create their own politics.

James Q. Wilson, among others, has focused on the particular *mix* of costs and benefits associated with a policy, identifying the incentives and opportunities created for supporters and opponents to mobilize. Policies that impose explicit costs, for example, on a narrow and well-defined constituency (such as cuts in Medicare reimbursements to physicians) and that provide benefits to the collective whole (such as overall cost savings for beneficiaries and taxpayers) are likely to stimulate active and vocal resistance from the former and little in the way of energetic encouragement from the latter, because the benefits spread among a vast population will be less recognized, making collective action difficult to activate.[23]

The political response to policy options also depends on the *timing* of benefits and costs. Programs with early, upfront costs (such as increased taxes or new premiums) and late-order benefits (such as the added security of coverage years later) focus attention on the costs, rather than the benefits, and agitate in particular those who will have to pay them.[24]

Finally, the political calculation of elected officials will be influenced by whether or not the benefit and costs are *traceable* to public actions that they have taken, such as roll-call votes. Can they claim credit for the benefits or avoid blame for the costs? Elected officials have at their disposal a variety of policy design choices and strategic actions to boost the traceability of what is good and hide what is bad, but these options are not always available. Overall, at the extreme, policy initiatives may be particularly attractive to policymakers if they produce obvious, early-order benefits for which one can assert responsibility and ambiguous, hidden, or late-order costs that are easily overlooked. "Repellent" policies, in contrast, inflict well-recognized, early-order costs and promise only ephemeral or future advantages.[25]

It does not take much imagination to figure out which types of policies are associated with triggering the third rail in Medicare. The MCCA offers a prime example of how not to draft politically effective policies with respect to benefits and costs. The main benefit of the program was to provide a sense of security for Medicare recipients, so that they would not be financially ruined by a lengthy, expensive illness. Such events are devastating for those who experience them. But because most Medicare recipients do not ever encounter such costs and the risks may be well into the future, the benefit is more psychological than concrete, and many of the more affluent Medicare beneficiaries already had that kind of coverage through supplemental private insurance. In addition, in the name of fiscal responsibility, Congress chose to delay the availability of the benefits to build up a cushion of revenues. That meant that the costs—the new premiums—were to be collected by the government immediately, well before the MCCA provided recipients with any sense of additional security. On top of being early-order, the costs were unmistakable. The new premiums were collected in annual payments on the recipients' 1040 tax forms, which also made them look like a tax. To make the politics even more untenable, for the first time in the program's history, all the costs were to be borne by only the Medicare beneficiaries themselves. And because there would be no funding from taxpayers in general, fairness dictated a progressive payment by beneficiaries, thereby imposing the highest premiums on upper-income seniors—the group easiest to mobilize politically.

Consider the contrasting design of the later Medicare Modernization Act of 2003 (MMA), which also included pharmaceutical coverage. Most of the costs are being shouldered not by beneficiaries but rather by taxpayers at large (more precisely, because the committed funding added to the federal deficit, payment would be the responsibility of future taxpayers yet to be born, a particularly hard group to mobilize politically in 2003!). Other potentially problematic programmatic changes included in the law, such as a demonstration project intended to shift Medicare toward a market model by requiring direct price competition for the fee-for-service program against private plans, which could be costly to beneficiaries, were scheduled for years later (and never actually materialized). The prescription discount cards made available during the first stage of implementation provided a salve before the beginning of the actual prescription drug coverage. Rather than requiring a large upfront deductible, the program delayed draconian patient cost-sharing until a beneficiary encounters the "donut hole" of no coverage, originally set between $2,250 and $5,100 in total drug charges. The politics of benefits and costs helps keep transformation of Medicare off the active legislative agenda.

## Path Dependency

The attributes I have been discussing foster the presence of the third rail. Together, they reinforce its long-term endurance and the constancy, thus far, of the Medicare social insurance status quo. This systematic characteristic of Medicare after 1965 comports with what a number of scholars have described as path dependency. Medicare was enacted at a "critical juncture" (John F. Kennedy's assassination, the 1964 landslide presidential and congressional elections, and, one might add, a robust economy) out of which the program's core features were forged. Once in place, the basic structural attributes of an established program can, under certain conditions, produce "increasing returns" such that the "costs of switching from one alternative to another will, in certain social contexts, increase markedly over time," leading to policymaking "inertia," with the "dead weight of previous institutional choices seriously limit[ing] . . . room to maneuver."[26] Medicare has the particular attributes that are most likely to produce the extreme kind of stability referred to as policy lock-in, including the creation of large institutions, organized constituencies, long-term commitments, and a broad penetration of many aspects of American social and economic life.[27] Policymakers who have had long experience grappling with Medicare would readily recognize these characteristics.

Path dependency, of course, is not absolute. The potential for policy change always exists. Jacob Hacker identifies two processes of policy shifts. In the first, subsequent policymakers enact adjustments in the program, but over time the range of options that would include structural changes becomes more limited as a result of the political dynamics of path dependency. Starting in the early 1970s, various aspects of the financing and organization of the program have been modified through a series of amendments. In the 1980s Congress and the executive branch made substantial changes in the way in which Medicare pays hospitals and doctors, moving from largely uncontrolled retrospective reimbursements to prospective payments to hospitals and a legally specified fee schedule for physicians. A number of omnibus budget reconciliation acts in the 1980s included provisions that cut Medicare expenditures in various ways.[28]

None of these, though, has challenged the social insurance paradigm of the program. Moreover, with the exception of single-payer plans offered by some members of Congress and advocacy organizations, no major comprehensive healthcare system reform proposal has included provisions that would affect Medicare other than at the very margin. Not Richard Nixon's Comprehensive Health Insurance Plan, not Jimmy Carter's public-private approach to reform, not Bill Clinton's Health Security Act, not Senator Daschle's American Health Security Plan on which I worked, nor even the Affordable Care Act (ACA) supported by Barack Obama. Policymakers rejected any call to incorporate the Medicare population in the reform initiative as touching the third rail—an act that would spell the nearly automatic death of reform and attract the wrath of beneficiaries.

The second kind of policy shift noted by Hacker, however, involves forces at play that "undermine the self-reinforcing trajectory" of path dependency.[29] Dramatic swings in the political context, major economic disruptions, and other momentous events could open the door for an entirely different policy direction. The ingredients for such a new and potentially disruptive political and policy setting seemed to emerge in the mid-1990s. Our next task is to determine whether the unusual social, political, and economic tides unleashed at that time have so altered the Medicare context as to shut down the third rail and put at serious risk the program's social insurance principles.

## POLITICAL EARTHQUAKE AND FISCAL PRESSURES: A DROP IN VOLTAGE?

A few years after I wrote the memos to Senator Daschle in response to Bush's proposed budget, everything changed. A political earthquake hit Washington, with long-lasting effects. This tremor arrived just at the moment that policymakers had begun to acknowledge the depth of Medicare's long-term financing problems created by the demographics of an aging population and relentless growth in healthcare costs. The Medicare trustees' had issued long-term projections indicating that, without significant policy adjustments, a sizable gap would emerge and grow between the program's revenues and expenditures. These events, in combination, offered the potential of a new "critical juncture" of the sort that could disrupt the settled—that is, path-dependent—arrangements of the past. In this new context, challenging the traditional Medicare program, at least in terms of formulating proposals that would represent significant departures from the established social insurance principles, appears to have lost its political edge. The third rail's voltage has dropped, at least in terms of the risks to an elected official's political survival. But the current has remained sufficient to keep transformative plans on paper from moving through the legislative process to adoption. Even so, some policies have been enacted that could become placeholders for more expansive disruptions of the status quo.

The 1994 congressional elections granted Republicans concurrent control of the House and Senate for the first time in 40 years. As a result, the politics of Medicare joined the country's larger politics of partisanship and ideological conflict.[30] Policy discourse, which suddenly embraced free market principles, had not been energized by new evidence of the market's superiority over social insurance in social policy. Rather, this shift grew from the simple political fact that the election replaced Democratic with conservative Republican majorities.[31] In the ensuing "age of polarization," healthcare coverage, in general, and Medicare, in particular, have become instruments for each party to either try to secure a long-term majority coalition or to eviscerate its opposition's future prospects.[32]

Once in command of Congress, Republican leaders like Speaker Newt Gingrich set out immediately to restructure Medicare into a defined-contribution voucher program. This policy strategy, whatever its substantive merits, would fragment the program's clientele and would break the ties of the middle-class electorate to Democratic government. Hence Democrats and liberals saw the imperative to strive for its defeat.[33] In 1995 the newly ascendant Republican leadership was in fact able to pass through Congress a plan for Medicare that would have explicitly transformed it from a publicly run, defined-benefit program befitting social insurance to a budgeted (capped) system of vouchers for the purchase of private insurance, shifting risks and costs to individuals. Moreover, Republicans kept control of Congress for more than a decade, during which time they kept a market-oriented approach to Medicare alive on the table. The 2006 election returned Democratic House and Senate majorities, but the GOP sailed back with a vengeance to the House following the 2010 walloping of their partisan opposition. By then the ideological gap between the two parties in both the House and Senate had become unprecedented, greater than at any time since 1879, mostly driven by the Republican flight to the Right.[34]

Medicare's financial pressures also created a potential political environment that would possibly permit fundamental policy change over any remaining fear of the third rail.[35] The impression that Medicare was in financial trouble grew more stark in the 1990s and beyond, as the 75-year projections required of the Medicare trustees in their annual reports showed expenditures rapidly exceeding revenues. Assuming no policy changes, the Part A hospital trust fund financed by payroll taxes would descend into "bankruptcy" at some point in the near future (sometimes projected to be in less than 10 years); the program overall would eat up vast expanses of the federal budget and would consume an ever-growing share of the national income. Why? The coming retirement of the baby boomers would double the number of beneficiaries, the ratio of taxpaying workers to beneficiaries was dropping, and overall costs of healthcare services were climbing.[36]

These projected trends have certainly created the perception of an ongoing fiscal crisis, even though Medicare's history has demonstrated the favorable impact of frequent policy adjustments. Very long-term projections are highly suspect and often wrong, and other studies suggest greater sustainability.[37] In combination with a long period of Republican control of Congress, six years of unified Republican government, an especially aggressive set of conservative Republican legislators and leaders, and the overall greater prominence of market approaches in health care, the fiscal pressures—whether real or illusory—have added impetus to a full-bore questioning of the sustainability of Medicare as a social insurance program.

The experiences of the last several years, then, have tempered the earlier assumption that politicians who touch the third rail of Medicare will suffer immediate electrocution. As noted previously, the Republican House and Senate in 1995 enacted legislation that would have cut Medicare spending substantially and would have profoundly altered the organization and administration of the program. Among many other changes, it would have turned the Medicaid program into a block grant to the states and repealed many environmental regulations. Although there were deep worries within what was then known as the Health Care Financing Administration (the predecessor to CMS) that President Clinton would yield and sign this legislation,[38] the aura of the third rail motivated the president to veto the bill. The proposed disruption of Medicare lent the most political leverage to the veto. Clinton also won the political battle that emerged over the ensuing shutdown of the federal government and was re-elected in 1996 despite a scandal that eventually led to his impeachment.[39]

But despite Clinton's victory in this skirmish, there were no third-rail deaths. The Republican Party held on to both its House and Senate majorities through the next five congressional elections. It was able to push successfully for the establishment of the National Bipartisan Commission on the Future of Medicare, which focused its attention on a voucher-style plan favored by Republicans (and some conservative Democrats). The plan failed, however, to attract the supermajority on the commission needed to make it an official recommendation. The co-chairs, Republican Representative Bill Thomas and Democratic Senator John Breaux, introduced bills based on the commission's plan, but neither progressed through Congress.[40] The one piece of significant legislation that did pass, on a bipartisan vote, was the Balanced Budget Act of 1997, which combined Democratic-style cuts in provider reimbursements with a promotion of private managed-care plans favored by Republicans. As implemented, however, the so-called Medicare+Choice approach ultimately reversed the growth of managed-care plans in Medicare.[41]

The election of President George W. Bush finally gave Republicans their best opportunity yet to restructure Medicare away from social insurance and toward a far more contained system of subsidized private coverage. Or so they thought. Bush wanted to provide drug coverage only to those beneficiaries willing to abandon traditional fee-for-service Medicare and join a private insurance plan, an incentive strategy intended, ultimately, to move all beneficiaries into competing private health plans as a long step on the path to a budgeted and privatized Medicare. The third-rail impulse, however, stood in the way. Republican Billy Tauzin, chair of the House Committee on Energy and Commerce, exclaimed, "you couldn't move my mother out of Medicare with a bulldozer. She trusts it, believes in it, it's served her well."[42] The final version of the Medicare Modernization Act of 2003 did not force this choice, but it did require those in fee-for-service Medicare to obtain their drug coverage from free-standing (and as yet nonexistent) private drug plans, a significant break from past approaches. Seniors initially had little enthusiasm for this approach to prescription drugs (in February 2004, two months after the law was signed, 55 percent had an unfavorable impression, with 17 percent favorable).[43] Nonetheless, Bush received a majority of the votes cast by Medicare beneficiaries a year later in the 2004 presidential election, and Republicans picked up a few seats in both the House and Senate.[44]

After regaining their majority in the House of Representatives in 2011, the Republicans voted overwhelmingly to support a far more dramatic plan released by House Budget Committee Chair Paul Ryan. Ryan's plan went the full distance to replace Medicare as a defined-benefit social insurance program with a form of private insurance vouchers for all beneficiaries (dubbed "premium support"). In addition, Ryan's plan set federal Medicare funding on a specific growth path regardless of whatever happened to healthcare and insurance premium costs, shifting substantial cost risks to the beneficiaries.[45] That vote neither cost the GOP its majority in the 2012 election (it lost only eight seats) nor kept Ryan off the Republican ticket as Mitt Romney's vice presidential nominee.

What explains this new version of Medicare politics, with no (political) pain but no (policy) gain? The many years of conservative Republican dominance of Congress since 1994, combined with six years of unified government by the GOP during the Bush administration, helped propel market models, private health plan competition, and personal "skin in the game" onto the overall healthcare agenda.[46] Medicare could hardly remain isolated from these trends, especially given the yearly long-term projections mandated from the Medicare trustees. This new context afforded an opening for opponents of social insurance to put forward a wholesale redesign of the program without the political risks of the past.

In a direct sense, however, they have succeeded substantively only at the margin. They have not been able to upend the social insurance architecture because of the same forces that have been at play since early in the life of Medicare. Campbell's Chapter 11 in this volume follows the program's sustained popularity, even as the alternative approach of "privatization" has been given a full and open hearing in public discourse. Fairly recent surveys, for example, show that the vast majority of people—72 percent overall and 88 percent of senior citizens—continue to hold positive views of Medicare.[47] Beyond public opinion, all of the factors that reinforce Medicare's staying power—interest groups and their stakes; the benefits, costs, and timing of policy change; and path dependency—remain largely in place, even as commercial insurance carriers and the pharmaceutical industry demand larger pieces of the action with far fewer federal constraints. That desire was readily apparent in their campaign finance support of George W. Bush and members of Congress who pushed the MMA, and the rewards in business, subsidies, and protections that these interests reaped from the law.[48]

There are nonetheless reasons for advocates of social insurance principles to be concerned about the future. To start, as discussed by Mark Schlesinger in Chapter 7 of this volume, there are a few signs that public support for traditional Medicare has begun to shift. For example, subtle changes in the design of Medicare could confuse beneficiaries and the broader public about the nature of Medicare and undermine allegiance to the program's mission and financing. Among individuals participating in 10 focus groups organized in California concerning the Medicare+Choice plans, seniors made clear their belief that enrollment in a managed-care plan meant that they were "no longer 'in Medicare.'"[49]

Beneficiaries who perceive themselves as outside the program may no longer feel connected to, nor sense a shared interest with, other Medicare recipients. Now called Part C "Medicare Advantage" plans, private plans currently include more than just managed care offerings; Part D drug coverage is also similarly provided through competing private plans. The perceptual implications of having private insurance providers for Parts C and D for the public's understanding of Medicare and the government's role in it are pronounced.[50]

To be sure, the international experience demonstrates that nations can have robust social insurance systems that incorporate the choice of private, even commercial, insurance carriers, as long as they remain universal and pool risks, provide comprehensive coverage of services, and retain payment by the population based on income and not medical need. Some policy changes in Medicare, such as the ACA filling in the pharmaceutical coverage "donut hole" and improving coverage of preventive care, have strengthened the program's underlying social insurance premises. Others, such as the strong encouragement of private plan competition within the program, have not *yet* subverted the program's social insurance character. But the question remains whether this movement toward privatization will ultimately undermine the public's decades-long support for Medicare in its current form and open the door to its replacement by a program that fragments the beneficiary population, subsidizes the purchase of private insurance, and puts more risks and costs on program participants. What we do know is that the third rail has lost enough shock value that the agenda of freely discussed alternatives is now open to a broad range of approaches, including complete abandonment of social insurance, at least in the abstract.

## The Policy Implications: Stability but Also Rigidity

In many other Western democracies, typically those with parliamentary institutions that can facilitate legislative coalition building, governments can move forward with even controversial initiatives and then be awarded or punished in the next round of elections.[51] In the United States, legislation to either launch new policy transformations or to institute substantial changes in some kinds of existing policy often requires something resembling a popular consensus, even on specific points of policy, to overcome the numerous veto points in the policymaking process. In the case of Medicare, such a consensus may be impossible to achieve given the complexity of the issues and the competing stakes involved.[52] The social insurance foundation of Medicare has been particularly resistant to fundamental redirection, even in the face of vast changes in the nation's political environment, the rise of the market model in health care, and perceptions of a coming fiscal crisis in the program. Many quite significant changes have been made, but as has been the case with social insurance programs abroad, which are routinely subject to nontrivial revisions, the core principles have remained in place. One clear signal of Medicare's vaunted place on the American landscape—a demonstration of the continued vitality of the third rail metaphor, even in the present ideologically polarized setting—came when Republicans in opposition to the ACA attacked it for, of all things, cutting Medicare funding.[53]

Given that Medicare is a healthcare program on which a particularly vulnerable population depends for timely access to much-needed medical services from trusted providers, this political resilience has been valuable. This stability is also important given the long-term commitment of everyone who starts paying the Medicare payroll tax from the moment they start their first jobs, decades before they themselves will be eligible for the program. From a policy-analytic perspective, however, stability—or at least the third-rail politics associated with it—can translate into undue rigidity that prevents thoughtful debate and the enactment and implementation of effective responses to changed circumstances. Those on the Left frame every proposal emanating primarily from conservatives as an existential threat to Medicare's social insurance principles, even though some are already in place in the well-regarded social insurance programs of other nations. Advocates of their own versions of reform from the Right contort themselves into a misleading rhetoric that suggests the best way to save Medicare is to replace it. Policy change of any sort can thus be stymied by both advocates on the Right (who want to bring market forces to Medicare) and the Left (who want to invigorate Medicare's social insurance commitment and perhaps expand the program to a larger population), resulting in stalemate, no matter the needs of the program. The result is that Medicare performs well below what would be possible without the third-rail shackles.

## Notes

1. Paul Krugman, "Health Care Realities," *New York Times*, July 30, 2009, http://www.nytimes.com/2009/07/31/opinion/31krugman.html.

2. Theodore R. Marmor, *The Politics of Medicare*, 2nd ed. (New York: Aldine de Gruyter, 2001); Jonathan Oberlander, *The Political Life of Medicare* (Chicago: University of Chicago Press, 2003).
3. Quoted in James A. Morone, *The Democratic Wish: Popular Participation and the Limits of American Government* (New York: Basic Books, 1990), 262, from "Ronald Reagan Speaks Out Against Socialized Medicine," LP audio recording, 1961.
4. Marmor, *The Politics of Medicare*. See also Oberlander, *The Political Life of Medicare*.
5. David Blumenthal and James A. Morone, *The Heart of Power: Health and Politics in the Oval Office* (Berkeley: University of California Press, 2010), ch. 5.
6. Joseph White, *Competing Solutions: American Health Care Proposals and International Experience* (Washington, DC: Brookings Institution Press, 1995), 215–217.
7. There is one glaring difference between Medicare and the international standard of the universal system abroad: because it is limited to only part of the population and remains embedded in a larger fragmented healthcare system well beyond its control, the federal government does not have real leverage to discipline cost growth.
8. "Medicare Enrollment: National Trends, 1966–2010," HISMI2010.pdf, https://www.cms.gov/Research-Statistics-Data-and-Systems/Statistics-Trends-and-Reports/MedicareEnrpts/downloads/HISMI2010.pdf.
9. Jill Bernstein and Rosemary A. Stevens, "Public Opinion, Knowledge, and Medicare Reform," *Health Affairs* 18, no. 1 (January/February 1999): 181–182.
10. Robert J. Blendon, Mollyann Brodie, and John Benson, "What Happened to Americans' Support for the Clinton Health Plan?" *Health Affairs* 14, no. 2 (May 1995): 12.
11. Richard Himelfarb, *Catastrophic Politics: The Rise and Fall of the Medicare Catastrophic Coverage Act of 1988* (University Park: Pennsylvania State University Press, 1995), ch. 5.
12. Annenberg Institutions of American Democracy Surveys of Congress (personal staffs, N = 252), August 4 to November 22, 2004, and of the Public (N = 1,500), December 18, 2004–January 18, 2005, conducted by Princeton Survey Research Associates International. The public was given the statement "The policy decisions that Congress makes are often negatively influenced by special interests" (I report here "Strongly agree/Agree"), and congressional staff were given the statement "Policies (are/were) distorted by pressure from special interests" (I report here "Very True/Somewhat True").
13. Oberlander, *The Political Life of Medicare*, 23; Andrea Campbell, *How Policies Make Citizens: Senior Political Activism and the American Welfare State* (Princeton, NJ: Princeton University Press, 2003).
14. Campbell, *How Policies Make Citizens*.
15. Campbell, *How Policies Make Citizens*; Lindsay Smith, "Top of the List: Associations," *Washington Business Journal*, November 1, 2010, http://www.bizjournals.com/washington/news/2010/11/01/top-of-the-list-associations.html?page=all. For the political significance of these interest group attributes, see Mark A. Peterson, "From Trust to Political Power: Interest Groups, Public Choice, and Health Care," *Journal of Health Politics, Policy, and Law* 26, no. 5 (October 2001): 1145–1163.
16. Marmor, *The Politics of Medicare*; Peterson, "From Trust to Political Power."

17. Peterson, "From Trust to Political Power."
18. Bruce C. Vladeck, "The Political Economy of Medicare," *Health Affairs* 18, no. 1 (January/February 1999): 27–30.
19. Vladeck, "The Political Economy of Medicare," 31.
20. Daniel Gitterman, Joanne Spetz, and Matthew Fellowes, "The Other Side of the Ledger: Federal Health Spending in Metropolitan Economies," discussion paper for The Brookings Institution Metropolitan Policy Program, Brookings Institution, Washington, DC, September 2004.
21. See Jacob S. Hacker, *The Divided Welfare State: The Battle over Public and Private Social Benefits in the United States* (New York: Cambridge University Press, 2002).
22. Campbell, *How Policies Make Citizens.*
23. James Q. Wilson, "The Politics of Regulation," in *The Politics of Regulation*, ed. James Q. Wilson (New York: Basic Books, 1980).
24. R. Douglas Arnold, *The Logic of Congressional Action* (New Haven, CT: Yale University Press, 1990).
25. Arnold, *The Logic of Congressional Action.*
26. Paul Pierson, "Increasing Returns, Path Dependence, and the Study of Politics," *American Political Science Review* 94, no. 2 (June 2000): 251, 263; Hacker, *The Divided Welfare State*, 54.
27. Hacker, *The Divided Welfare State*, 55.
28. Marilyn Moon, *Medicare: A Policy Primer* (Washington, DC: Urban Institute, 2006); Oberlander, *The Political Life of Medicare.*
29. Hacker, *The Divided Welfare State*, 54.
30. Oberlander, *The Political Life of Medicare*, 6.
31. Mark A. Peterson, "The Limits of Social Learning: Translating Analysis into Action," *Journal of Health Politics, Policy, and Law* 22, no. 4 (August 1997): 1077–1114.
32. Mark A. Peterson, "The Politics of Health Care Policy: Overreaching in an Age of Polarization," in *The Social Divide: Political Parties and the Future of Activist Government*, ed. Margaret Weir (Washington, DC, and New York: Brookings Institution Press and Russell Sage Foundation, 1998), 181–229.
33. Peterson, "The Politics of Health Care Policy"; Theda Skocpol, *Boomerang: Clinton's Health Security Effort and the Turn Against Government in U.S. Politics* (New York: W. W. Norton, 1996).
34. Matt Eckel and Jeb Koogler, "Yes Virginia, They Really Are More Extreme," Foreign Policy Watch (fpwatch.com), August 17, 2011; "The Polarization of the Congressional Parties," updated January 19, 2014, http://voteview.com/political_polarization.asp; Theda Skocpol and Vanessa Williamson, *The Tea Party and the Remaking of Republican Conservatism* (New York: Oxford, 2013), 169.
35. Oberlander, *The Political Life of Medicare*, 146.
36. *Annual Report[s] of the Boards of Trustees of the Federal Hospital Insurance and Federal Supplementary Medical Insurance Trust Funds*; Moon, *Medicare*, 29–46; Oberlander, *The Political Life of Medicare*, 83–106.
37. Theodore R. Marmor, "Report from the Field: How Not to Think about Medicare Reform," *Journal of Health Politics, Policy, and Law* 26, no. 1 (February 2001): 107–117; Moon, *Medicare*, 45; Joseph White, "Uses and Abuses of Long-Term Medicare Cost Estimates," *Health Affairs* 18, no. 1 (January 1999): 63–79.

38. Personal conversation with Bruce Vladeck, administrator, Health Care Financing Administration.
39. Peterson, "The Politics of Health Care Policy."
40. Marilyn Moon, ed., *Competition with Constraints: Challenges Facing Medicare Reform* (Washington, DC: Urban Institute, February 1, 2000).
41. Moon, *Medicare*, 54–87; Oberlander, *The Political Life of Medicare*, 107–135; Nancy-Ann DeParle, "As Good as It Gets? The Future of Medicare+Choice," *Journal of Health Politics, Policy, and Law* 27, no. 3 (June 2002): 495–512.
42. Robert Pear and Robin Toner, "Bush Medicare Proposal Urges Switch to Private Insurers," *New York Times*, March 5, 2003, http://www.nytimes.com/2003/03/05/politics/05MEDI.html.
43. Kaiser Family Foundation/Harvard School of Public Health, "The Medicare Drug Benefit: Beneficiary Perspectives Just Before Implementation," Chartpack November 2005, Chart 2.
44. Robert J. Blendon et al., "Voters and Health Care in the 2004 Election," *Health Affairs* web exclusive, March 1, 2005: W5–93, doi:10.1377/hlthaff.w5.86.
45. US Congressman Paul Ryan, Committee on the Budget, US House of Representatives, "A Roadmap for America's Future," Health Care Security, www.roadmap.republicans.budget.house.gov/plan/#Healthsecurity; "Long-Term Analysis of a Budget Proposal by Chairman Ryan," Congressional Budget Office, Washington, DC, April 5, 2011.
46. Kimberly J. Morgan and Andrea Louise Campbell, *The Delegated Welfare State: Medicare, Markets, and the Governance of Social Policy* (New York: Oxford University Press, 2011), ch. 4; Mark A. Peterson, ed., *Healthy Markets? The New Competition in Medical Care* (Durham, NC: Duke University Press, 1999); James C. Robinson, *The Corporate Practice of Medicine: Competition and Innovation in Health Care* (Berkeley: University of California Press, 1999).
47. Robert J. Blendon and John Benson, "The Public and the Conflict over Future Medicare Spending," *New England Journal of Medicine* 369, no. 11 (September 12, 2013), 1067, 1070; Ross White, "Reforming Medicare: Public Opinion," The Hastings Center Health Care Cost Monitor, February 14, 2011.
48. Thomas R. Oliver, Philip R. Lee, and Helen L. Lipton, "A Political History of Medicare and Prescription Drug Coverage," *Milbank Quarterly* 82, no. 2 (June 2004): 283–354.
49. Bernstein and Stevens, "Public Opinion, Knowledge, and Medicare Reform," 184.
50. Morgan and Campbell, *The Delegated Welfare State*, ch. 7.
51. A good example is shown in Robin D. C. Gauld, "Big Bang and the Policy Prescription: Health Care Meets the Market in New Zealand," *Journal of Health Politics, Policy, and Law* 25, no. 5 (October 2000): 815–844.
52. Sven Steinmo and Jon Watts, "It's the Institutions, Stupid! Why Comprehensive National Insurance Always Fails in America," *Journal of Health Politics, Policy, and Law* 20, no. 2 (Summer 1995): 329–372.
53. John McDonough, "Republican Medicare Hypocrisy," Health Stew blog, December 3, 2012, http://www.boston.com/lifestyle/health/health_stew/2012/12/republican_medicare_hypocrisy.html.

# 9

# MEDICARE INNOVATIONS IN THE WAR OVER THE KEY TO THE US TREASURY

## UWE E. REINHARDT

Medicare evokes conflicting images within the community of health-policy analysts. Those ideologically positioned to the left of center usually view the program as a major achievement in social policy and a great success. Those to the right of center usually view the program as archaic, rigid, and lacking in innovation.[1] In between are the American people, among whom the program remains highly popular—including those Medicare beneficiaries who otherwise want government off their backs.[2] Andrea Campbell, in Chapter 11, demonstrates the strong support for Medicare across all groups of Americans.

A central point of contention between these two groups concerns what prices Medicare should pay for its services. While in office as the administrator for the Centers for Medicare and Medicaid Services (CMS), Thomas Scully described Medicare as a "dumb price fixer."[3] Scully, who had been appointed to that post by President George W. Bush, looked askance at

Medicare's pricing policies. It is true, of course, that Medicare is a "price fixer." By necessity, the prices that Medicare pays for healthcare services and products must be set. Medicare must set them in a way that both healthcare providers and patients can accept as equitable, and it must do so through a public and open process.[4] The resulting prices must be public as well.

Private health insurers, by contrast, have the luxury of working out the prices they pay with healthcare providers through an opaque negotiating process, out of the public's view. The prices they agree on do not have to be either horizontally fair or efficient. As part of an agreement between providers and insurers, these prices are kept as a jealously guarded trade secret—an approach unheard of in any other economic sector and one that makes a mockery of the idea that the private healthcare system is a properly functioning market.

How "dumb" Medicare is in determining the prices it will pay for health care, relative to how prices are determined in the private health insurance sector, is a debatable question.[5] To begin to get a sense of the issue, consider the range of prices that two private health insurers in New Jersey and California, respectively, paid for a number of standard procedures in 2007 (Figure 9.1; Table 9.1). The price variations do not reflect different levels of quality or value to patients, or even differences in costs, but merely the relative bargaining strength between insurers and providers, which vary from market area to market area. Furthermore, within a market area the same commercial insurer may pay Hospital A much more than it pays Hospital B for one procedure, but the obverse may be true for another procedure.

Overall, there seems to be no rhyme or reason driving the enormous price variations in the private insurance sector. It is not clear, then, why anyone would believe that private health insurers' mechanisms for pricing health care are any more rational—less "dumb"—than Medicare's. Even Michael Porter and Elizabeth Omsted Teisberg—business school faculty hardly known as critics of the private sector—in their book *Redefining Health Care*, have criticized how private insurers in the United States pay for health care.[6]

The remainder of this chapter will review briefly the history of price setting in the Medicare program, the innovations Medicare has brought to this process, the program's performance in controlling the growth of healthcare costs, and the crossroads at which the program now finds itself.

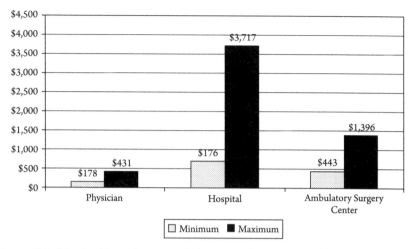

FIGURE 9.1 Price Paid for a Screening Colonoscopy by Private Health Insurer in New Jersey, 2007.

Source: New Jersey Commission on Rationalizing Health Care Resources, *Final Report*, January 24, 2008, Table 6.3.

## COMPROMISES MADE UPON MEDICARE'S ESTABLISHMENT

Although Medicare as originally conceived has been mainly a single-payer system, it has not generally acted as one. In 1965, physicians and the hospital industry acquiesced in the enactment of Medicare only on the condition that the program as an insurer not exercise the market power that single-payer systems usually have, or interfere in any way with how hospitals were constructed

TABLE 9.1 Variation in Actual Payments Made by One Large Commercial Insurer to Different Hospitals in California, 2007

|  | Appendectomy[a] | CABG[b] |
|---|---|---|
| Hospital A | $1,800 | $33,000 |
| Hospital B | $2,900 | $54,600 |
| Hospital C | $4,700 | $64,500 |
| Hospital D | $9,500 | $72,300 |
| Hospital E | $13,700 | $99,800 |

Adapted from New Jersey Commission on Rationalizing Health Care Resources, *Final Report* (2009), Chapter 6, Table 6.5.
[a]Actual payment per case (DRG 167).
[b]Coronary bypass with cardiac catheterization (DGR 107); tertiary hospitals only.

and operated or medicine was practiced. While some changes in hospital and medical practice did inevitably occur anyway (for two examples, see Chapter 2 by David Barton Smith and Chapter 3 by Rashi Fein in this volume), medical practitioners maintained a surprising amount of autonomy. As Wilbur Cohen, one of the chief architects of Medicare, ruefully put it later on:

> The sponsors of Medicare, myself included, had to concede in 1965 that there would be no real controls over hospitals and physicians. I was required to promise before the final vote in the Executive Session of the House Ways and Means Committee that the Federal Agency [to be in charge of administering Medicare] would exercise no control.[7]

Part of this remarkable deal was that Medicare simply adopted the then-ruling payment polices of the Blue Cross and Blue Shield plans.

Here it must be noted that the hospital industry originally created the nationwide system of private, not-for-profit Blue Cross hospital insurance plans during the 1930s mainly as a stable conduit of money to that industry. At that time, the state-based Blues plans typically *reimbursed* each hospital for the costs it had incurred in treating patients. I emphasize the word "reimbursement" here because it produces a rather different management style than does the word "payment." The hospitals understood the concept of "reimbursement" to mean that each hospital could incur whatever costs it wanted to provide good quality health care, and that the Blues plans then owed each hospital reimbursement for whatever its costs happened to be.

By contrast, the word "payment" suggests that a hospital's top line (its revenue) is highly constrained by the payment system, and that hospitals have to manage their line-item costs against that external constraint. It is how businesses should be managed. That so many hospitals and physicians still use the word "reimbursement" today suggests how much they still cling to the old management model. The wide range of fees paid by insurers, mentioned above, demonstrates how passively private insurers, and employers behind them, still honor that old management style with their payments.

The state-based Blue Shield plans—as distinct from Blue Cross plans—had similarly been created, this time by physicians, to assure a steady money flow to that sector. Typically, the Blue Shield plans paid each individual physician his or her "usual, customary, and reasonable (UCR)" fee, which meant that different physicians in the same area could receive vastly different fees for identical services.

Both types of Blues plans thus operated as more or less passive conduits of money from households and employers to healthcare providers, rather than as guardians of the premium-payers' purses.[8]

Medicare's original structure merely adopted this inherently inflationary system. Thus, Medicare was required to reimburse each individual hospital (and certain other inpatient facilities) *retrospectively* a pro rata share for all the money that the individual facility reported to have spent on capital investments in structures and medical equipment. Medicare also was to reimburse each facility a pro rata share for whatever its operating costs might be. This structure guaranteed a rate of return on equity to investor-owned facilities; not surprisingly, the investor-owned hospital business grew apace as a result. Investing in hospitals required little entrepreneurial talent or stomach for risk-taking, because an investor-owned hospital literally could not fail under this odd payment system.

Just as under the Blue Shield plans, physicians (and certain other professionals) were to be paid by Medicare according to their "customary, prevailing, and reasonable (CPR)" fees for each particular service.[9] The "reasonable" fee to be paid the individual physician for a particular service was determined as the lowest of three fees:

1. The physician's actual charge for the service,
2. The median of the frequency distribution of the fee he or she had charged in the previous year (the "customary" fee), or
3. The seventy-fifth percentile of all "customary" charges for all physicians performing that service in the relevant market area.

This CPR system was not invented for Medicare. It instead reflected the payment practices of private insurers at the time.

In effect, then, in return for acquiescing in the passage of Medicare into law in 1965, healthcare providers extracted the key to the US Treasury from Congress. Its sponsors in Congress and the Johnson administration, eager to see the program enacted, conceded to this brazen condition. As health policy scholar Rick Mayes puts it, "With hospitals and physicians in control of American medicine, those who paid the bills they charged had little-to-no means of questioning either the legitimacy or the necessity of the care that patients received."[10] One has to be mindful of this surrender of the key to the US Treasury—and, earlier, of the keys to the treasuries of employers—to understand the subsequent history of US health policy.

Starting in the mid-1970s, that history has included an endless war between the providers of health care and the US government, which has sought to retrieve its keys to the treasury. It is no small irony that the leading generals on the government's side have been Republican stalwarts, who usually style themselves as the healthcare industry's ostensible friends. In their own ways, Presidents Nixon, Ford, Reagan, and George H. W. Bush each sought to bring the hospital and physician sectors to their knees, in ways that Democrats would never dare to do. What's more, these Republican stalwarts have each copied tactics straight from the Democrats' war manual.[11]

## EARLY ATTEMPTS AT COST CONTROL: MEDICARE AS INNOVATOR

The sponsors of Medicare clearly understood that their surrender to the healthcare industry could not be defended on any reasonable economic grounds. They also understood that the payment structure would be highly inflationary, and that it would not be sustainable over the longer run. One would assume that the providers of health care understood this as well, but hoped to make hay, so to speak, while the sunshine lasted. As sociologist Paul Starr has noted, American medicine soon lapsed into irresponsible excess.[12]

That the payment system for hospitals was both inflationary and unfair is self-evident. The system did not put any brake on the cost incurred by individual hospitals in constructing and operating their facilities, and it paid different hospitals vastly different prices for the same procedures. Payments to hospitals for the same service could vary widely simply because the hospitals differed in their managerial behavior vis-à-vis costs. Between 1966 and 1975, total US spending on hospitals more than doubled, after adjustment for the GDP deflator. Real Medicare spending on hospitals rose even faster, in part, of course, because the program ramped up during that period.

Alarmed by the pace of general price inflation during the 1970s, and particularly by rising healthcare costs, President Nixon sought to stem the tide through economy-wide price controls, a move that lasted longest in the healthcare sector. In what came to be known in the industry as Section 223 regulations, the Nixon administration also enacted payment limits on the portion of hospital operating costs considered "routine"—mainly the hotel-like costs of a hospital stay—and enumerated some outlays—for example, country-club memberships—that would not be reimbursed at all.

During the late 1970s, the Carter administration proposed new measures to control the growth in hospital spending by Medicare. To ward off this legislation, the hospital industry promised to achieve the same goal of cost control through what was called the "Voluntary Effort," that is, a voluntary effort by hospitals to control spending. This amounted to a promise to voluntarily bill Medicare less than they could in principle. That promise was either hopelessly naïve or utterly cynical. In any event, it failed after but a year or two, as many health policy analysts had predicted.

So when President Reagan took the helm and contemplated the healthcare cost crisis facing his administration, he immediately noticed Medicare's violation of core business principles. The very idea of *retrospective full-cost reimbursement*, an approach that would look strange to anyone accustomed to normal business practices, particularly vexed the administration. After the predictable collapse of the Voluntary Effort, the Reagan administration found in the Democratic Congress widespread, bipartisan support for switching, over the period of 1983 to 1986, from "reimbursement" to a system of prospectively set diagnosis-related "payments"—albeit for Medicare only, and not for Medicaid or the VA health system.[13] Initially, policymakers arranged medical conditions into slightly over 500 so-called diagnosis-related groups, or DRGs. Since then, that number has been raised to 745.

DRGs constituted a truly revolutionary innovation. The approach has subsequently been copied by many countries around the world, notably France, Australia, and Germany, but has also been adopted on a more experimental basis by Taiwan and in China. Indeed, eventually even the private US health insurance system, which for many years after Medicare's introduction of DRGs had steadfastly clung to either fee-for-service payments to hospitals or to per diems, grudgingly accepted it.

The concept of the DRGs was based on research funded by Medicare. Its development started with research undertaken by Yale University professor of public health and hospital administrator John D. Thompson and his colleague Robert B. Fetter, a professor of operations research and administration. They had originally planned to develop not a means of reforming hospital payments, but rather a cost-accounting tool for the internal management of hospitals. In the process, however, they had statistically demonstrated the possibility of assigning the huge array of services produced by the typical hospital to a relatively small set of diagnosis-related groupings whose average cost-per-patient (within a given DRG) had a relatively low variance.

From this breakthrough in purely managerial economics, it was but a short jump to using a case-based costing system as the platform for a new prospective hospital payment system. The idea would be to pay hospitals a preset fixed sum per case at a level permitting the hospital to cover its costs, with some margin on top. With the help of the Yale team, the State of New Jersey decided to experiment with that approach in the 1970s and 1980s, with evident success. Federal legislators leaned on that experience in scaling up the concept to the entire federal Medicare system.

But as a base for paying for inpatient health care, the DRG case payments system carried a danger and a flaw. The danger consisted of the incentive that hospitals might have to skimp on the resources going into an inpatient treatment—for example, discharging patients "quicker and sicker" after surgery. Subsequent research, however, has shown that the system has served mainly to wring the excess from hospital costs, rather than to under-serve patients.

The flaw in the DRG system lies in its basis on what are actually *relative costs* incurred in producing the various DRG cases, rather than on the *relative value* to patients or to society as a whole of the services covered by the DRGs. Although to economists, the difference between a "relative value scale" and a "relative cost scale" is crucial, non-economists may see the distinction as splitting hairs. In many cases a medical condition—for example, lower back pain—can be addressed through either medical or surgical therapies, yielding the same clinical outcome. That outcome will have a value to the patient or to society. But if the surgical approach costs relatively more than the medical approach, it is reasonable to compensate the surgical approach at a higher dollar value than that accorded the medical approach. Clearly, an ideal payment system would base its payments on the relative values of different procedures provided to patients or society, not their relative costs.

Unfortunately, this shortcoming of the DRGs, or of any payment system based on relative costs, is not easily remedied. This is the case because no one—not even economists—knows the relative values of different DRG cases, value being an inherently subjective concept. In any event, the cost-based case-payment system is surely no worse than the relative values produced by the chaotic, opaque, and discriminatory price system we observe in the private health insurance sector to this day.

The CPR system for physicians produced a similarly inflationary effect on healthcare costs. It gave all physicians the incentive to inflate their actual charges in year one to push up their "usual fees" for year two. That tactic, in turn, would push the frequency distribution of fees charged by all physicians in the relevant market area to the right, so that the upper bound set for a "reasonable fee"—the seventy-fifth percentile of that frequency distribution—would increase as well. As early as 1973, Congress therefore passed legislation limiting the growth in a region's "prevailing" physician fees to the growth of an index that reflects general earnings trends in the economy, general price inflation, and a price index for the practice inputs typically purchased by physicians.

By the mid-1980s, more and more of the physicians treating Medicare patients saw their "customary and reasonable" fees bump into this ceiling. This upper constraint thus caused the CPR system to stumble toward something resembling a fee schedule of sorts, but one with fees set entirely haphazardly. Fees could still vary considerably among market areas and even among physicians within the same market area—often within the same medical arts building—for reasons not related to either practice costs or the quality of services rendered.

Recognizing the absurdity of such a system, in the mid-1980s the Medicare administration funded a major study on the relative costs of providing various physician services. The Harvard-based research term, working with input and assistance from the American Medical Association (AMA), asked a large, stratified, random sample of physicians to identify the time, skill, and risk involved in treating a large number of distinct medical vignettes.[14] The responses furnished the basis of the infelicitously named "resource-based relative value scale" (RBRVS).

The research team submitted its report to Medicare in 1988. Researchers in the Medicare administration, with the advice of the newly established Physician Payment Review Commission, added an estimated allocation of medical-practice costs (staff, rent, supplies, etc.) and malpractice expenses to the Harvard team's costs. Thus, at the behest of the administration of George

H. W. Bush, Congress in 1989 passed legislation calling for a new Medicare physician fee schedule based on the RBRVS. To this day, the RBRVS underlies the annually adjusted monetary fee schedule that Medicare uses to compensate physicians for a list of some 7,000 distinct services.

During a four-year period from 1992 to 1996, the new physician fee schedule was gradually blended with the existing CPR system. By 1996, then, the CPR system had vanished from Medicare's payment system. Like the DRG system, the Medicare fee schedule is, in effect, a system of administered prices set for the entire country by the federal government, albeit with a number of geographic adjustors for variations in labor costs, malpractice premiums, and the cost of the space (rental or capital cost) needed for the practice.[15]

While solving one problem, the Medicare fee schedule creates another one. As a payment system that perpetuates the traditional fee-for-service base of payment—embracing, as noted, some 7,000 distinct services—it provides an incentive for over-treatment. At the behest of the George H. W. Bush administration, Congress attempted to address this problem by incorporating a prospectively set global Medicare budget for physician services in the form of the so-called Volume Performance Standard (VPS). The VPS was linked to the growth in GDP, but also was adjusted for the growth in medical-practice costs and an assumed allowance for productivity growth. In a nutshell, the system required a reduction in the fees that would otherwise be paid physicians if, in the previous year, actual Medicare spending on physician services exceeded the budgeted VPS. In 1997, that system was modified into the Sustainable Growth Rate (SGR) system, with similar intent. That budgeting system has been highly controversial among physicians and has, in fact, been routinely disregarded by Congress, save for a year or two after 2000. Most recently, it has been the focus of what is widely referred to as the "doc fix."[16]

Private health insurers in the United States soon adopted the innovative Medicare physician fee schedule as a basis for their negotiations with individual physicians. The Medicare fee schedule thus represents a second Medicare-initiated innovation flowing from Medicare to the private insurance sector, in addition to the DRGs.

Like the DRG system, the RBRVS system is based on *relative costs*, not *relative values*. A more honest name might have been the Resource-Based Relative Cost Schedule (RBRCS). Unfortunately, the value of particular health services is inherently subjective. To this day, neither Medicare nor private insurers truly base their payments to providers on the value of services rendered. Instead, Medicare and private insurers have recently begun to experiment with sundry pay-for-performance (P4P) schemes that they call "value-based pricing." Again, however, the name is misleading. These third-party payers simply pay a little more for slightly better outcomes, not for the total value of these outcomes.

## THE LEVERAGE OF MEDICARE OVER US HEALTH CARE

In 2012, Medicare accounted for about 20 percent of total national health spending, at $572.5 billion of a total of $2.793 trillion.[17] The percentage can be larger for healthcare providers. For hospitals, for example, the average was 27 percent; for physicians, 23 percent. This circumstance gives Medicare considerable leverage over the provider community.

As such, Medicare has become a natural leader in payment reform for both public and private healthcare spending, as discussed above. Indeed, private health insurers argue that the market and geographical fragmentation of the private insurance industry makes it difficult for any one of them to deviate too much from the pack in payment methods. They have therefore come to look to Medicare for taking the lead in payment reforms.

As an illustration, consider the much-bemoaned shortage of primary-care physicians in this country. The situation is usually explained, at least in part, as a consequence of the low fees paid to primary-care physicians relative to payments to other specialists. Private insurers have argued that they cannot unilaterally increase these medical payments without upsetting their business models. If they did so without cutting specialists' fees, the insurers' costs and premiums would rise to uncompetitive levels; if, on the other hand, an insurer cut fees to specialists to keep total costs and premiums constant, then the specialists might refuse to accept that insurer's patients. The alternative—acting in unison—is barred by antitrust laws. Medicare, in contrast, has more flexibility.

Medicare's leading role in US health care makes it critical that the program continue to experiment with innovations in payments and other factors likely to enhance the efficiency of healthcare delivery. That thought was the impetus for including an Innovation Center within the Centers for Medicare and Medicaid Services (CMS) as part of the passage of the

Affordable Care Act (ACA).[18] The Innovation Center funds demonstration projects for novel ideas thought to either enhance the quality of health care without raising costs, or lowering costs without lowering quality. Change in Medicare is difficult, as Mark Peterson's Chapter 8 in this volume has explored, but not impossible.

## WILL MEDICARE BE SUSTAINABLE IN THE FUTURE?

Figure 9.2 depicts the role of Medicare and Medicaid in the overall federal budget. In 2013, the total federal budget stood at $3.5 trillion, of which Medicare accounted for $492 billion.[19] Medicare consumes a sizable fraction of the total federal budget, but not as large as defense spending or outlays on Social Security.

Critics of the Medicare program typically argue that the program is "not sustainable" because its costs are "out of control." By logical extension, the federal deficit is therefore largely a Medicare problem. Those who see government as an inept manager of anything seem to find this line of thought particularly appealing. A reasonable response is to ask what these critics mean by "sustainable." The relative success of cost control by Medicare, compared to that of private health insurers in the past and in the foreseeable future, raises serious questions about this criticism.

In their latest annual report, the trustees of the Medicare program estimate that, by 2050, total Medicare expenditures as a percentage of GDP

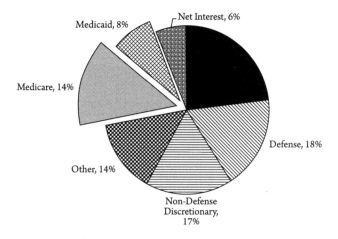

FIGURE 9.2 Medicare and Medicaid as a Share of the Federal Budget, 2013.
Source: Kaiser Family Foundation, "The Facts on Medicare Spending and Financing," July 28, 2014, Exhibit 1.

could be somewhere between 6 to 7 percent, compared to current levels of about 3.5 percent.[20] The report assumes that real (inflation-adjusted) GDP per capita will grow at an average annual rate of 1.7 percent during this period.[21] The question, then, is whether spending 6 to 7 percent of GDP on Medicare in 2050 is "sustainable."

Consider the situation through the light of per capita spending. In 2013, US GDP per capita in 2009 dollars was about $50,000. Of that total, 3.5 percent, or $1,700 per capita, went to Medicare, so that $48,250 of GDP remained for non-Medicare spending. Let us assume that real (inflation-adjusted) GDP per capita between now and 2050 will grow at only 1.5 percent per year (rather than the more optimistic 1.7 percent assumed by the Medicare Trustees in their report).[22] At that growth rate, real GDP per capita in 2050 in 2009 dollars would be $86,740. If, say, Medicare consumed 7 percent of GDP—the upper bound of the Trustees' estimates—this would still leave over 93 percent of $86,740, or $80,670, for non-Medicare spending (Figure 9.3).

Put another way: future generations will be richer. What part of this picture is not sustainable from a macro-economic perspective? After all, Medicare spending is part of GDP and is mirrored in jobs. If our current generation can afford to look after its elderly citizens, why cannot future,

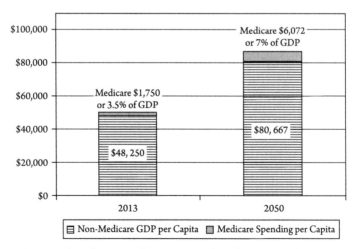

FIGURE 9.3 Projected Real Non-Medicare GDP and Medicare Spending per Capita to 2050.

Source: Sisko, et. al., Health Affairs 33 (October 2013), Exhibit 3.

richer generations? In short, the argument that Medicare is not economically sustainable is not convincing.

Political sustainability, as distinct from economic sustainability, refers to
the willingness of citizens in the upper strata of the nation's distribution of
income and wealth to help finance, through taxes and transfers, the health
care needed by citizens in the lower income strata.

Medicare is fully financed by taxes and transfers. Although Medicare beneficiaries have been led to believe that they pre-funded their own healthcare
in old age through payroll taxes paid during their younger working years,
research well known to health policy analysts has shown that this pre-funding falls significantly short of the total burden that most seniors place on
Medicare.[23] Medicare is therefore at least partially a tax-and-transfer, pay-
as-you-go form of social insurance. The question arises, then, to what extent
future American taxpayers will be willing to fill the pre-funding gap in
Medicare with their taxes—particularly as the number of Medicare recipients as a fraction of the population grows.

The current debate on US fiscal policy clings to the notion that the fraction of overall government spending as a percentage of GDP must be kept
at or below a given percentage—20 percent is often mentioned—regardless
of the funds needed for the nation's defense, of the aging of the population, or to address the growing income inequality in our society. *This* is the
idea that is unsustainable. If there is even a pretense that our health system
should operate on a roughly egalitarian basis, if the United States seeks to
remain the militarily strongest nation on earth, and if Americans continue
their habit, as they have for decades, of receiving more services from the
government than they are willing to pay for in taxes, then an ever larger fraction of the federal budget is absorbed by net interest charges. Larger interest
charges, in turn, leave less money for everything else to be financed by the
federal budget.

As the federal budget data displayed in Figure 9.2 shows, net interest at
6 percent of the total has already become an entitlement almost as large as
Medicaid (8 percent). Citizens sometimes forget that contracted interest
on the federal debt is an entitlement even more unalterable *ex post* than are
entitlements to human services. Much of that entitlement to interest payments accrues to foreign lenders.

A second set of criticisms center on the claim that it is more expensive to
provide health services under government health insurance programs than

it would be to provide the same services under private health insurance. Medicare spending, in other words, is out of control.[24]

This assertion is usually made in a data-free context, apparently on the assumption that it is intuitively obvious. It seems equally intuitive to many economists, who generally are beholden to the theory that government is inherently inefficient. The theory is particularly appealing in the case of Medicare, whose governing statutes forbid certain cost-containment tools—for example, selective contracting—open to private health insurers.

Medicare can, of course, avail itself of the cost-containment techniques available to private insurers by delegating the purchasing of beneficiaries' health care to private health insurers under the Medicare Advantage program (Part C of Medicare). Remarkably, however, to be competitive with government-run Medicare, the private plans so far have demanded and received from Medicare (i.e., from taxpayers) *more* money per beneficiary choosing to enroll in a private plan than those beneficiaries would have cost taxpayers under the traditional, fee-for-service Medicare program.[25] With the extra payment, the private plans have been able to cover more services than traditional Medicare, which gives them their competitive edge. But the net effect is that Part C of Medicare certainly has not been a route to cost savings for taxpayers.

Another version of this argument points to the fact that traditional Medicare—not including Medicare Advantage—can only control prices, not the volume of services. Indeed, one frequently sees distinguished health economists advancing this very argument.

Data published by CMS's Office of the Actuary (OACT) can shed light on this issue.[26] The data in Table 9.2 are taken directly from the latest in an annual series of data releases on national health expenditure data released by that office.[27] The OACT is the originator of the official statistics on national health spending, broken down in detail by object and source of funding. To control for changing benefit packages, which have changed over time for both private and public insurers, the actuaries provide a column entitled "Common Benefits," which makes spending under Medicare and private health insurance more comparable.

As Table 9.2 suggests, Medicare spending per beneficiary during most periods actually appears to have risen *more slowly* than has per-capita spending under private health insurance. Policy scholars and the Congressional Budget Office have reached similar conclusions.[28]

TABLE 9.2 Annual Growth Rate in Per-Capita Health Spending, 1969–2012

| Period | All Benefits (as percent increase) | | Common Benefits (as percent increase) | |
|---|---|---|---|---|
| | Medicare | Private Insurance | Medicare | Private Insurance |
| 1969–2012 | 8.4 | 9.7 | 7.7 | 9.2 |
| 1969–1993 | 10.9 | 12.8 | 10.7 | 12.2 |
| 1993–1997 | 7.2 | 4.3 | 5.9 | 2.0 |
| 1997–1999 | −0.4 | 6.2 | 1.6 | 4.6 |
| 1999–2002 | 6.4 | 8.5 | 5.6 | 8.0 |
| 2002–2007 | 7.8 | 6.7 | 4.7 | 7.2 |
| 2007–2012 | 2.8 | 4.7 | 2.2 | 5.2 |

Adapted from Office of the Actuary, CMS, HHS, *National Health Expenditures 1960–2012*, Table 21, http://www.cms.gov/Research-Statistics-Data-and-Systems/Statistics-Trends-and-Reports/NationalHealthExpendData/Downloads/tables.pdf.

The statutory limits on Medicare's cost-containment techniques raise the question of how Medicare has achieved this level of cost control. The answer is straightforward: price control. The prices that Medicare pays its health-care providers tend to be significantly lower than the comparable price paid by private insurers.

Private insurers allege that they must absorb the consequences of government underpayment in the form of higher prices charged to private insurers by healthcare providers, a phenomenon known as *cost shift*. On that theory, the cost of government-sponsored health care is actually larger than what is reported because a part of that cost is assumed by private payers.

Many economists, the current author included, question the validity of the theory of cost shift, arguing that the observed price differentials between Medicare and private insurers' fees merely reflect the standard price discrimination present in many industries. Indeed, as was noted earlier in connection with the huge price variations within the private insurance sector, even more significant cost shifts would be seen from large insurers able to bargain for lower prices to less powerful ones who are charged higher prices.[29] The Medicare Payment Advisory Commission, established by Congress to advise it on paying providers of healthcare under Medicare, also questions the cost-shift theory.[30]

Indeed, one must caution private health insurers not to lean on the cost-shift theory in defense of their higher costs, as it amounts to a confession of impotence in the market for healthcare services. If providers find it so easy to shift costs to private payers when government is the alleged culprit of underpayment, then what would stop providers from also shifting to private payers the cost of excess capacity, duplicative expensive medical equipment, or other inefficiencies? If the cost-shift theory were valid, how could society ever trust private insurers to exercise adequate cost control on patients' behalf?

## FUTURE DIRECTIONS

The federal Medicare program for America's elderly citizens, along with the federal-state Medicaid program for the nation's poor, was conceived and put in place by a generation of Americans who had suffered through the Great Depression and had joined, rich and poor, to fight shoulder-to-shoulder in World War II in Europe, North Africa, and in the Pacific. They are the Americans whom journalist Tom Brokaw famous celebrated as "the Greatest Generation."[31]

These Americans had come to know that much success in life was the product of luck or bad luck. To them it made sense that the financial consequences of the misfortune of illness should be shared among the peoples in a nation. Medicare represented a vision that eventually foresaw that all Americans should have the same healthcare experience when sick, on equal terms, regardless of their ability to pay for their own health care, without undue stress on the family's household budget. This was the vision of social insurance, pure and simple, long ago adopted by most other industrialized nations.

Very quickly, Medicare helped pull millions of elderly Americans out of poverty.[32] Very quickly, these Americans also gained access to the kind of health care other Americans—especially those with employment-based private health insurance—enjoyed. And very quickly, Medicare helped to eliminate the formal racial segregation of healthcare facilities then still dominant in many states of the union (see David Barton Smith's Chapter 2 in this volume),[33] although not all forms of racial discrimination are reported to have disappeared from US health care.[34] It seems inconceivable that the private healthcare sector could have accomplished so much, so quickly, on the agenda of a civilized nation.

One should think that today's healthcare providers—notably organized medicine and the hospital industry—would blush at the dubious conditions their predecessors imposed on Medicare in return for allowing Congress to enact that program. Doctors and hospitals required nothing less than the surrender of the key to the US Treasury, a truly audacious demand by any standard. Everything that followed in the history of these two social programs can be viewed as an endless set of skirmishes between government and the providers of health care over ownership of those keys. The war continues unabated.

Limited by statute and by the monetized lobbying permitted by our system of governance, Medicare has had to be inventive in its fight to get the key back. As this chapter has sought to argue, so it has been. Currently both Medicare and the private health insurance industry are experimenting with yet other approaches to payment reform, notably evidence-based bundled payments for entire medical treatments (inpatient or ambulatory) and linking payments to the quality of care produced.

At the moment, Medicare stands at a crossroads. One branch of this path would grant Medicare greater freedom to employ the same arsenal of tools that private health insurers can use to control the growth of health spending and to assure that good quality health care is delivered in return for money. It might allow Medicare, for example, to limit the providers with whom it works to high-quality providers of care. Medicare would remain a *defined-benefit* program.

The alternative branch confines Medicare to the task of extracting the financing of health care for the elderly from US households and channeling those funds to private health insurers. Those insurers would, in turn, perform (hopefully prudently) the purchasing of beneficiaries' health care. This might be in the form of a program similar to the current Medicare Advantage, but with more explicit competitive bidding for Medicare business by private insurers. A truly competitive bidding process might trigger stiffer competition among private health plans for the Medicare business, although one wonders how much mileage can be had this way when a fragmented health insurance industry negotiates prices with an ever more consolidated supply side of health care. If adopted, that approach would convert Medicare into a *defined-contribution* program. But a defined-contribution approach would be, inter alia, an ideal platform to shift more of the financial burden of health care into the budgets of Medicare beneficiaries, should pressures in the federal budget call for it.

The next decade will reveal on which branch Medicare will travel.

NOTES

1. Robert E. Moffit and Alygene Senger, "Medicare's Outdated Structure—and the Urgent Need for Reform," The Heritage Foundation Backgrounder # 2777 (March 22, 2013), http://www.heritage.org/research/reports/2013/03/medicares-outdated-structureand-the-urgent-need-for-reform.
2. Harris, A Nielson Company, "Medicare, Crime-Fighting, Social Security, Defense—the Most Popular Federal Government Services," January 14, 2010, http://www.harrisinteractive.com/vault/Harris_Interactive_Poll_Politics_Gov_Services_2010_01.pdf; Karen Davis and Sara Collins, Medicare at Forty," Health Care Financing Review 27, no. 2 (Winter 2005–6): 53–62; Catherine Rampell, "Keep Your Government Hands off My Government Programs!" New York Times Economix blog, February 11, 2011, http://nyti.ms/1cX4zxX.
3. Uwe E. Reinhardt and Thomas Scully, "The Medicare World from Both Sides: A Conversation with Tom Scully," Health Affairs 22, no. 6 (2003): 167–174.
4. In this regard, see Payment Basics for Medicare, published annually by the Medicare Payment Advisory Commission (Medpac), http://www.medpac.gov/payment_basics.cfm.
5. Uwe E. Reinhardt, "The Pricing of U.S. Hospital Services: Chaos Behind a Veil of Secrecy," Health Affairs 25, no. 1 (January 2006): 57–69.
6. Michael E. Porter and Elizabeth Olmsted Teisberg, Redefining Health Care (Boston, MA: Harvard Business School Press, 2006), 65–66.
7. Cited in Rick Mayes, "The Origins, Development, and Passage of Medicare's Revolutionary Prospective Payment System," Journal of the History of Medicine 62 (January 2007): 25.
8. In the intervening years, Blue Cross plans have become more like regular commercial insurers who, when they can, try to confront providers with countervailing market power.
9. Richard Buddin and Joyce Mann, Medicare Reimbursement Differentials by Physician Experience (Santa Monica, CA: Rand Corporation, 1992), http://www.rand.org/content/dam/rand/pubs/monograph_reports/2006/MR147.pdf.
10. Rick Mayes, "Origins, Development, and Passage," 3.
11. Joseph Antos, "Confessions of a Price Controller," The American, October 30, 2010, http://www.american.com/archive/2010/october/confessions-of-a-price-controller.
12. Paul Starr, The Social Transformation of Medicine: The Rise of a Sovereign Profession and the Making of a Vast Industry (New York: Basic Books, 1982), 379.
13. For a crisp description of how that system works today, see Medicare Payment Advisory Commission, Hospital Acute Inpatient Services Payment System, October 2013, http://www.medpac.gov/documents/MedPAC_Payment_Basics_13_hospital.pdf.
14. American Medical Association, History of the RBRVS, http://www.ama-assn.org//ama/pub/physician-resources/solutions-managing-your-practice/coding-billing-insurance/medicare/the-resource-based-relative-value-scale/history-of-rbrvs.page.

15. For a description of this modus operandi, see Medicare Payment Advisory Commission, *Physician and Other Professionals Payment System*, October 2013, http://www.medpac.gov/documents/MedPAC_Payment_Basics_13_ Physician.pdf.

16. See Mary Agnes Carey, "Congress Is Poised to Change Medicare Payment Policy: What Does That Mean for Patients and Doctors?" *Kaiser Health News*, January 16, 2014, http://www.kaiserhealthnews.org/stories/2014/january/16/ congress-doc-fix-sustainable-growth-rate-sgr-legislation.aspx; and Paul H. Keckley et al., "Understanding the SGR: Analyzing the 'Doc Fix,'" Deloitte Center for Health Solutions, 2012, http://www.deloitte.com/assets/Dcom-UnitedStates/ Local%20Assets/Documents/us_dchs_Sustainable%20Growth%20Rate%20 _102912.pdf.

17. US Department of Health and Human Services, Centers for Medicare and Medicaid Services, Office of the Actuary, "National Health Expenditures 1960–2012, Table 3," http://www.cms.gov/Research-Statistics-Data-and-Systems/Statistics-Trends-and-Reports/NationalHealthExpendData/Downloads/tables.pdf.

18. US Department of Health and Human Services, Center for Medicare and Medicaid Services Innovation, http://innovation.cms.gov/.

19. Kaiser Family Foundation, *The Facts on Medicare Spending and Financing*, July 28, 2014, Exhibit 1, http://kff.org/medicare/fact-sheet/medicare-spending-and-financing-fact-sheet/.

20. The Board of Trustees, Federal Hospital Insurance and Federal Supplementary Medical Insurance Trust Funds, *2014 Annual Report* (July 28, 2014), Figure I.1:5, http://www.cms.gov/Research-Statistics-Data-and-Systems/Statistics-Trends-and-Reports/ReportsTrustFunds/downloads/tr2014.pdf.

21. Board of Trustees, *2014 Annual Report*, Table II.C.1: 14.

22. Prior to the financial collapse in 2007, real GDP per capita had grown at a long-run average of about 2 percent.

23. Louis Jacobson, "Medicare and Social Security: What You Paid Compared with What You Get," *PolitiFact.com*, February 1, 2013, http://www.politi-fact.com/truth-o-meter/article/2013/feb/01/medicare-and-social-security-what-you-paid-what-yo/.

24. For an example of this sort of claim, and my response, see Sally Pipes, "Employer Health Insurance: A Bargain Compared to Government-Sponsored Coverage," *Forbes*, July 28, 2014, http://www.forbes.com/sites/sallypipes/2014/07/28/employer-health-insurance-a-bargain-compared-to-government-sponsored-coverage/, and Uwe E. Reinhardt, "Employment-Based Health Insurance 'Cheaper' Than Government-Sponsored Insurance? Say What?" *Forbes*, August 4, 2014, http://www.forbes.com/sites/theapothe-cary/2014/08/04/employer-based-health-insurance-cheaper-than-government-sponsored-insurance-say-what/.

25. Uwe E. Reinhardt, "The Complexities of Comparing Medicare Choices," *New York Times* Economix blog, January 13, 2013, http://nyti.ms/1pQYnin.

26. Cited in Uwe E. Reinhardt, "Medicare Spending Isn't Out of Control," *New York Times* Economix blog, December 21, 2012, http://nyti.ms/1lVlOpg.

27. Office of the Actuary, *National Health Expenditures*, Table 21.

28. Cristina Bocutti and Marylin Moon, "Comparing Medicare and Private Insurers: Growth Rates in Spending over Three Decades," *Health Affairs* 22, no. 2 (2003): 230–237; Congressional Budget Office, *The 2014 Long-Term Budget Outlook* (June 2014), Table 2-1, http://www.cbo.gov/sites/default/files/cbofiles/attachments/45471-Long-TermBudgetOutlook_7-29.pdf.

29. A very thorough review of the evidence on the cost-shift theory can be found in Austin Frakt, "How Much Do Hospitals Cost Shift? A Review of the Evidence," *Milbank Quarterly* 89, no. 1 (March 21, 2011): 90–130, doi:10.1111/j.1468-0009.2011.00621.x.

30. Medicare Payment Advisory Commission, *Report to the Congress* (March 2009), Ch. 2, http://medpac.gov/chapters/Mar09_Ch02A.pdf.

31. Tom Brokaw, *The Greatest Generation* (New York: Random House, 2001).

32. Amy Finkelstein and Robin McKnight, "What Did Medicare Do? The Initial Impact of Medicare on Mortality and Out-of-Pocket Medical Spending," *Journal of Public Economics* 92 (2008): 1644–1668.

33. P. Preston Reynolds, "Professional and Hospital Discrimination and the U.S. Court of Appeals Fourth Circuit, 1956–67," *American Journal of Public Health* 94, no. 5 (2004): 710–720, http://www.ncbi.nlm.nih.gov/pmc/articles/PMC1448322/; and David Barton Smith, "Racial and Ethnic Health Disparities and the Unfinished Civil Rights Agenda," *Health Affairs* 24, no. 2 (March 2005): 217–224.

34. Hooch Zheng and Chao Zhou, "The Impact of Hospital Integration on Black–White Differences in Mortality: A Case Study of Motor Vehicle Accident Death Rates," December 2008, http://artsandscience.usask.ca/economics/research/pdf/ChaoZhouBUMarch2509.pdf.

# 10

# MEDICAID RISING

## *THE PERILS AND POTENTIAL OF FEDERALISM*

### FRANK J. THOMPSON

Though often viewed as a down-at-the-heels second cousin to Medicare, Medicaid has become an increasingly important pillar in the American healthcare system. Despite occasional attempts to retrench Medicaid, the program has not only endured but expanded in terms of expenditures and enrollees, and has now become a key component of the Affordable Care Act (ACA). Over its 50 years, policymakers have separated Medicaid from its origins as "welfare medicine." Medicaid's evolution testifies to the growing importance of the executive branch and the administrative presidency in the American separation-of-powers system. In each of these themes, we see ongoing tensions and collaborations between the states and the federal government—the question, in other words, of federalism.

This chapter tells the story of how Medicaid has grown over four historical periods to become a pillar of the American health insurance regime. It reveals how the rise of waivers and executive federalism, giving states more power to experiment with the program, particularly during the Clinton years, stoked Medicaid's ascendance. While over these years Medicaid lost its image as "welfare medicine," struggles persisted among the federal government, states, and various interest groups surrounding provider payments, and these battles have reinforced its status as second-tier health care. Yet Medicaid has also persisted. The chapter closes by considering how this story of Medicaid's unlikely rise could conceivably become, in years ahead, one of decline, depending on how the political debate unfolds over debt, taxes, and entitlement reform.

This chapter opens with a brief assessment of three historical periods. The first (1965–1980) featured the birth of Medicaid, followed by a series of congressional amendments that established the basic template for the program. The second (1981–1992) manifested extraordinary congressional entrepreneurship and involvement by the courts to expand Medicaid, delink it from welfare, and bolster provider payments (for more on the role of the judiciary, see Chapter 6 by Sara Rosenbaum in this volume). The third (1993–2008) featured the growing importance of executive branch action in transforming Medicaid, with waivers looming large as a policy tool. I then turn to a more detailed treatment of a fourth period (2009–2015) that witnessed passage of the Affordable Care Act (ACA) and a new era of Medicaid expansion. Here, I look closely at two cases. The first involves the Obama administration's response to federal court decisions on Medicaid provider payment, which provided an opportunity to mitigate the program's status as second-tier care. A second focuses on the Obama administration's strategies for achieving the ACA's coverage goals in the wake of a Supreme Court decision making state participation in the Medicaid expansion voluntary.

## LINKAGE AND THE INCREMENTAL POLITICS OF LONG-TERM CARE (1965–1980)

In working to create Medicaid in 1965, Representative Wilbur Mills, a Democrat from Arkansas, anticipated that states' responses to the program might well resemble their lukewarm reaction to its predecessor, the Kerr-Mills program.[1] As a result, the original Medicaid legislation gave states wide latitude to determine eligibility for the program. It sought to head off state foot-dragging through a provision that required them to make a "satisfactory showing" in the "direction of broadening the scope of . . . care" and "liberalizing the eligibility requirements" by 1975.[2] Most states lived up to Mills's expectation that Medicaid would not lead to runaway costs. About half did not launch Medicaid programs in 1966; many of the states that did were guarded in their extension of benefits and eligibility. But what Mills and others failed to anticipate was the degree to which a handful of liberal states—especially California and New York—would move rapidly to establish capacious Medicaid programs. In early 1966, for instance, New York's Republican governor, Nelson Rockefeller, pledged to forge a Medicaid program that might conceivably cover 45 percent of the state's population. Increasingly, congressional critics came to view New York and other expansive states as pursuing an "irresponsible junket in which vast public sums were being dissipated."[3]

This prompted Mills to forge amendments to curb state ambitions in 1967. The amendments firmly established Medicaid as "welfare medicine," linking eligibility for the program to that for Aid to Families with Dependent Children (AFDC). (For more on Medicaid's origins as welfare medicine, see Chapter 5 by Jill Quadagno in this volume.) AFDC eligibility criteria, over which states possessed vast discretion, not only constrained Medicaid services to the poor; they also limited who could qualify as "medically needy."

While the 1967 congressional amendments transformed Medicaid's leitmotif from expansion to retrenchment, the 1965–1980 period nonetheless featured significant program growth. This partly reflected the increasing number of states choosing to participate in Medicaid. By the end of 1972, all states, except Arizona, had signed up, with federal and state outlays for Medicaid from 1968 through 1972 nearly doubling (in constant dollars).[4] Medicaid's subsequent growth in this period substantially reflected an "unchecked incrementalism" that greatly enlarged the program's role in providing long-term institutional care for the elderly and people with disabilities.[5]

The Medicaid statute had required participating states to provide skilled nursing home care. Medicaid's founders had envisioned that this care would have a substantial medical component and would not extend to those who principally needed "custodial" services. In 1967, however, Congress gave states the option to obtain Medicaid funds to serve people in intermediate care facilities (ICFs), which had a much lower medical component than skilled nursing homes. This institutional expansion continued in 1971, when Republican Senator Henry Bellmon, from Oklahoma, crafted an amendment that made ICFs serving the "mentally retarded" eligible for Medicaid reimbursement. In 1972, Congress also permitted states to extend Medicaid coverage to individuals in psychiatric hospitals. Policymakers in many states welcomed these measures as a source of fiscal relief. Whereas in the past states had to spend their own monies to assist people with disabilities, they could now obtain a hefty federal subsidy to do so.[6]

State policymakers were less pleased when the Nixon administration persuaded Congress to create the Supplemental Security Income program (SSI) to provide cash assistance to the aged, blind, and disabled in 1972. The legislation also made SSI beneficiaries eligible for Medicaid. In the face of opposition from certain governors, Congress provided some loopholes to ease cost pressures on states. But over time the SSI cohort joined AFDC recipients as a cash-assisted (albeit less stigmatized) group covered by state Medicaid programs.

The expansion of benefits to people with disabilities and the elderly fueled the rapid growth of Medicaid spending during the 1970s. Federal and state outlays grew by 34 percent from 1972 to 1976 and another 18 percent during the Carter administration (in constant dollars). By the end of the decade, the elderly and people with disabilities annually absorbed 75 percent of Medicaid spending—nearly 10 percentage points more than in later periods. Expenditures on people with intellectual disabilities housed in ICFs became the fastest growing budget item.[7]

## The Triumph of Congressional Entrepreneurship (1981–1992)

Ronald Reagan's arrival in the White House and the Republican takeover of the Senate in 1981 unleashed a concerted attempt to revamp and cut Medicaid. During its first term, the Reagan administration aggressively pursued several initiatives that would vitiate Medicaid as an open-ended entitlement to the states.[8] Ultimately, however, the White House achieved only modest, temporary retrenchment. Congress went along with shifting more costs to the states by lowering the federal match rate for three years—by 3 percent in 1982, 4 percent in 1983, and 4.5 percent in 1984. Despite this measure and Republican control of the White House throughout the 1981–1992 period, federal and state Medicaid spending grew substantially—by 16 percent during the first term of the Reagan administration, by 27 percent in its second term, and by a whopping 66 percent under

President George H. W. Bush (in constant dollars). Meanwhile, the number of Medicaid enrollees grew apace.

Medicaid's expansion largely stemmed from the extraordinary policy entrepreneurship of Representative Henry Waxman, a California Democrat. Throughout this period, the Democrats enjoyed substantial majorities in the House of Representatives, with Waxman chairing a subcommittee overseeing Medicaid. In this position, he skillfully exploited his role in the budgetary process to preserve Medicaid as an entitlement. While the program was under siege in 1981, Waxman planted seeds for expansion by obtaining approval for a legislative amendment establishing Medicaid's Disproportionate Share Hospital program (DSH).[9] Under DSH, states could direct Medicaid monies to hospitals that served uncommonly high numbers of the uninsured and Medicaid enrollees. Starting in the mid-1980s, certain states rushed to secure DSH subsidies for these hospitals. Many of them used DSH as a platform for fiscal gimmicks associated with provider taxes and donations that eventually increased the federal share of Medicaid costs from the 57 percent embedded in the statute to well beyond 60 percent. DSH expenditures grew rapidly, consuming over 11 percent of all Medicaid spending by 1992.[10] Waxman also successfully fought the Reagan administration's efforts to extend the cuts in the Medicaid match rate beyond 1984.

Subsequently, Waxman turned his efforts to expanding eligibility for Medicaid. A Waxman two-step emerged, in which Congress first gave states the option to insure children, pregnant women, and certain other adults with incomes above AFDC poverty thresholds, and then mandated that they do so. In these and other ways, the delinkage of Medicaid eligibility from AFDC gained momentum. The elderly and people with disabilities also benefited from Waxman's efforts. In the late 1980s, Congress passed measures that required state Medicaid programs to pay the Medicare premiums and cost sharing for significant numbers of "dual eligibles"—those who met enrollment criteria for both programs.

While Medicaid's growth from 1981 through 1992 substantially reflected the commitment and legerdemain of Henry Waxman, other stakeholders also played pivotal roles. Acting individually and through their associations, governors did much to shape Medicaid's evolution.[11] The National Governors Association assiduously resisted the Reagan administration's efforts to restructure Medicaid and cap its funding. Waxman's success in enlarging coverage for pregnant women and children depended heavily on strong support from Southern Democratic governors. Only toward the end of the period did the governors become uneasy with federal eligibility mandates (especially those requiring states to subsidize the dual eligibles). At that point, all the governors, except Mario Cuomo, a Democrat from New York, signed a letter urging Congress to cease imposing unfunded Medicaid mandates on the states.

The 1981–1992 period also witnessed greater involvement by the federal courts. Again, Waxman did much to set the table for this development. In the last year of the Carter administration, Senator David Boren, a Democrat from Oklahoma, had secured congressional approval of a Medicaid payment provision directed at long-term care institutions. His amendment required states to establish Medicaid rates that were "reasonable and adequate to meet the costs which must be incurred by efficiently and economically operated facilities" to provide appropriate care and services.[12] In 1981, Waxman engineered the extension of this "Boren amendment" to hospitals. As Rosenbaum has discussed in Chapter 6, the provision opened the gates for hospitals to sue states over "inadequate" Medicaid payment rates. Provider victories in the courts, along with other factors, helped make inpatient hospital services the leading contributor to Medicaid expenditure growth as this period ebbed.[13]

## Delinkage and the Rise of Executive Federalism (1993–2008)

Medicaid during the Clinton and George W. Bush years underwent a major transformation on several fronts. President Clinton's comprehensive reform proposal to expand insurance coverage would have consigned Medicaid to being a long-term care program. When his proposal failed, however, he successfully resisted Republican efforts to convert Medicaid to a block grant. As in the prior period, congressional action played an important role in further distancing Medicaid from welfare medicine. In 1996, President Clinton and Republican leaders in Congress reached an accord on welfare reform, replacing the increasingly stigmatized AFDC with Temporary Assistance to Needy Families (TANF). TANF beneficiaries continued to be eligible for Medicaid. But the number on welfare fell by over 60 percent in the decade following TANF's inception.[14] Welfare recipients thereby comprised an increasingly smaller portion of the ever-expanding number of Medicaid enrollees. The approval of the Children's Health Insurance Program in 1997 further attenuated the link between cash assistance and Medicaid eligibility.

While delinkage distanced Medicaid from its image as second-tier coverage, other congressional and court actions had the opposite effect. In 1997, Congress repealed the federal payment provisions targeting hospitals and long-term care institutions that Senator Boren and Representative Waxman had successfully promoted in 1980 and 1981. This repeal seriously undercut provider leverage to challenge state payment rates in the federal courts. Provider prospects in the courts took an additional turn for the worse in 2002 when the Supreme Court in *Gonzaga v. Doe* limited the circumstances under which private parties could sue for relief against actions by state governments.[15]

While Congress and the courts played significant roles in the 1993–2008 period, the surging importance of the executive branch was the dominant governance theme. In essence, a pattern of *executive federalism* emerged, under which presidents and their appointees facilitated transformations in Medicaid without congressional authorization.[16] The significant changes that occurred hinged less on who dominated Congress than on control of the presidency and key governorships. The soaring use of a particular administrative tool, program waivers, reflected the rise of executive federalism.

Waivers are a congressional delegation of authority to the executive branch to permit states to deviate from the ordinary requirements of federal law. Medicaid waivers assume two basic guises: demonstrations and more targeted initiatives focused on long-term care. The demonstration waivers derive from Section 1115 of the Social Security Act, which Congress approved in 1962. This provision gives the federal executive broad authority to experiment with alternative state approaches to social programs. The second category of more targeted waivers emanates from congressional action in 1981. These waivers, rooted in Section 1915(c) of the Social Security Act, seek to rebalance Medicaid long-term care away from nursing homes and other large institutions toward home and community-based services (HCBS). When approved by federal administrators, these waivers allow states to circumvent Medicaid law related to HCBS by targeting specific geographic areas in a state, altering eligibility criteria and capping enrollment.

Prior to 1993, concerns about the "cost-neutrality" of waivers and other factors undercut federal willingness to approve them. Federal administrators had approved about 50 demonstration waivers since Medicaid's birth and had seldom renewed them. The Reagan and George H. W. Bush administrations had been more willing to approve HCBS waivers. By 1992, states had received 155 waivers, which accounted for about 15 percent of all Medicaid spending on long-term care. But states often found negotiations with the federal bureaucracy to obtain approval of HCBS waivers to be arduous and protracted.

The arrival of the Clinton administration galvanized an outpouring of Medicaid waivers. Clinton initiated a series of administrative measures that made it much easier for states to obtain waivers, and the George W. Bush administration followed suit. Well over 100 Section 1115 demonstrations won approval from 1993 through 2008.[17] Over 40 states operated some facet of their program under a demonstration waiver as of 2008. Many of these waivers were comprehensive and transformational. For instance, a bevy of states used them to move Medicaid enrollees into managed care while expanding coverage to new adult populations (further delinking the program from welfare). Of particular note, negotiations between Republican Massachusetts Governor Mitt Romney and the George W. Bush administration over a Medicaid waiver yielded a plan for near-universal coverage in that state in 2006. The Massachusetts model became the template for the ACA. HCBS waivers also proliferated, with about 280 in effect by the time the Obama administration took office. All states used waivers to cover at least some HCBS, which had grown to account for nearly 45 percent of all Medicaid spending on long-term care.

Overall, Medicaid expanded substantially during the Clinton and George W. Bush years. The first term of the Clinton administration witnessed an increase in federal and state outlays of 26 percent and the second term another 20 percent (in constant dollars). This growth rate increased to 32 percent during the first term of the George W. Bush administration before falling sharply to 4 percent in his second term. It also deserves note that Medicaid spending and enrollments per poor person rose in all 50 states during this period.[18]

HEALTH REFORM AND CONTENTIOUS FEDERALISM
(2009–2015)

The 2008 election gave the Democrats control of the presidency and Congress with majorities not seen since the late 1970s. In contrast to the

Clinton reform initiative, the ACA assigned Medicaid a pivotal role in the coverage expansion. Half of the more than 30 million projected to gain insurance would do so via Medicaid. Approved on a straight party-line vote, the ACA mandated that with certain exceptions, all non-elderly, non-disabled people with incomes of up to 138 percent of the poverty line would qualify for Medicaid. It called for the federal government to pick up the entire tab for the newly eligible as of 2014. Starting in 2017, this federal match will gradually decline, leveling off at 90 percent in 2020. Medicaid's appeal to policymakers largely stemmed from its ability to pare the overall price tag of the ACA. The Congressional Budget Office estimated that it would cost 50 percent more per enrollee to insure the poor on the ACA's insurance exchanges than it would through Medicaid.[19]

After the 2010 election, gridlock—rooted in a three-decade trend toward partisan polarization—sidelined Congress from additional legislative action directed at Medicaid. Republicans, who regained control of the House of Representatives in 2011, repeatedly attempted to repeal the ACA, to derail its implementation, and to eviscerate funding for Medicaid. Faced with deeply entrenched Republican hostility in Congress, the Obama administration had to rely on executive branch action to get the ACA off the ground.

Following passage of the ACA, the federal courts did more than Congress to reshape the implementation playing field for the Medicaid expansion. The most publicized case involved the June 2012 Supreme Court decision that effectively made state participation in the Medicaid expansion voluntary. But prior to assessing that case, the Obama administration's response to federal court action dealing with a major source of Medicaid's status as second-tier health care deserves attention.

## The Obama Administration and Medicaid Payment Rates

During the debate over the ACA in 2009, Republican senators pilloried the proposed Medicaid expansion as a feeble overture to the uninsured. Senator John Cornyn (Texas) cited research to the effect that Medicaid's "lousy" payment rates were only 72 percent of those provided by Medicare and even less compared to employer insurance. Senator Mike Enzi (Wyoming) asserted that poor pay meant that 40 percent of doctors would not see Medicaid enrollees. Senator John Kyl (Arizona) summed up by declaring that all this meant that the Medicaid expansion would "promise folks care that we are not going to be able to deliver."[20]

Sensitive to these criticisms, Democratic lawmakers took some steps to ameliorate access issues for Medicaid enrollees. The ACA temporarily elevated Medicaid payment levels for primary care practitioners in 2013 and 2014. It expanded the number of community health centers, which receive more generous Medicaid reimbursement. The ACA also enlarged the role of the Medicaid and CHIP Payment and Access Commission, which would now be responsible for issuing an annual report on barriers to access affecting children and adults. On balance, however, Congress did little to alter the intergovernmental dynamics that had long shaped provider payment. These dynamics had forged a pattern in which the federal government establishes upper limits on Medicaid payment levels, but defers to the states on minimum rates.

Federal Medicaid law provides only general guidance on the minimum amounts that states can pay providers. In 1968, Congress passed an amendment affirming that provider payments should promote the goals of efficiency, economy, and quality. In 1972, it eliminated the requirement that state payment rates to hospitals mirror those of Medicare.[21] In 1989, Henry Waxman attempted to address the disparity between Medicaid and Medicare rates by pushing through an amendment that identified "access" as another goal of Medicaid payment policy. More specifically, the amendment affirmed that Medicaid payment rates had to be "sufficient to enlist enough providers so that care and services are available . . . at least to the extent that such care and services are available to the general population in a geographic area."[22] However, no presidential administration had ever issued a federal rule defining and enforcing this access provision. States submitting changes in payment rates for federal review and approval typically furnished little data to support their claims that access would be preserved.[23]

This pattern of federal deference to the states did not change with the great migration of Medicaid enrollees to managed-care plans in the 1990s.[24] In 2002, the Centers for Medicare and Medicaid Services (CMS) issued regulations requiring that state contracts with managed-care organizations be "actuarially sound."[25] This generally implied that these organizations had to pay enough to establish provider networks that could adequately serve their Medicaid enrollees. But in approving state managed-care plans, CMS deferred so heavily to state assessments of actuarial soundness that the Government Accountability Office criticized the agency for lax oversight.[26]

Litigation in California put the issue of Medicaid payment on the decision agenda of the Obama administration. In February 2008, California policymakers submitted Medicaid plan amendments that would reduce payments to certain providers by 10 percent. Before CMS took action on the request, providers and other stakeholders filed a series of lawsuits in the federal courts asserting that the rates failed to assure adequate access to care. The various suits led the Ninth Circuit Court of Appeals to block the proposed rate cuts. California officials promptly appealed the circuit court rulings to the Supreme Court, which agreed to hear the case. (Sara Rosenbaum's Chapter 6 in this volume describes the ensuing developments in the courts.)

The Ninth Circuit decisions forced the Obama administration to make a political "Hobson's choice" between two competing constituencies. The first was the intergovernmental lobby consisting of state and local officials (especially governors) and the associations that represent them. The legacy of deference to the states on Medicaid payments largely represented the triumph of this lobby over the decades. The circuit court rulings now fueled concern among state officials that they had failed to put a "stake in the heart" of the "vampire" of federal intervention.[27] The intensity of state opposition to court supervision of their payment rates partly reflected the enormous fiscal pressures they faced in the wake of the Great Recession. Moreover, maintenance-of-effort provisions in the ACA had closed other avenues for paring Medicaid costs (e.g., reducing eligibility for the program). In this context, a survey conducted in early 2011 found that 33 states planned to cut Medicaid provider payments and 16 more to freeze them.[28]

While the Obama administration faced strong pressure from the states to fend off court intervention on Medicaid matters, liberal supporters of the program pushed in the opposite direction. These included advocates for the disadvantaged, Democrats in Congress, and former top officials in the federal government. They saw court intervention as a counterweight to the legacy of deference to the states that had reinforced Medicaid's status as second-tier insurance. A brief filed in the Supreme Court by a dozen former administrators from the Department of Health and Human Services cogently presented this view.[29] Arguing that providers should be able to sue under the Supremacy Clause of the constitution, the brief portrayed CMS as a virtual captive of the states on payment issues. It noted that the agency is "under far more political pressure from the states than from private parties" and that expecting CMS to single-handedly enforce payment and access requirements was completely unrealistic.[30] The brief underscored that CMS lacked the basic capacity to supervise state payment practices. It noted that the agency had "fewer than 500 federal employees" focused on Medicaid, most of them "out of necessity" devoted to "bookkeeping and routine financial management."[31] Given these circumstances, the brief argued that adequate review of state payment practices would only occur if the system of CMS review was supplemented by private enforcement through the federal courts.

Finding itself between a rock and a hard place, the Obama administration's response played out on several fronts. The administration initially argued that there was no need for the Supreme Court to rule on the Supremacy Clause.[32] But when the court rejected this argument, the Obama administration sided with the intergovernmental lobby rather than its liberal allies. In May 2011, the Justice Department filed a brief with the Supreme Court that rejected the applicability of the Supremacy Clause to Medicaid payments and urged that the Ninth Circuit rulings be overturned because they infringed on the authority of the Secretary of Health and Human Services. Not surprisingly, the filing sparked intense criticism. Henry Waxman said he was "bitterly disappointed" by the administration's brief, denouncing it as "wrong on the law and bad policy."[33] Bruce Vladeck, the administrator responsible for Medicaid and Medicare under President Clinton, subsequently coauthored an editorial in the *New York Times* called "Killing Medicaid the California Way." The piece condemned the Obama administration for being "complicit in eviscerating Medicaid."[34]

Having sided with the states in this case, the Obama administration simultaneously pursued two strategies to signal its commitment to more effective oversight of state payment practices. In November 2010, CMS rejected California's proposed rate cuts on grounds that state officials had failed to provide adequate documentation. It then engaged in extensive negotiations with California officials over how to demonstrate that the rate reductions would not impair access to care. California administrators subsequently submitted access studies for each of the services targeted for payment cuts. They also presented an 82-page monitoring plan, which identified 23 different measures they would regularly assess to ensure that the rate reductions did not erode beneficiary access. In the face of this documentation and California's willingness to withdraw certain of the proposed cuts, CMS approved the other reductions in October 2011.[35]

The Obama administration also promised to issue what three prior presidential administrations had failed to promulgate—a formal rule interpreting Waxman's 1989 equal access provision. The proposed rule that CMS published in May 2011 applied to Medicaid fee-for-service payments, not the burgeoning managed-care sector.[36] It pointed to certain data that states should present when they wanted to modify their payment rates (e.g., metrics on the utilization patterns of Medicaid recipients and the number of providers accepting new Medicaid enrollees). It also required states to have a "public process" to afford Medicaid providers and stakeholders ample opportunity to comment on rate changes. It mandated that states monitor the impact of rate reductions on enrollee access and, when necessary, craft corrective action plans. In addition to targeting changes in payment rates, the regulation proposed that states analyze access for a subset of Medicaid services each year and publicize the results.

In a period of intense partisan polarization, the proposed regulation united red and blue states in their opposition. Republican governor Scott Walker's top Medicaid official in Wisconsin denounced the proposal as a "federal power grab" and branded it as yet "another example of how distant and disconnected the administration is from what is happening across the country." In turn, the Medicaid director in the administration of Washington Governor Christine Gregoire, a Democrat, asserted that the Obama "administration had gone overboard, creating a system of access review that is far too complex, elaborate, and burdensome."[37]

The Obama administration planned to publish the final rule by December 2011, but delayed in the face of state resistance. Then, in June 2012, the Supreme Court ruled that the ACA's Medicaid expansion amounted to unconstitutional federal coercion of the states. The ruling prohibited the federal government from defunding a state's existing Medicaid program if it failed to implement the expansion, thereby making state participation voluntary.[38] With the administration now needing to persuade states to participate, its appetite for aggravating them by issuing a rule on payment and access plummeted. As of late 2014, CMS had not published the rule and is highly unlikely to do so in the foreseeable future. This inaction, combined with the victory of the Obama administration in the courts (described by

Sara Rosenbaum in Chapter 6), reinforced the legacy of federal deference to the states on Medicaid payments.

## THE ADMINISTRATIVE PRESIDENCY AND PARTISAN FEDERALISM

The contentious federalism that characterized the Obama administration's dealings with the states over provider payment was business as usual.[39] Throughout Medicaid's history, state policymakers from both parties had sought autonomy to set payment rates. In sharp contrast, the contentious federalism that marked state decisions on whether to participate in the ACA's Medicaid expansion had deep roots in a three-decade trend toward partisan polarization. Polarization fueled an ideological model of federal-state interaction in program implementation. This model features key party and ideological elites at the national level striving to promote a *vertical partisan coalition* in which state policymakers face pressure to act as loyal party members in the implementation process. The partisan identities of state policymakers drive their behavior more than pragmatic policy and administrative considerations about the advantages and disadvantages of a federal program for their jurisdictions.

Thus, the Obama administration needed to persuade Republican policymakers in the states to defect from the vertical partisan coalition to achieve the ACA's coverage goals. This turned out to be a formidable challenge. As 2013 dawned, Republicans controlled the governorship and both houses of the legislature in 24 states. In 6 of the 13 states with divided governments, Republicans occupied the governor's mansion. Faced with the need to coax state participation, the Obama administration pursued four primary strategies.

*First, it preserved an all-or-nothing approach to the expansion.* The June 2012 Supreme Court ruling kindled efforts by Republican governors to reinterpret many of the ACA's Medicaid provisions. Of particular importance, some governors expressed interest in partial expansions under which they would receive the 100 percent federal match to cover a subset of the newly eligible, rather than all those up to 138 percent of poverty. Despite pressure from Republican governors and their congressional allies, CMS announced in December 2012 that it would not approve partial measures. In essence, the Obama administration gambled that the

ACA's generous federal match, as well as lobbying pressures from providers and others, would ultimately encourage most, if not all, states to expand fully.

*Second, the Obama administration reassured states that it would preserve the ACA's financial commitment to them.* This required the administration to backtrack. In mid-2011, President Obama's quest to achieve a "grand bargain" with Republicans over the budget deficit prompted him to propose a "blended" match rate for Medicaid. Rather than have a different match for the newly eligible under the ACA and those in the existing Medicaid program, the Obama administration would devise a common rate that would yield some federal budget savings. Discussions of the blended rate stirred unease among state policymakers. During a meeting with President Obama in early December 2012, the chair of the National Governors Association, Jack Markel, a Democrat from Delaware, stressed that any uncertainty about Washington's financial commitment to the states would undercut the Medicaid expansion.[40] In response, the Obama administration assured the governors that it would no longer pursue the blended rate or other significant reductions in Medicaid spending.

*Third, the Obama administration sought to incentivize interest groups to pressure state policymakers to expand Medicaid.* Hospitals comprised a particularly important target. Major hospital lobbies had supported the ACA largely on grounds that it would reduce the amount of uncompensated care they delivered to the uninsured. In recognition that hospitals would face less fiscal stress from this source, the ACA cut funding for Medicaid's DSH program by 20 percent from 2014 to 2020. With the court ruling making the Medicaid expansion voluntary, hospital lobbyists now wanted DSH cuts pared or eliminated in nonparticipating states. The Obama administration, however, grasped that this would reward recalcitrant states with more federal funds and would reduce the incentive for hospital lobbyists in these states to press for the Medicaid expansion. Thus, when Secretary of Health and Human Services Kathleen Sebelius met with leaders of major hospital groups in July 2012, she offered no relief from the DSH cuts. Instead, she urged them to solve the problem by lobbying vigorously in their states for the expansion.[41] State hospital associations generally responded as the Obama administration had hoped. Their support for the Medicaid expansion often rested on well-publicized studies documenting its economic benefits to the states.

*Fourth, the Obama administration employed waivers to persuade states to launch Medicaid expansions.* The ACA provided CMS with comprehensive waiver authority, starting in 2017. In the meantime, the Obama administration used Section 1115 waivers to serve its aims. While the White House used waivers in multiple ways, its flexibility in considering premium-assistance and other market-based initiatives is especially notable.[42] The Medicaid statute had long given states the option to cover program enrollees through private insurance, and a few had launched modest initiatives. To pursue the ACA's Medicaid expansion via premium assistance, however, state policymakers sought flexibility that only waivers could provide.

In 2013, two states with divided partisan control of their governments obtained CMS approval to pursue the Medicaid expansion via premium assistance. Arkansas aimed to enroll its entire expansion population, except for those with special medical needs, in private plans offered on the insurance exchanges. Iowa in turn targeted a more limited Medicaid cohort, those with incomes from 101 to 138 percent of poverty, for enrollment in the exchange or, if available, through employer insurance. The following year, Pennsylvania, with a unified Republican government, also received approval for a waiver expanding Medicaid through premium assistance. Meanwhile, Republican policymakers in other states, including Florida, Indiana, New Hampshire, and Utah, expressed interest in the approach.

Republican proponents of premium assistance portray it as a market-oriented, "conservative" alternative to the traditional "broken" Medicaid program. They contend that it holds down costs by empowering beneficiaries to choose among private plans competing on the exchanges to enroll them. The premium assistance model also has elements that liberals like. The private plans on the exchanges tend to pay providers more than Medicaid, thereby enhancing enrollee access to "mainstream" care. Use of the exchanges might also reduce churning—people moving between Medicaid and the exchange plans due to fluctuating incomes. It might therefore bolster participation rates among the Medicaid expansion group and foster continuity of care. Little wonder that in responding favorably to a Republican premium assistance proposal in Florida, a Democratic state senator observed: "A rose by any other name is still a rose."[43]

Though this approach was appealing to the Obama administration as a way to defuse the Medicaid expansion as a polarizing partisan issue, the potential price tag of premium assistance was a concern. Demonstration waivers are supposed to be budget-neutral, costing no more than the regular Medicaid program. But the Congressional Budget Office had estimated that it cost 50 percent more to insure a person on the exchanges than through Medicaid. Over the short term, however, the Obama administration's interest in accommodating Republican policymakers overrode cost concerns. Federal administrators have bent over backwards to accept sanguine state estimates that their waivers are budget-neutral.

Overall, the Obama administration has made some headway in defusing Republican resistance in the states. Table 10.1 presents an overview of state participation in the Medicaid expansion as of September 2014 by partisan control of state government. At this point 27 states had opted to expand, along with the District of Columbia. As befits an intensely polarized time, only 22 percent of states where Republicans controlled the governorship and the legislature (Arizona, Michigan, North Dakota, Ohio, and Pennsylvania) chose to participate, while all states controlled by the Democrats signed up. Of states with divided government, 70 percent expanded Medicaid.

TABLE 10.1  States Expanding Medicaid by Partisan Control of State Government (September 2014)

| Partisan Control, 2013–2014 | Total | Number Participating | Percent Participating |
|---|---|---|---|
| Unified Republican | 23 | 5 | 22 |
| Unified Democrat[a] | 15 | 15 | 100 |
| Divided | 10 | 7 | 70 |
| Other[b] | 2 | 0 | 0 |
| Total | 50 | 27 | 54 |

Source: Kaiser Family Foundation.
[a] This cohort includes Rhode Island, where the governor switched his allegiance to the Democratic Party in mid-2013. It also incorporates New York and Washington, where Democrats held a majority in each state senate, but a bipartisan coalition led each.
[b] This includes Virginia, which switched from being unified Republican to divided in January 2014; it also includes Nebraska, which formally has a nonpartisan legislature.

Three central conclusions emerge from Medicaid's evolution over the last half-century. First, Medicaid has grown over four historical periods to become a pillar of the American health insurance regime. Several factors have interacted through time to fuel supportive policy feedbacks leading to growth.[44] Medicaid's open-ended *funding formula* allows each level of government in the federal system to leverage money from the other when it enlarges the program. Elected policymakers at both levels can take political credit for expanding Medicaid while paying only part of the tab. So too, a panoply of *service providers and other advocates* (e.g., hospitals, nursing homes, managed-care organizations, and disability rights organizations) has staunchly defended the program. Movement toward a *more positive social construction of the program's enrollees* has also bolstered Medicaid.[45] Its image as "welfare medicine" has faded as a shrinking share of its non-disabled enrollees receives cash assistance. Instead, Medicaid has emerged as a program for working people and as a safety net for middle-class individuals who need long-term care for themselves or loved ones due to aging or disability. With occasional lapses by Republican governors, the *intergovernmental lobby* has protected and promoted Medicaid as an open-ended entitlement to the states. In addition, *skilled policy entrepreneurship* by Democrats in Congress, especially during the 1980s and in the politics triggering the ACA's passage, contributed to Medicaid's expansion.

The *rise of waivers and executive federalism* has also stoked Medicaid's ascendance. The increased willingness of the executive branch to grant these waivers has facilitated state eligibility expansions (most dramatically, Romneycare in Massachusetts) and has kindled the growth of home and community-based services. In cooperation with key gubernatorial allies, presidents can employ waivers to overcome barriers to adaptation and innovation rooted in the supermajority bias of American governance, especially under divided government and intense partisan polarization. The more permissive federal stance on waivers has enriched the stream of Medicaid policy "solutions" and has opened new policy windows for state officials. By reshaping state policy dynamics in these ways, waivers have also have signaled to governors that they can obtain flexibility to reshape Medicaid without backing block grant proposals.

Second, while delinkage from cash assistance has distanced Medicaid from "welfare medicine," the intergovernmental dynamics surrounding provider payments have reinforced its status as second-tier health care. To be sure, considerable evidence supports the view that Medicaid coverage enhances access to care and desirable health outcomes.[46] Still, Medicaid provider payment levels, while varying among states, tend to afford less access to a range of providers than Medicare and employer insurance. In theory, federal administrators could insist that states do more to assure the adequacy of these rates. But as the behavior of the Obama administration attests, federal policymakers are extremely reluctant to do so. Keeping the courts at bay on provider payment heightened the ability of the president to use payment as a bargaining chip, a kind of loss leader, to obtain state support on other Medicaid matters.

Finally, the story of Medicaid rising could conceivably become, in years ahead, one of Medicaid stymied or falling. The growing federal debt, resistance to tax increases, and rising healthcare prices continue to spawn proposals to pare Medicaid as a part of "entitlement reform." Partisan polarization and the movement of the Republican Party to the right also threaten Medicaid. In this regard, the degree to which Republican-dominated states continue to resist the Medicaid expansion bears watching. By the end of 2014, 26 states had moved to expand Medicaid, a pace of state participation similar to that after passage of the original Medicaid law in 1965.[47] It took until the end of 1970 for 48 states to initiate the original Medicaid program. If the number of states expanding Medicaid by the end of 2017 appreciably trails that number, it will point to the potency of the partisan ideological model of federalism in impeding Medicaid growth.

Medicaid's reversal of fortune could be even more severe if the 2016 elections leave Republicans in control of the presidency and Congress. Since its birth, Medicaid has spent only four years under unified Republican government—2003 through 2006. During that time, the George W. Bush administration tried to convert Medicaid to a block grant, but the proposal won little support among Republican governors and died in Congress. More recently, however, Republicans in the House of Representatives have for four consecutive years (2011–2014) passed budget resolutions that would not only repeal the ACA but convert Medicaid to a block grant with massively reduced funding. The Romney-Ryan ticket ran on this anti-Medicaid platform in 2012. Whether a Republican government would in fact retrench Medicaid remains an open question. The severity of any such retrenchment would diminish to the degree that Republican governors lobby federal policymakers to preserve the program.

## NOTES

My thanks to Joel Cantor, Jennifer Farnham, David Mechanic, and the editors of this book for helpful comments on a prior draft.

1. Shanna Rose, *Financing Medicaid: Federalism and the Growth of America's Health Care Safety-Net* (Ann Arbor: University of Michigan Press, 2013), 27. Passed in 1960, Kerr-Mills provided federal matching grants to the states to deliver health care to the elderly.

2. Rose, *Financing Medicaid*, 48.

3. Robert Stevens and Rosemary Stevens, *Welfare Medicine in America* (New York: Free Press, 1974), 91–92.

4. Data on Medicaid expenditure growth primarily come from the Office of the Actuary, Centers for Medicare and Medicaid Services, Department of Health and Human Services. Calculations are based on constant 2012 dollars. See http://www.cms.gov/Research-Statistics-Data-and-Systems/StatisticsTrendsandReports/NationalHealthExpendData/NationalHealthAccountsHistorical.hmtl.

5. David G. Smith and Judith G. Moore. *Medicaid Politics and Policy, 1965–2007* (New Brunswick, NJ: Transaction Publishers, 2008), 134.

6. Smith and Moore, *Medicaid Politics*, 78–79, 104–105.

7. John Holahan and Joel Cohen, *Medicaid: The Trade-off Between Cost Containment and Access to Care* (Washington, DC: Urban Institute, 1986), 1, 37, 87.

8. Rose, *Financing Medicaid*, 78.

9. Smith and Moore, *Medicaid Politics*, 168–169.

10. Michael K. Gusmano and Frank J. Thompson, "Safety-Net Hospitals at the Crossroads: Whither Medicaid DSH?" In *The Health Care Safety Net in a Post-Reform World*, ed. Mark A. Hall and Sara Rosenbaum (New Brunswick, NJ: Rutgers University Press, 2012), 156, 161.

11. Rose, *Financing Medicaid*, 78–129.

12. Smith and Moore, *Medicaid Politics*, 130.

13. Theresa A. Coughlin, Leighton Ku, and John Holahan, *Medicaid since 1980* (Washington, DC: Urban Institute Press, 1994), 23–27.

14. Frank J. Thompson, *Medicaid Politics: Federalism, Policy Durability, and Health Reform* (Washington, DC: Georgetown University Press, 2012), 72.

15. *Gonzaga University et al. v. Doe* (01-6679), 536 US 273 (2002).

16. See Thomas Gais and James Fossett, "Federalism and the Executive Branch," in *The Executive Branch*, ed. Joel D. Aberbach and Mark A. Peterson (New York: Oxford University Press, 2005), 486–524; see also Thompson, *Medicaid Politics*, 101–166.

17. Thompson, *Medicaid Politics*, 134–166.

18. Thompson, *Medicaid Politics*, 60–65.

19. Leighton Ku, "Medicaid Expansion Using Private Plans: The Role of Premium Assistance." Health Reform GPS, April 8, 2013, http://healthreformgps.org/resources/medicaid-expansions-using-private-plans-the-role-of-premium-assistance-and-cost-sharing.

20. US Senate Committee on Finance, *Executive Committee Meeting to Consider Health Care Reform*, http://finance.senate.gov/hearings/hearing/id+d812a4e-bc6b-dc2c3-8b31-49ec4efd1824 2009, 361, 407, 411, 416–417.

21. Stevens and Stevens, *Welfare Medicine in America*, 339.

22. US Medicaid and CHIP Payment and Access Commission, *Report to the Congress on Medicaid and CHIP* (Washington, DC, 2011), 160, http://www.macpac.gov/reports/MACPAC_March2011_web.pdf?attredirects=0&d=1.

23. US Department of Health and Human Services, "Medicaid Program: Methods for Assuring Access to Covered Medicaid Services; Proposed Rule." *Federal Register* 76, 88 (May 6, 2011), 26348–26349.

24. By 2010, nearly 70 percent of Medicaid enrollees were in these plans. States contracting with managed-care organizations typically pay the plans a fixed monthly rate per Medicaid enrollee (a procedure known as capitation). See Michael Sparer, *Medicaid Managed Care: Costs, Access, and Quality of Care* (Princeton, NJ: Robert Wood Johnson Foundation, 2012).

25. US Department of Health and Human Services, "Medicaid Program; Medicaid Managed Care; New Provisions," *Federal Register* 67, 115 (June 14, 2002): 40989.

26. US Government Accountability Office, *Medicaid Managed Care: CMS's Oversight of State Rate Setting Needs Improvement* (Washington, DC: GAO-10-810, 2010).

27. John Wilkerson, "States Worry Upcoming CMS Rate-Setting Reg Could Bust Budgets," March 18, 2011, http://insidehealthreform.com/201103182358310/Health-Daily-News/Daily-News/states-worry-up.

28. Rachana Dixit, "Many States Turn to Provider Payment Cuts, Raising Taxes or Fees to Sustain Medicaid," June 7, 2011, http://insidehealthreform.com/201106072366274/Health-Daily-News/Daily-News/providers.

29. *Brief of Former HHS Officials as Amicus Curiae in Support of Respondents, in the Supreme Court of The United States, Tony Douglas v. Independent Living Center of Southern California et al.,* Nos. 09-958, 09-1158, and 10-283 (2011).

30. *Brief of Former HHS Officials,* 4, 12.

31. *Brief of Former HHS Officials,* 19.

32. US Department of Justice, *Brief for The United States as Amicus Curiae, in the Supreme Court of the United States, Maxwell-Jolly v. Independent Living Center of Southern California, Inc. et al.,* No. 09-958 (2010).

33. Robert Pear, "Administration Opposes Challenges to Medicaid Cuts," *New York Times,* May 28, 2011, http://www.nytimes.com/2011/05/29/us/29medicaid.html.

34. Bruce C. Vladeck and Stephen I. Vladeck, "Killing Medicaid the California Way," *New York Times,* October 14, 2011, http://www.nytimes.com/2011/10/14/opinion/killing-medicaid-the-california-way.html.

35. US Court of Appeals for the Ninth Circuit, *Managed Pharmacy Care et al. v. Sebelius et al.,* No. 12-55067, D.C. No.2: 11-cv-09211-CAS-MAN (2012), 19–20.

36. US Department of Health and Human Services, "Medicaid Program: Methods for Assuring Access," 2011, 26342–26362.

37. Robert Pear, "Rule Would Discourage State's Cutting Medicaid Payments to Providers," *New York Times,* May 2, 2011, http://www.nytimes.com/2011/05/03/us/politics/03medicaid.html.

38. *National Federation of Independent Business v. Sebelius* ("NFIB"), 132 S. Ct. 2566 (2012).

39. This section draws on Frank J. Thompson and Michael K. Gusmano, "The Administrative Presidency and Fractious Federalism: The Case of Obamacare," *Publius: The Journal of Federalism,* 44, no. 3 (2014): 426–450.

40. Rachana Dixit and Amy Lotven, "NGA Chair Tells Obama Medicaid Cuts Eyed in Fiscal Debate Put Expansion in Jeopardy," December 4, 2012, http://insidehealthreform.com/201212112441/Health-Daily-News/Daily-News/nga.
41. Rachana Dixit, "HHS urges Hospitals to Push States on Medicaid Expansion But Doesn't Show Hand on DSH Cuts," July 26, 2012, http://insidehealthreform.com/20120762405684/Health-Daily-News/Daily-News/hhs-urg.
42. Thompson and Gusmano, "The Administrative Presidency." Some states, such as Michigan and Indiana, pursued waivers that stressed cost sharing and health savings accounts for enrollees, along with rewards for healthy behaviors.
43. Lizette Alvarez, "In Reversal, Florida Says It Will Expand Medicaid," *New York Times*, February 20, 2013, http://www.nytimes.com/2013/02/21/us/in-reversal-florida-says-it-will-expand-medicaid-program.html.
44. For elaboration, see Thompson, *Medicaid Politics*, 207–222.
45. Public opinion surveys reveal substantial support for Medicaid, e.g., Rose, *Financing Medicaid*, 19–20.
46. Thompson, *Medicaid Politics*, 12–14.
47. Kaiser Commission on Medicaid and the Uninsured, *A Historical Review of How States Have Responded to The Availability of Federal Funds for Health Coverage* (Washington, DC, 2012).

# 11

# INDEPENDENCE AND FREEDOM

## PUBLIC OPINION AND THE POLITICS OF MEDICARE AND MEDICAID

ANDREA LOUISE CAMPBELL

A half-century after their passage, the two large government health insurance programs, Medicare and Medicaid, occupy unique positions in the public mind. Medicare, along with Social Security, has proven one of the most popular government programs since its inception five decades ago. Medicaid is the most highly regarded social assistance program, and trails the big social insurance programs in public support fairly closely. Beyond their popularity, what sets Medicare, and even to a certain extent, Medicaid, apart from many other issue areas and government programs is their wide appeal across societal groups. With some variation, support for Medicare is high among rich and poor, young and old alike. Differences across political and ideological groups are more muted than in most areas of public policy as well. Support for Medicaid shows more variation across groups, but with surprisingly little range compared to the usual patterns in American public opinion.

What distinguishes these programs as attitude objects is the role of personal experience. Because Medicare is a universal social insurance program that addresses an essential but otherwise hugely expensive and unattainable need—health insurance in old age—the vast majority of Americans grasp its importance. They know they will rely on it when they retire. They know their parents rely on it now and would need help with their healthcare costs if Medicare didn't exist. Thus public regard for Medicare arises from its obvious and tangible role in providing intergenerational financial stability and independence.

As a means-tested rather than universal program, Medicaid may be less visible than Medicare, but the program covers an even larger number of Americans. As a result of the program's wide reach, plenty of ordinary citizens recognize its importance as a safety net and personally know people who are benefiting from the program, including some in their own families.

Thus, despite handwringing at the elite level about the cost of these programs, particularly among fiscal conservatives, opinion surveys consistently indicate that the public remains bullish on them because of their widespread and very personal effects. Even in an atmosphere of budget cuts and retrenchment, these positive public attitudes have helped prevent deep cuts or structural change.

## Medicare: A History of Strong Public Support

In most scholarly accounts of Medicare's origins and founding, elected politicians, social insurance advocates and bureaucrats, and stakeholder groups star in leading roles. Public opinion plays a bit part. While public opinion generally supported government health insurance for older Americans, it was not necessarily the key impetus to program creation. Ted Marmor summarizes this view well when he says that public opinion was not "decisive" but "permissive."[1]

That said, public opinion has proven a vital resource for the program since its inception. In Larry Jacobs's account of the program's origins, opinion polling induced John F. Kennedy to emphasize Medicare during his 1960 presidential campaign.[2] Certainly the publicly available data from that period demonstrates the popularity of public health insurance for older Americans (particularly in light of the failure of national health insurance under President Truman). In his compilation of survey data from the early

1960s, Michael E. Schiltz finds strong support for extending the payroll tax to fund health insurance for older Americans; three-fifths to two-thirds of survey respondents supported the idea.[3] Moreover, the Social Security–type government insurance program out-polled a private insurance alternative.

The available data indicate that the general public clearly regarded senior citizens, the target of the legislation, as a sympathetic group, having the highest health expenses but the lowest incomes and the least access to private health insurance.[4] Although policymakers would later debate the suitability and wisdom of using the payroll tax for health insurance (compared to using it for Social Security, which is more actuarially predictable), the mechanism had an advantage, in that ordinary Americans knew and were comfortable with it. The main dimensions of Medicare support emerged during this era: the desirability of providing health insurance to this needy and sympathetic group; the embrace of the contributory funding model; and the elevation of Medicare, along with Social Security, to near-sacred status.

Public support for Medicare has remained high since that founding era, even as the program has faced numerous fiscal and political challenges. During its first three decades, Medicare experienced an "era of consensus" among national-level policymakers, during which time the program enjoyed a muted politics, and policy changes were incremental, consensual, and bipartisan.[5] All of this changed when fiscal difficulties in the Medicare program coincided with the rise of the conservative Right during the 1990s, resulting in challenges including proposed spending cuts and structural changes (see also Chapter 8 by Mark Peterson in this volume). Such proposals gained new life with the large budget deficits arising from the Great Recession that began in 2007, which conservatives used to catapult proposals for long-term structural change in entitlement programs onto the political agenda.

When we examine various aspects of public opinion toward Medicare, however, the turmoil over the program among political elites fades from view. Such events and critiques do appear to undermine the public's confidence in Medicare's future, but Americans' fundamental support for the program remains unshaken. Broad swaths of the public readily recognize the importance of Medicare to individuals' financial stability in retirement, indeed to entire families' economic situations, which would be threatened by a lack of government health insurance for senior citizens. So central are Medicare's supports that the differences in attitudes across income, age, and political groups that typify American public opinion narrow considerably with regard to the program. Among the public, crises such as the Great Recession do not inspire calls for cuts, as they do among conservative politicians, but instead underscore the importance of entitlement programs. Medicare and Social Security stabilize senior citizens' financial footing and their health insurance situations. These programs, moreover, serve as the safety net for elders' adult children, who have few safety nets of their own in the circumscribed American welfare state. Positive personal experiences with Medicare blunt the usual skepticism toward government and elicit broad program support across a variety of societal groups.

Of these two programs—Social Security and Medicare—we have far less polling on Medicare. There is, for example, no decades-long series on Medicare attitudes to facilitate an examination of opinion trends over time. Nevertheless, surveys going back to the mid-1990s, when elite challenges to the program had already begun, demonstrate a steady pattern of high salience and support for seniors' government health insurance among the public, a support often at odds with the tumultuous Washington politics of the program.[6]

For example, since 1997, one polling organization has asked national survey respondents about their priorities for the president and Congress at the beginning of each year. Through 2013, the proportion of respondents saying that taking steps to make the Medicare system financially sound should be a "top priority" has never fallen below 50 percent, and has typically been over 60 percent.[7] Although some policymakers wish to trim Medicare spending to address the federal budget deficit—Medicare is, after all, one of the largest components of federal spending—the public is particularly hostile to such proposals. When asked in October 2013 about "some government programs whose spending could be cut to reduce the federal budget deficit," a remarkable four out of five *National Journal* poll respondents said they did not want Medicare cut at all.[8] Similarly, when asked in December 2013 about their fiscal priorities, more than two-thirds of Pew respondents ranked keeping Social Security and Medicare benefits unchanged higher than taking steps to reduce the budget deficit—a level of support that crept up nearly 10 points from mid-2011, when Pew first asked the question. Less than one-quarter thought deficit reduction should take priority.[9] Indeed, rather than reduce the deficit on the back of Medicare, 58 percent of September 2012

Kaiser Health Tracking Poll respondents said that "if policymakers made the right changes, they could reduce the federal budget deficit without reducing Medicare spending."[10]

In public opinion, the major entitlement programs also win out against defense spending: when asked which of the "largest items in the federal budget" they would be willing to change in order to cut spending, about half of survey respondents single out defense for spending cuts, while only one in five mentions Medicare and one in six, Social Security.[11] Given the chance to consider whether the federal government should even be in the business of providing health insurance to older and poorer Americans, poll respondents embrace the programs wholeheartedly. Fully 86 percent of respondents to a January 2014 Pew Center poll said that the government should "continue programs like Medicare and Medicaid for seniors and the very poor." A mere 12 percent said the government should "not be involved in providing health insurance at all."[12]

Of course, survey respondents have little at stake when they say they want spending on this or that program to continue, particularly when poll questions do not mention the taxes required to support that spending. Even when taxes are mentioned, however, support for Medicare remains strong. More than two-thirds of respondents to CBS News Polls in 2011 and 2014 agreed that the "benefits from Medicare are worth the cost of the program for taxpayers." Just 21 percent said the program was not worth it.[13]

Despite high levels of support for the Medicare program, public confidence in the future of the program and in its ability to sustain current benefits are low, and have been for decades, mirroring a pattern seen in attitudes regarding Social Security.[14] In February 2013, only 14 percent of Bloomberg National Poll respondents said that they thought Medicare would "definitely be there" for them in retirement; 43 percent said it would probably be there, while a large proportion—39 percent—said it would "probably not" or "definitely would not" be there for them at retirement age.[15] Similarly, 53 percent of USA Today/Gallup Poll respondents in September 2012 were pessimistic that "twenty years from now, the Medicare program will still provide all Americans over age sixty-five with adequate health care coverage," compared to 43 percent who were optimistic that it would do so.[16] In May 2013, just 8 percent of Harvard School of Public Health survey respondents said that in 15 years, Medicare would pay a higher level of benefits than it does now, while

18 percent thought it would pay about the same, 38 percent said it would pay a lower level, and 32 percent—almost one-third—thought Medicare would no longer exist at that point.[17]

Low confidence in Medicare's future has a long history. When 57 percent of January 2011 Kaiser Poll respondents said that they were "very concerned" that the Medicare benefits seniors have today will not be available for them when they retire, with another 25 percent saying that they were "somewhat concerned," they were repeating virtually the same responses that the public gave when first asked the question in April 2003.[18] Indeed, a time-series of Medicare confidence polls going back to 1996 shows that the proportion of respondents skeptical about the program's future—the share who are "not too confident" or "not at all confident" that the Medicare system will continue to provide benefits at least equal to current benefits—has never fallen below half. Confidence peaked in 2003, with the addition of the prescription drug benefit; that year, a mere 54 percent said that they were not too confident or not at all confident in Medicare's future. That proportion had been 70 percent in 1996, shortly after the trust fund crisis of that decade, and rose back up to 66 percent in 2013, after the Great Recession and considerable talk about entitlement spending and the size of the budget deficit.[19]

But while confidence in the Medicare system has waxed and waned, support for the program as a whole remains strong. One important factor is the crucial role that Medicare plays in individuals' and families' financial security. Survey questions reveal that Medicare figures prominently in individuals' retirement plans, providing independence for beneficiaries and financial freedom for adult children, who would otherwise have to help pay for their parents' health care.

Very large majorities of Americans recognize the centrality of Medicare's health insurance benefit for retirees. Two-thirds of respondents to an August 2012 AP-GfK Poll said that Medicare would be "very important" or "extremely important" to their financial security in retirement. Just one in six respondents said it would be just slightly or not at all important.[20] In a July 2011 NPR survey of respondents aged 50 and over who were retired or on the cusp of retirement, 70 percent reported that Medicare was "very important" to their golden years, with another 18 percent saying "somewhat important." Just 3 percent said that Medicare was not very important or not at all important.[21]

Moreover, Medicare matters to entire families, not just to retirees themselves. In a January 2011 Kaiser/Harvard poll, 55 percent of respondents said that Medicare is "very important" to themselves *and their family*, while another 22 percent said that it is "somewhat important."[22] The program spells financial emancipation for the adult children of Medicare beneficiaries. A May 1995 Gallup/CNN/*USA Today* poll asked respondents with older parents: What would happen if their parents or in-laws no longer received Medicare? Sixty-five percent said it would be necessary for them to help their parents pay their medical bills; just 29 percent it would not be necessary.[23]

Typically preferences about public policy differ significantly across age, income, gender, race, and political groups in the United States. Attitudes about Medicare, however, demonstrate strikingly little difference across subgroups. To be sure, women are generally more supportive of Medicare than men;[24] people with low income more so than high income; African Americans more than whites; Democrats more than Republicans; and liberals more than conservatives. Age differences in support depend on the precise question and its interaction with position in the life cycle (see Table 11.1). For the most part, however, these differences in attitudes are far smaller than we usually observe, particularly across partisan and ideological lines.

Some survey responses vary quite a bit by age: while 81 percent of seniors say that Medicare benefits are worth the cost to taxpayers, only 55 percent of those under 30 agree (Table 11.1, line 2). Similarly, three-quarters of seniors say that Medicare is very important to them and their families, while only 34 percent of the youngest group agree (Table 11.1, line 5). However, age groups are on the same page when it comes to reform: large majorities of all groups say Medicare should not be cut to address the federal budget deficit, and two-thirds or more of each age group wishes to keep Medicare as it is today, rather than switch to a fixed dollar-amount, or voucher, system (Table 11.1, lines 1 and 7).[25] The high levels of support for the program among non-seniors may be attributable to the financial emancipation effect: 64 to 70 percent of those under 65 say that they would have to pay for their parents' or in-laws' health care if not for Medicare (Table 11.1, line 6).

Income, too, often divides American public opinion, but again, attitudinal differences across class are muted when it comes to Medicare. Although high-income respondents tend to have more conservative attitudes on social welfare issues,[26] they, even more than lower-income respondents, say

TABLE 11.1  Medicare Attitudes across Select Demographic and Political Groups

| | | Age | | | | Income | | | | Race | | Party | | | Ideology | | |
|---|---|---|---|---|---|---|---|---|---|---|---|---|---|---|---|---|---|
| | | 18–29 | 30–49 | 50–64 | 65+ | <$30K | $30–49.9K | $50–74.9K | $75K+ | W | B | R | I | D | Lib | Mod | Con |
| Support | (1) MC spending should not be cut at all to reduce deficit | 81 | 84 | 82 | 77 | 86 | 83 | 87 | 74 | 80 | 89 | 71 | 80 | 90 | – | – | – |
| | (2) MC benefits worth cost to taxpayers | 55 | 63 | 76 | 81 | 68 | 67 | 66 | 73 | – | – | 63 | 69 | 73 | 75 | 75 | 62 |
| Confidence | (3) Very concerned today's MC benefits not there when you retire | 51 | 61 | 59 | – | 63 | 62 | 63 | 48 | 57 | 65 | 58 | 58 | 56 | 57 | 59 | 55 |
| Personal Importance | (4) Raising MC age would affect financial situation: a great deal | 18 | 18 | 34 | 15 | 29 | 17 | 21 | 22 | 22 | 33 | 20 | 21 | 24 | – | – | – |
| | Some | 26 | 36 | 27 | 9 | 21 | 19 | 39 | 27 | 24 | 20 | 25 | 26 | 25 | – | – | – |
| | (5) MC very important to you and your family | 34 | 52 | 64 | 77 | 67 | 64 | 49 | 41 | 53 | 66 | 50 | 55 | 60 | 56 | 52 | 56 |
| | (6) If no MC would have to pay for parents' & in-laws' health care | 70 | 64 | 70 | 57 | 74 | 64 | 65 | 54 | 64 | 72 | 59 | 67 | 69 | – | – | – |
| Structural Reform | (7) MC continue as today (not change to fixed $ amount) | 69 | 66 | 71 | 76 | 80 | 71 | 70 | 61 | – | – | 53 | 71 | 83 | 81 | 71 | 61 |

Sources: (1) United Technologies/National Journal Congressional Connection Poll, October 3–6, 2013; (2) CBS News Poll, June 3–7, 2011; (3) Kaiser/Harvard The Public's Health Care Agenda for the 112th Congress Survey, January 4–14, 2011; (4) Pew Research Center for the People & the Press Poll, December 13–16, 2012; (5) Kaiser/Harvard The Public's Health Care Agenda for the 112th Congress Survey, January 4–14, 2011; (6) Gallup/CNN/USA Today Poll, May 1995; (7) Kaiser Health Tracking Poll, February 13–19, 2012.

Note: Age categories for item (1) are 18–34, 35–54, 55–65, and 65+; for item (4) are 18–34, 35–44, 45–64, and 65+; and for item (7) are 18–29, 30–49, 50–59, and 60+. Figures in table indicate percentages.

that Medicare benefits are worth the cost to taxpayers (Table 11.1, line 2). Moreover, they are more likely to say that raising the Medicare retirement age would affect them "a great deal" (Table 11.1, line 4). The more affluent do worry less about Medicare not being there when they retire, and voice fewer objections to reforms that would cut Medicare spending or change the structure of the program. That said, while the higher-income group evinces slightly less support for traditional Medicare than lower-income groups, nonetheless large majorities of the more affluent reject cutting Medicare, or adopting a voucher system.

What's most interesting about Medicare opinion is the agreement among partisans. In contemporary opinion surveys, Republicans and Democrats, and conservatives and liberals, are often poles apart in their views. Medicare surveys demonstrate some of these familiar patterns, particularly those survey items that evoke such deeply politicized proposals as cutting Medicare to address the deficit or switching to a voucher system, where Republicans and conservatives are 20 to 30 points more supportive than Democrats and liberals (Table 11.1, lines 1 and 7). When it comes to general support for the program, confidence in its future, and personal importance, however, differences across political groups dwindle. Only 10 points separate Republicans and Democrats on the worth of Medicare to taxpayers, the importance of Medicare to one and one's family, and whether one would have to pay for one's parents' health care in the absence of Medicare (Table 11.1, lines 2, 5, and 6). Partisan and ideological differences disappear altogether in level of concern about Medicare being there for one's own retirement and in the impact of an increase in the eligibility age (Table 11.1, line 3 and 4).

## THE WORLD THAT MEDICARE CREATED

Medicare helped create a world in which large majorities support government provision of health insurance to older Americans. The public recognizes and acknowledges the crucial role that Medicare plays in retirees' financial security. Majorities of every political and ideological group and most income groups say that Medicare is "very important" to them and their families. Large proportions of the public recognize that they would be on the hook for their parents' healthcare costs if the program did not exist. And an overwhelming share of Americans say that Medicare spending should not be cut in the face of the budget deficit—including 71 percent of

Republicans. Majorities—including 62 percent of conservatives and 63 percent of Republicans—say that Medicare is worth the cost to taxpayers. Most Americans reject burdening Medicare recipients with greater cost sharing: majorities say seniors already pay enough of their healthcare costs.[27] And despite many predictions to the contrary, age-related dissatisfactions and intergenerational conflict have never emerged in public opinion polls.[28] Political elites may argue about Medicare's purpose, structure, and future, but the public embrace is warm and widespread, owing largely to the substantial, clear, and tangible effects Medicare has on beneficiaries and their families.

### MEDICAID: THE MOST POPULAR MEANS-TESTED PROGRAM

If Medicare has enjoyed an unusual and politically propitious career in the public mind, so too has Medicaid, the government health insurance program for the poor. Medicaid had a serendipitous birth, tacked onto the Medicare bill at the last minute by House Ways and Means Chairman Wilbur Mills.[29] It has also exhibited a surprisingly robust politics and trajectory: unlike many means-tested programs that have completely withered on the vine, most notably cash benefits to poor families (now known as Temporary Assistance to Needy Families) and public housing, Medicaid has enjoyed strong growth over time.[30]

Although scholars typically attribute Medicaid's resilience to strong support from crucial stakeholders such as hospitals and governors,[31] public opinion also matters. Even less polling exists on Medicaid than on Medicare, but the existing data support the notion of a permissive stance among the public, or at least greater openness to Medicaid than other means-tested programs. And as with Medicare, personal experience turns out to have important effects on program attitudes.

The most extensive cross-program study of public opinion appeared 20 years ago and indicated that Americans are relatively more supportive of Medicaid than other targeted programs. Although respondents were less supportive of increased spending on Medicaid than on Medicare, Supplemental Security Income, or Social Security, they were more supportive of Medicaid than of unemployment insurance, Aid to Families with Dependent Children cash assistance, or food stamps.[32] Other survey items indicated that the relatively favorable ranking of Medicaid could be due to perceptions of the deservingness of the target beneficiaries. When asked to rank their willingness to help various groups with financial assistance or food programs, respondents listed the disabled elderly, poor elderly, and poor children—three of Medicaid's main constituencies—at the top, with poor adults (excluded from Medicaid in many states) ranking far behind.

More recent surveys continue to reveal high levels of support for Medicaid compared to other means-tested programs and government responsibilities. When asked in a January 2013 Kaiser poll whether they would support spending reductions for various programs to reduce the federal budget deficit, the majority of respondents rejected cuts for public education, Medicare, and Social Security. Medicaid came next, with just under 50 percent desiring no cuts to that program; it fared better than aid to farmers, defense, food stamps, unemployment insurance, federal government salaries and benefits, Afghanistan, and foreign aid, where greater proportions embraced minor or major reductions.[33] A May 2011 Kaiser Health Tracking Poll asked the same question and similarly found very little support for cutting Medicaid spending—53 percent said they wanted no reductions at all. Another 30 percent supported minor reductions, and only 13 percent said they would support major reductions in Medicaid spending to reduce the budget deficit.[34]

High levels of support for Medicaid may be due in part to perceptions of the personal importance of the program. Nearly half of respondents to the May 2011 Kaiser poll said that Medicaid was very important or somewhat important to their family. The poll asked respondents *why* Medicaid was important to them: 71 percent said they like knowing Medicaid exists as a safety-net protection for low-income people; 63 percent said they think they or a family member will rely on Medicaid in the future; 58 percent know someone who has received Medicaid; and 43 percent know someone who has received nursing home or long-term care services through the program.

The May 2011 Kaiser poll additionally asked respondents whether they would enroll in Medicaid if they were uninsured, needed health care, and qualified for the program—what we might term "hypothetical personal interest." A majority of respondents responded affirmatively, with no meaningful differences across age groups. Republicans were much less likely than Democrats to be willing to enroll in Medicaid (67 percent vs. 91 percent), although the proportion was somewhat higher among lower-income

Republicans (78 percent of Republicans with household incomes below $40,000 said they would enroll under those circumstances).

As with Medicare, public opinion on Medicaid displays less of the variation across societal groups and political views commonly seen for other issues. The availability of individual-level data for the May 2011 Kaiser Health Tracking Poll enables us to examine attitudes across demographic and political groups (Table 11.2).

Similar to Medicare, support for Medicaid holds steady across age groups, with 50 to 60 percent of each age group preferring no cuts in the program for the sake of deficit reduction. The pattern of personal importance of the program does differ from that of Medicare: while older Americans were most likely to say that Medicare is very important to them (Table 11.1), it is the under-35 group that is most likely to say that Medicaid is very important or somewhat important to themselves or their family (Table 11.2), reflecting Medicaid's role as an insurer of low-income children and, depending on the state, some of their parents.

Attitudes regarding Medicaid differ more across income and partisan groups, as we might expect for a means-tested program (in contrast to a universal social insurance program). Whereas only 12 points separated high- and low-income groups in their support of Medicare spending (Table 11.1), the groups are 23 points apart—twice as much—when it comes to Medicaid spending (Table 11.2, line 1). Similarly, while Democrats were 19 points more likely than Republicans to say that Medicare shouldn't be cut at all (Table 11.1), they are 37 points more likely to say that Medicaid spending shouldn't be cut (Table 11.2).

These greater differences in Medicaid attitudes across income and partisan groups may result from greater differences in the personal importance of the program. While higher-income and Republican respondents considered themselves somewhat less dependent on Medicare than their lower-income and Democratic counterparts, the gaps grow when it comes to Medicaid. Among those with incomes over $75,000, 41 percent said Medicare was "very important" to them and their families, but just 10 percent say the same of Medicaid. Similarly, 50 percent of Republicans describe Medicare as very important to them, while a mere 8 percent said the same of Medicaid.

The personal importance of the program plays a strong role when it comes to attitudes about its potential reform. The same May 2011 Kaiser poll asked respondents whether they wanted to "keep Medicaid as is, with

TABLE 11.2  Medicaid Attitudes across Select Demographic and Political Groups

| | | Age | | | | Income | | | | Race | | Party | | |
|---|---|---|---|---|---|---|---|---|---|---|---|---|---|---|
| | | 18–34 | 35–44 | 45–64 | 65+ | <$30K | $30–49.9K | $50–74.9K | $75K+ | W | B | R | I | D |
| Support | (1) Medicaid spending should not be cut at all to reduce deficit | 50 | 60 | 52 | 51 | 67 | 51 | 49 | 44 | 51 | 67 | 32 | 53 | 69 |
| Personal Importance | (2) How important for you and your family is Medicaid: Very important | 32 | 31 | 24 | 22 | 54 | 20 | 16 | 10 | 23 | 55 | 8 | 29 | 40 |
| | Somewhat important | 30 | 22 | 21 | 14 | 17 | 29 | 28 | 20 | 22 | 21 | 21 | 22 | 23 |
| Structural Reform | (3) Prefer keep Medicaid as it is | 63 | 61 | 61 | 57 | 77 | 62 | 56 | 47 | 58 | 82 | 39 | 57 | 79 |
| | Or fixed amount to each state | 33 | 36 | 37 | 35 | 21 | 34 | 41 | 49 | 38 | 17 | 57 | 36 | 18 |

Source: Kaiser Health Tracking Poll, May 12–17, 2011.
Note: Figures in table indicate percentages.

the federal government guaranteeing coverage and setting minimum standards for benefits and eligibility," or "change Medicaid so that the federal government gives states a fixed amount of money and each state decides who to cover and what services to pay for"—the so-called block grant proposal frequently proposed by conservatives to limit the federal government's outlay for Medicaid. Respondents overall supported the status quo over the block grant proposal, at 60 percent to 35 percent, about the same ratio of status quo to support for structural change observed for Medicare.

Age differences in support of structural reform were again muted (Table 11.2, line 3), while partisan differences were pronounced. Democrats supported the status quo at higher rates than Republicans (79 to 39 percent), while Republicans preferred block grant reform (57 percent, compared to 18 percent among Democrats; Figure 11.1). That said, personal experience with Medicaid blunts Republican support for block granting considerably. Among those who said that Medicaid was "very" or "somewhat important" to them or their family, support for the block grant reform fell to 33 percent among Republicans, and only 20 points separated Democrats and Republicans, half the gap between Democrats and Republicans overall.

## Medicaid: The Widely Recognized Safety Net

Thus personal experience matters for both Medicare and Medicaid: those who believe the programs are important to them or their families are more supportive. The main difference between the programs is that so many more Americans are accepting of the universal social insurance program than the targeted means-tested program. However, as Medicaid has expanded extensively over time, both in the groups served and the numbers of Americans covered, large and growing proportions of Americans have observed the program benefiting family members or others in need. As a result, public opinion, while not the chief factor in Medicaid's expansion, has at least been permissive, and more so than for other means-tested programs.

Public opinion has long been strongly supportive of Medicare, and, to a lesser but still impressive extent, Medicaid. Even though Medicare has funding sources well beyond the payroll tax, unlike Social Security, Medicare nonetheless enjoys status as an earned entitlement and a crucial benefit for a still-sympathetically viewed population. Public opinion has been influential

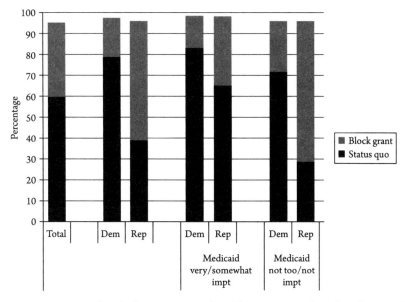

FIGURE 11.1 Support for Block Granting Medicaid by Party ID and Medicaid Personal Importance, 2011.
Source: Author calculations from Kaiser Health Tracking Poll, May 12–17, 2011.
Note: Figure shows percentages.

on policy outcomes in a broad sense: despite fiscal pressure over the years, the basic benefit hasn't been reduced, and has even been expanded with the addition of prescription drug coverage. For its part, Medicaid benefits politically from being the most popular means-tested program, one which many Americans see their family and friends benefiting from, and one for which they can project their own need in old age.

Thus the public's stance toward both programs depends on the role of personal experience. As two of the largest federal spending items, Medicare and Medicaid invite attention from budget cutters who wish to go where the money is. Thus far, however, positive public opinion has helped prevent deep cuts or structural change, in large part because of the freedom and independence these programs afford beneficiaries and their families.

## NOTES

Thanks to Sara Chatfield and Blair Read for research assistance and to Fay Lomax Cook, the editors, and conference participants for helpful suggestions.

1. Theodore R. Marmor, *The Politics of Medicare*, 2nd ed. (New York: Aldine de Gruyter, 2000), 75–76.
2. Lawrence R. Jacobs, *The Health of Nations: Public Opinion and the Making of American and British Health Policy* (Ithaca, NY: Cornell University Press, 1993), 94–99.
3. Michael E. Schiltz, *Public Attitudes toward Social Security, 1935–1965*, Social Security Administration, Office of Research and Statistics, Research Report No. 33 (Washington, DC: US Government Printing Office, 1970), 140.
4. Robert M. Ball, "What Medicare's Architects Had in Mind," *Health Affairs* 14, no. 4 (1995): 62–72.
5. Fay Lomax Cook, "Navigating Pension Policy in the United States: From the Politics of Consensus to the Politics of Dissensus about Social Security," *The Tocqueville Review* 26, no. 22 (2005): 37–66; and Jonathan Oberlander, *The Political Life of Medicare* (Chicago: University of Chicago Press, 2003).
6. Except where indicated otherwise, all poll results were accessed from the iPoll database at the Roper Center for Public Opinion Research, University of Connecticut.
7. Greg M. Shaw and Sarah E. Mysiewicz, "The Polls—Trends: Social Security and Medicare," *Public Opinion Quarterly* 68, no. 3 (Fall 2004): 395–423; and as updated through 2013 by the iPoll database at the Roper Center. Since 2002, Medicare has been outscored as a top priority by strengthening the nation's economy, improving the job situation, defending against terrorism, improving education, and securing Social Security, but has outscored other issues such as reducing healthcare costs, reducing crime, helping the poor and needy, protecting the environment, dealing with the nation's energy problem, strengthening the military, dealing with moral breakdown or dealing with global warming. See Pew Research Center for the People and the Press, "Thirteen Years of the Public's Top Priorities," January 27, 2014, http://www.people-press.org/interactives/top-priorities/.
8. United Technologies/*National Journal*, Congressional Connection Poll, October 3–6, 2013.
9. Pew Research Center for the People & the Press, Political Surveys, December 3–9, 2013; and June 15–19, 2011.
10. Kaiser Family Foundation Health Tracking Poll, September 13–19, 2012, available at http://www.pollingreport.com/health3.htm.
11. Results from CBS News/*New York Times* Poll, April 24–28, 2013 and September 19–23, 2013; CBS News Poll, October 19–21, 2013.
12. Pew Research Center for the People & the Press, Political Polarization and Typology Survey, January 23–March 16, 2014.
13. CBS News Poll, June 3–7, 2011; and January 17–21, 2014.
14. On such patterns in Social Security, see Lawrence R. Jacobs and Robert Y. Shapiro, "Myths and Misunderstandings about Public Opinion toward Social Security," in *Framing the Social Security Debate*, ed. R. Douglas Arnold, Michael J. Graetz, and Alicia H. Munnell (Washington, DC: National Academy of Social Insurance, 1998).
15. Bloomberg National Poll, February 15–18, 2013, http://www.pollingreport.com/health3.htm.
16. *USA Today*/Gallup Poll, September 16–17, 2012, http://www.pollingreport.com/health3.htm.

17. Harvard School of Public Health, Public Health Survey, May 13–16, 2013.
18. Kaiser/Harvard, The Public's Health Care Agenda for the 112th Congress Survey, January 4–14, 2011; Kaiser Family Foundation and Harvard School of Public Health, Public's Views on Medicare Survey, April 25–June 1, 2003.
19. Retirement Confidence Survey, yearly, 1996–2013. Similarly, two-thirds of 1990 Gallup respondents said that Medicare would not provide the same level of benefits it does today when they retired. See Gallup/EBRI Poll, January 1990.
20. AP-GfK Poll, August 16–20, 2012, available at http://www.pollingreport.com/health3.htm.
21. NPR/Robert Wood Johnson Foundation/Harvard School of Public Health, Retirement and Health Survey, July 25–Aug 18, 2011.
22. Kaiser/Harvard, The Public's Health Care Agenda for the 112th Congress Survey, January 4–14, 2011.
23. Gallup/CNN/USA Today Poll, May 11–14, 1995.
24. Because of space constraints, gender differences are not shown in Tables 11.1 and 11.2. Depending on the survey item, women are generally 5 to 8 points more pro-Medicare than men.
25. Although responses do vary with question wording, most polls conducted between 1995 and 2012 show only minority support for changing Medicare to a voucher or premium support model—usually around one-third of respondents—and typically strong majorities favoring the status quo. See Kaiser Family Foundation, "Polling on Medicare Premium Support Systems over Time: From 1995 to 2012," Data Note, October 2012.
26. Martin Gilens, Affluence and Influence: Economic Inequality and Political Power in America (New York: Russell Sage Foundation; and Princeton, NJ: Princeton University Press, 2012).
27. Pew Research Center Poll, June 15–19, 2011, http://www.pollingreport.com/health4.htm.
28. For a review of intergenerational conflict arguments, see Jill Quadagno, "Generational Equity and the Politics of the Welfare State," Politics and Society 17 (1989): 253–276, and Mark Schlesinger's Chapter 7 in this volume.
29. Julian Zelizer, Taxing America: Wilbur D. Mills, Congress, and the State, 1945–1975 (New York: Cambridge University Press, 1998).
30. Lawrence D. Brown and Michael S. Sparer, "Poor Program's Progress: The Unanticipated Politics of Medicaid Policy," Health Affairs 22, no. 1 (2003): 31–44; and Shanna Rose, Financing Medicaid: Federalism and the Growth of America's Health Care Safety Net (Ann Arbor: University of Michigan Press, 2013).
31. Brown and Sparer, "Poor Program's Progress"; Rose, Financing Medicaid.
32. Fay Lomax Cook and Edith J. Barrett, Support for the American Welfare State: The Views of Congress and the Public (New York: Columbia University Press, 1992), 62.
33. Kaiser/RWJ/Harvard School of Public Health, The Public's Health Care Agenda for the 113rd Congress, January 3–9, 2013.
34. Kaiser Health Tracking Poll, May 12–17, 2011.

# PART IV

# THE ROAD TO AFFORDABLE CARE

The world that Medicare and Medicaid created is not merely a world of beneficiaries, but also of the doctors, hospitals, nursing homes, and healthcare industries that rely on payments from those programs. The world that Medicaid made stretches into every state in the union, as some governors and state legislatures ask whether they can afford to keep the program, while others wonder whether they can afford *not* to keep it. Given Medicaid's origins as a smaller and weaker program than Medicare, and given that Medicare was once seen as the steppingstone toward coverage expansion, there is great irony in the fact that Medicaid, rather than Medicare, has expanded systematically over time to become one basis for the Affordable Care Act's expansion of coverage.

In Chapter 12, Keith Wailoo examines how, despite the rising rhetorical criticism of "big government" on the Right and Left in American politics, both Republicans and Democrats, from Richard Nixon and Ronald Reagan to George W. Bush, and from Bill Clinton to Barack Obama, have supported such expansions as kidney dialysis coverage, prescription drug coverage, and children's healthcare coverage. Looking beyond rhetoric, he finds that both parties have become increasingly responsive not only to the primary beneficiaries of those government programs but also to the secondary beneficiaries, including doctors, dialysis companies, pharmaceutical companies, and so on, who had grown dependent on them. Yet despite this record of expansion, as Judith Feder observes in Chapter 13, the US social insurance system as it developed over the past half-century is missing an important piece of coverage: Medicare does not cover long-term care, a major need for an aging population, and Medicaid serves only as a "last resort" back-stop for middle-class seniors who exhaust their financial assets. Feder examines how this gap came about and assesses the likelihood of action on this front. Jacob Hacker writes in Chapter 14, as concerns about costs persist and as ACA implementation continues, Medicare has become a powerful potential engine of cost control. He focuses on how Medicare went from being a servant of the medical-industrial complex to its master, and explores what perils may exist as governments wield that power in the future.

# 12

# THE ERA OF BIG GOVERNMENT

## *WHY IT NEVER ENDED*

### KEITH A. WAILOO

Facing the Republican takeover of Congress in January 1995, President Bill Clinton conceded that "the era of big government is over." With the defeat of his ambitious national health insurance plan a few months earlier and the subsequent Republican takeover of Congress, Clinton's declaration seemed to draw the curtain on 30 years of federal activism in health reform. The mid-1990s promised to bring a dire thirtieth anniversary for Medicare and Medicaid. Yet, within a year, the Republican-controlled Congress itself was embracing healthcare reform and expansion. By 1997, it had passed (and Clinton had signed) a new Children's Health Insurance program. Six years later, in 2003, Clinton's successor, Republican George W. Bush, would be the architect of another expansion—a new prescription drug benefit for Medicare recipients. And then Bush's successor, Democrat Barack Obama, would continue the trend by using Democratic control of both houses of Congress in 2010 to push through the Affordable Care Act (ACA) by the thinnest of margins. In truth, then, 20 years of big government activism followed Clinton's concession. It was also the case that both parties, often regardless of ideology, have embraced expansion and so-called bigger government.[1]

This chapter examines why Medicare and Medicaid have expanded despite enduring anti-government rhetoric and serious threats of retrenchment over the past five decades, and particularly since the rise of the political Right. While other chapters (Chapter 8 by Mark Peterson and Chapter 16 by Paul Starr) in this volume focus on why Medicare has proven so resistant to change, I turn, instead, to the political calculations on the Left and Right that have fueled the growth of both Medicare and Medicaid. Even Ronald Reagan—who famously announced in his 1981 inaugural address, "in the present crisis, government is not the solution to our problems, government IS the problem"—would oversee growth in both programs. Reagan expanded Medicaid eligibility and, toward the end of his second term, set in motion the ill-fated Medicare catastrophic care coverage provisions.[2] If one paid attention only to fierce and rising anti-government political discourse, these expansionary trends in Medicaid and Medicare's 50-year history might be surprising.

To understand the apparent paradox, we must distinguish between political rhetoric, on one hand, and the pragmatics of governance, on the other. Political rhetoric during campaigning usually creates stark binaries—Republican Party rhetoric, for example, has long hinged on the virtues of independence and freedom versus dependence on government programs, the value of hard work versus welfare, and the benefits of the private sector versus what its adherents see as the abuses of big government. Democratic rhetoric, on the other hand, has emphasized the capacity of government to help the most vulnerable, while framing conservatism as a hard-hearted and compassionless ideology aligned with business interests over people in true need. These easy and appealing "yin versus yang" frameworks have had enduring utility in politics for a half-century; yet, when faced with the challenge of governing, Republicans and Democrats alike often have governed differently than they have campaigned. When faced with political contingencies, with the task of mobilizing important constituents for coming elections, and with the pragmatics of working with Congress and the states, the stark binaries often fade. Instead, the challenge of administering social programs takes hold, and expansion has often followed.

The expansionary logic of governing becomes clear when we consider four moments in Medicare and Medicaid program reform: (1) the Nixon and Carter-era establishment and growth of a renal disease entitlement to Medicare in the 1970s; (2) the Reagan-era expansion of both Medicaid eligibility and Medicare benefits in the 1980s; (3) the Clinton-era passage of Children's Health Insurance Programs in the 1990s; and (4) the George W. Bush-era "modernization" of Medicare by adding a new prescription drug benefit. This chapter argues that for both Republicans and Democrats in power, particular challenges of governance and managing the expectations of voters and constituents have led to expansions in these programs—and almost inevitably toward bigger government and broader healthcare coverage and eligibility. At crucial stages in the last half-century, narrow political calculations by lawmakers (rather than scripted ideology) became central to the logic of expansion.

## RENAL DISEASE IN THE AGE OF ENTITLEMENT

Six years after Medicare and Medicaid had become law, two states had still not yet signed on to Medicaid; half the states that had implemented Medicaid offered only non-medical assistance. Even with these low levels of state participation, concerns about cost were already palpable and growing, casting a shadow over any future expansion.[3] By 1972 costs were becoming a "driving force" in Medicare and Medicaid policy. For much of these programs' history, then, the intense liberal goal of building on these programs—moving incrementally toward a truly national health insurance plan—met with strong resistance based on rising fiscal concerns.

In the face of continuing political pressure for national health insurance from powerful Senators like Edward Kennedy, modest expansion appealed to Republican President Nixon. As his Secretary for Health, Education, and Welfare explained, rather than allow Democrats to dictate the policy debate, "the administration sought to seize the initiative on the healthcare issue that the Democrats gained last year when they threw their support behind compulsory national health insurance…. [But] we see no need to introduce a massive nationalized health insurance program."[4] One of the moderate initiatives that Nixon supported was kidney disease legislation—expanding publicly financed access to kidney dialysis to anyone diagnosed with end-stage renal disease (ESRD). At the time, active government still retained a broad and positive meaning. "It is hard to remember," David Zarefsky has written, "but before President

Reagan and Bush redefined liberalism once again, the view of an activist government was often positive, because it had the energy to improve the human condition. Even Republican Presidents Eisenhower and Nixon felt constrained not to dismantle the major programs of the New Deal and its progeny."[5] The ESRD law emerged from this earlier era, just a few years after Medicare and Medicaid, when modest expansion still had political appeal.

*New York Times* physician/columnist Howard Rusk framed the case of Medicare expansion not as a story of big, bad government but as good government intervening in a stark drama of life and death.[6] Thousands of lives could be saved if all Americans were given access to kidney dialysis. "The fate of the 6,000 Americans with kidney disease who now die each year is squarely in the hands of those responsible for these budget cuts."[7] For such observers, renal dialysis coverage was but another incremental step in insurance coverage. For many, it foreshadowed things to come. It raised hope that, in the wake of ESRD coverage, national health insurance might someday cover other such catastrophic and expensive illnesses.[8]

The costs of the ESRD entitlement rose year by year; and as others in this volume have noted, the 1970s witnessed rising concern about spiraling costs. As US policymakers turned their attention to the goal of fiscal restraint, the ESRD program became seen in retrospect not as the next step toward wider coverage but as an outlier—a unique, diagnosis-based, special case of Medicare entitlement unlikely to serve as model for future expansion.[9] By 1978, legislators admitted to "having second thoughts" about the program's size and began searching for savings.

Costs had increased to $1 billion per year, but legislators soon discovered that such programs had become vital not only to the people it covered but also to the medical industry it underwrote. In a few short years, ESRD had created dialysis businesses and vocal constituencies who benefited from the largesse of government. Legislators discovered this fact when, for example, they considered one cost-saving proposal to move away from institution-based dialysis and toward home dialysis (purported to be less expensive than institutional care). When Congress took up this reform, lawmakers discovered that a powerful constituency—not just the elderly, but also the private dialysis marketplace and the nursing homes—quickly mobilized. Budgetary reform ran up against this new reality: the powerful health services industries that had grown as a result of the ESRD entitlement.

In part, then, the world that Medicare had created was a world of such private interests. As one observer noted, 90 percent of Americans underwent dialysis in institutions because "the United States is an island of socialism in a sea of free enterprise."[10] Reformists blamed lobbyists working for institutional dialysis for blocking changes that might have reined in costs. Even those who instinctively decried big government understood that this government expansion had benefited free enterprise. Former campaign manager for California Governor Ronald Reagan (turned Washington lobbyist) John Sears pressed congressional representatives to stand against home dialysis with one argument: "What's wrong with making a profit?"[11] Critics of big government might point to the renal dialysis program as an example of government waste and the need for cost containment, but reining in those costs would be difficult now that a private industry benefited from the program.[12]

Meanwhile, Medicaid was also in transition; by 1975, lawmakers had begun to watch with concern its expanding cost and coverage. Initial anxiety over ensuring that states signed on to Medicaid gave way to increasing worries (by 1976) about waste, fraud, abuse, and proper eligibility (see Chapter 10 by Frank Thompson in this volume).[13] In time, as Medicaid consumed more and more of state budgets, governors and state legislatures pushed for (and gained) greater control to shape the scope and coverage of the poverty program.[14] This devolution of power became a mantra of the Reagan years, with the belief that granting power to the states would lower the cost of Medicaid and also bring smaller government.

## Making Government Bigger and Better in the Reagan Years

When he was elected president, Ronald Reagan seemed unlikely to expand either Medicare or Medicaid, let alone both. In the early 1960s, he had famously decried Medicare as a fundamental assault on human freedom; his skepticism about the program endured through several campaigns for president. As president, he continued to assail big government programs, noting in the midst of the 1982 recession, "historically, whenever the economy hit a slowdown or recession in the past, the hounds of big government started their ritualistic baying, and there were demands for all sorts of pump-priming, make-work programs, public-service jobs, increased spending, and bigger deficits."[15]

In the early 1980s, Reagan's heated rhetorical assaults on social welfare programs moved the nation toward a greater hostility for big government. Indeed, during his administration the growth of domestic spending was constrained by lower tax revenues—but only somewhat. Judged by the rhetoric of the Reagan Revolution, it promised to be a turbulent time for Medicare and Medicaid. In retrospect, however, although social programs faced constant public criticism, it was a quiet time; but by the end of Reagan's second term, expansion was again in the air.

In 1987, Reagan surprised many with a vigorous call for adding Medicare Catastrophic Care (MCCA) legislation; when signed into law a year later, in his final year in office, the MCCA was characterized as the largest expansion of Medicare since the program's implementation. However, as Mark Schlesinger and Mark Peterson have explored earlier in this volume, the MCCA soon ran into political trouble and would be repealed within a year. The very mechanism that made this expansion easy for Republicans to embrace—having the beneficiaries pay for the new benefit themselves—was harshly lambasted as balancing the budget on the back of the elderly.[16] In the end, even after the MCCA's repeal (as numerous scholars like Brown and Sparer have noted), "much of what survived expanded Medicaid."[17] While the MCCA debacle has often been used to highlight the political dangers of angering Medicare recipients, the story carries another lesson: it shows that when faced with the right confluence of political pressures, even the small-government conservatives of the Reagan administration fostered healthcare expansion.

Medicaid expansion followed a different logic in the Reagan years, as the economic winds of the 1980s placed new pressures on the administration. Driven by recession and rising poverty rates, the proportion of low-income children without insurance, for instance, was rising rapidly. As one author has noted, "In 1977, about 21 percent of children living in families with incomes below 200 percent of poverty were uninsured; by 1987, this figure had climbed to nearly 31 percent."[18] Between 1984 and 1990 (spanning the Reagan and Bush years), Congress expanded Medicaid eligibility to poor and low-income children (and pregnant women) in a series of legislative actions—considered to be "among the major health policy initiatives of the late 1980s"[19] (see also Chapter 5 by Jill Quadagno in this volume.)

As a result, between 1988 and 1993 the number of children receiving Medicaid-covered services would expand by just over 50 percent.[20] In these years, these expanded programs were developing an active corps of supporters and advocates in the health and human services of both state and federal bureaucracies who served as an additional constituency.[21]

In summary, larger economic and political trends (recession, rising poverty, criticism from liberal Democrats, as well as events completely unconnected to health care) put great pressure on the Reagan administration to expand Medicare; the administration held its ground for many years, until the last year of Reagan's then-embattled presidency. As sociologist Debra Street notes, by the end of Reagan's first term, it was clear that Medicare payments were failing to keep pace with the rising costs of medical care for the elderly.[22] The appointment of a new Secretary for Health and Human Services, physician Otis Bowen, provided a catalyst for change. Some have even argued that the impetus came from elsewhere—from the administration's need for new policy initiatives in the face of the continued Iran-Contra arms-for-hostages scandal, which had cast a cloud over the Reagan presidency.[23] Others have argued that, with a growing crisis of rising numbers of uninsured and amid liberal pressure for reform, expanding coverage for catastrophic care was the easiest and least costly problem to solve because (conservatives hoped) it would be financed not by new taxes but largely by increased premiums paid by beneficiaries.[24]

The rhetoric of small government aside, expansion and spending were the norm in the Reagan years. As one scholar noted, "neither Americans nor even Republican politicians were ultimately weaned from dependence on big government. Under a Republican Congress, from 1994 to 2006, the number of earmarks for special federal spending projects tripled."[25] These expansions in eligibility during the 1980s set the stage for the establishment of the CHIP program during the Clinton administration, as the number of uninsured children continued to grow.

## EXPANSION IN THE NAME OF CHILDREN

Until the passage of the Affordable Care Act, one group has been particularly important in catalyzing the expansion of Medicaid: children. As political scientist Theodore Marmor noted in the 1970s, "Children rightly have political appeal as promising recipients of our medical dollars."[26] Indeed, throughout the century, rhetorical appeals to children's health have under-pinned health legislation—from the 1920s-era Sheppard Towner Act and the Children's Bureau through the post–World War II polio era.[27] Through the last half-century, the concern with the fate of poor children continued to be a powerful rhetorical force for Democrats, on the defensive and seek-ing to counter the conservative assault on "big government." As such, as Oberlander and Marmor discuss in Chapter 4 of this volume, children's health care became an appealing focus for expansion in the decade after Medicare and Medicaid's passage; and the plight of children became a continuing premise for expansion through the Reagan years and into the Clinton era.

In the wake of the defeat of Bill Clinton's healthcare plan, congressional Republicans cheered that expansive new programs crafted in the mold of the 1965 Medicare and Medicaid law were dead. Clinton's 1995 admission that the era of big government was over rang out like a public apology—not only for his first two years in office but also for Democrats' initiatives over the last 30 years. Little wonder, then, that when the prospects for a children's health insurance law emerged a few years later, Senate Majority Leader Trent Lott dismissed the scheme as "a big government program" that would have little chance of passing through a Republican-controlled Congress.[28] As it hap-pens, Lott had miscalculated the power of the appeal of children.

The history of the Children's Health Insurance Program (CHIP) pro-vides a case study of the politics of expansion even amidst retrenchment in the wake of the Clinton health plan's demise and the Republican take-over of Congress in 1996. Rhetorical calls for smaller government per-sisted, particularly after Republicans gained control of both the Senate and the House. Leaders of the party signaled that a new austere era had arrived when, in one single day in October 1996, Bob Dole (running to replace Clinton) "told one audience that he had voted against Medicare at its inception and Speaker Newt Gingrich told another that he expected to see the agency that administers Medicare 'wither on the vine.' "[29] In the face of such outright challenges to Medicare, and also because the prospect of losing these programs was so real, the imperative to protect them also gained a political foothold.

A year after Clinton's 1996 re-election, a Congress chastened by the pub-lic perception of its hostility to children's health care authorized $24 billion in federal funding for five years of the State Children's Health Insurance

Program (CHIP). The program extended health insurance to some 2.3 million children in 1998, according to the Congressional Budget Office. At the same time, President Clinton proposed another expansion that went nowhere—to allow individuals aged 62 to 64, as well as older displaced workers (those aged 55 to 64) to buy into Medicare. It became impossible to move this Medicare entitlement in a Republican Congress; however, the initiative in the name of children became, in time, the basis for a significant new expansion.[30]

This new benefit rested on a strategy of financing it without raising taxes, a concession to Republican control—but with a clever liberal twist. In the 1990s, the fight against big tobacco created a political opportunity: the idea of using tobacco taxes to fund the program. This mechanism for funding public programs had been adapted from the states. The CHIP proposal additionally acceded to the conservative case for "devolving" power from the federal government, giving more flexibility to the states in determining eligibility and administration. CHIP's design depended heavily on anti-tobacco campaigns: the program would be financed through either tobacco tax dollars or funds from tobacco settlements. Proposing the child bill in the Senate in 1997, Senator Edward Kennedy—the liberal powerhouse on social welfare issues—put the case bluntly to his fellow Senators: "Whose interest do you care about—the interests of the big tobacco companies? Are you for Joe Camel and the Marlboro Man, or millions of children who lack adequate health care?"[31] The argument stung Republicans who, although fully in control of Congress, were wary of standing alongside the cartoon figure that had been used in advertisements to increase the appeal of cigarettes among children.

The impetus for expanding children's health insurance also came from another corner: welfare reform. Clinton's success at moving more families from welfare to work had robbed conservatives of a powerful rhetorical issue; but it had also put more children, removed from the protection of welfare, at risk. As one study noted, "In the aftermath of welfare reform and the failure to implement comprehensive healthcare reform in the mid-1990s, pressure grew to move incrementally to broaden coverage for at least children."[32] All of these factors—the aftermath of welfare reform, the victimization of children by Joe Camel, the tobacco settlements, and the broader ideological battles of the 1990s—created fertile soil for expansion in the name of children.

It took rhetorical effort for Republicans in Congress to spin CHIP as anything other than bigger government. Looking past expansion, some conservatives praised CHIP for giving states the opportunity to experiment with market-based solutions to health care.[33] In practice, however, the federal monies expanded coverage and cost. In Texas, for instance, Republican Governor George W. Bush refused at first to accept the bargain offered by the federal initiative, waiting for his state legislature to act first. Bush asked legislators to fund families only to 150 percent of federal poverty levels, rather than 200 percent as the federal government requested. Bush's effort to hold firm against too much expansion and to speak for smaller government failed; in the end he lost his battle and the legislature voted to finance the expansion of the $180 million program with tobacco settlement money. As Bush turned to run for president, it was difficult for anyone to know exactly how the governor, and future president, would act when faced with similar challenges in national office. Perhaps the Texas skirmish over S-CHIP (as it was called in the early days) was all symbolism and electoral staging, noted one observer: "It's ... possible that Bush was trying to appease right-wingers in the Texas legislature or that he shared their concern that S-CHIP amounted to creeping Hillarycare."[34] The term (a forerunner to the term "Obamacare") was meant, of course, to disparage the CHIP program by association with First Lady Hillary Clinton, whose close involvement in the failed Clinton healthcare reform was well known.

Epithets aside, CHIP had bipartisan origins. Moreover, it was remarkable that within a year of Clinton's eulogy for big government, CHIP had arisen—in no small part owing to the skillful work of senators on the Left like Edward Kennedy, a Democrat from Massachusetts, and those on the Right such as Orrin Hatch, a Republican from Utah and a powerful congressional policy entrepreneur situated to move or hold back legislation.[35] CHIP greatly expanded Medicaid, extending health insurance to 8 million children at a cost of $40 billion. As many observers have noted, despite the tensions between healthcare expansion and contraction, in its first three decades Medicaid had gone from an add-on welfare program to the largest single insurer of children in the nation.[36] The Medicaid program also had acquired an ever-broadening constituency (with physicians, hospitals, community health centers, and others with strong interests in its preservation). In short, just as the Medicare and ESRD constituencies had grown beyond just beneficiaries to include healthcare providers, so too the Medicaid program had grown to be far more than merely a "poor person's program."[37]

## MEDICARE EXPANSION AND THE DREAM OF A DURABLE REPUBLICAN MAJORITY

Pundits and policy analysts alike often characterize the George W. Bush administration's embrace of a Medicare prescription drug benefit as the moment when small-government conservatism ran aground. Twenty years after Clinton's famous admission, it was Bush's turn to turn the rhetoric of small government on its head. By the time Bush left office, many on the Right who had once supported him now roundly criticized him as a "big government conservative."[38]

Bush's transformation was quicker and more calculated than Reagan's. He had been elected, in part, by voicing skepticism about the Clinton-era healthcare reform and the CHIP initiative. As Texas governor, he had been slow to accept the CHIP expansion. On the campaign trail, Bush used careful rhetoric—decrying big government (for its regulations, for its bureaucracy, for its restrictions on the states), but not decrying the *goals* of big government, particularly regarding expanding access to health care. As a self-styled "compassionate conservative," he noted a month before the 2000 election: "As a governor, I witnessed firsthand how the S-CHIP program has been burdened with regulations that restrict the ability of states to create innovative programs for their uninsured.... In a Bush administration, the federal government will not act as a regulatory roadblock and instead [will] work with states so that they have the freedom to innovate and create programs that reflect the needs of their uninsured populations, especially children." But on the campaign trail in search of votes in states with large elderly populations, promises to expand coverage also took center stage. Both Bush and his opponent, Vice President Al Gore, promised better and more effective government, but both also promised while campaigning in Florida to add a new prescription drug benefit to the Medicare program.[39]

Elected on the thinnest of electoral margins, and wary of the role of Florida in his future re-election battle, Bush acted on his promise to deliver on a drug benefit early in 2003; but he sought, like Reagan, to do it while upholding conservative principles of privatization. He commented, "we want to modernize Medicare to make sure that seniors can choose the coverage that fits them best, including coverage for prescription drugs." The most controversial part of the plan was linking expansion to privatization or, as one reporter noted, "the possibility of requiring the elderly to move from the traditional Medicare program to a private health insurance plan if they want prescription drug coverage, a benefit long promised to the elderly."[40] As in other Republican administrations, Bush's offer of healthcare expansion came as part of a larger bargain—a gambit to give liberals and the elderly what they wanted in order to make conservative gains. Government financing to increase access to prescription drugs, of course, would also aggrandize the companies that produced those drugs.

As uproar rose from the political Left over privatizing Medicare benefits, the Bush administration proposal evolved; on the defense for seeking to transform a popular program, his situation was not unlike Gingrich's and Dole's as they moved from minority party critics to confronting the challenge of governing as they took control of Congress in 1996. As Michigan's Democratic Senator Debbie Stabenow put it, "Instead of updating Medicare to include prescription drugs, the president is requiring seniors to join an H.M.O. to get the help they need paying for their medicines."[41] Some Republicans voiced concern over the electoral cost of this proposal, while others called for even more conservative principles (market-friendly reforms) in the Bush proposal. As one journalist commented on the ensuing fray, "While ideology and partisanship are important, healthcare in the end is an intensely local, pragmatic affair."[42]

The rhetoric of small government had one meaning to politicians seeking office; it had another meaning altogether to a politician like Bush fighting to remain president. Heading into a re-election fight against Senator John Kerry, Bush's goal of delivering results for constituents and stakeholders took precedence over the rhetoric of "small government."

In Bush's case, a powerful underlying electoral strategy to secure a permanent Republican majority also drove his administration toward expansion. The prescription drug benefit was perhaps the boldest articulation of this logic. In 2003, with Republicans controlling both houses of Congress, then, Bush signed Medicare Part D into law, even with dire predictions from the Right about looming costs. The rhetoric of small government was, apparently, only rhetoric. Conservatives decried the law as "the largest expansion of the welfare state since the creation of Medicare in 1965." As the *Wall Street Journal* noted, Bush had come to town "promising to fix Medicare and

Social Security so they would remain solvent when the baby boomers retire. But . . . the White House decided that the politics of a new drug entitlement are so good that the actual policy doesn't matter."[43] It was, the newspaper objected, an "exercise in senior pandering [designed to] win a permanent Republican majority." The president and his campaign advisor Karl Rove had their eyes, of course, on securing elderly voters in the 2004 election and in many other elections to come.

Who then is the party of big government? By and large it has been the Democrats; but, perhaps surprisingly, sometimes it's Republicans from Nixon to Reagan and Bush. It is tempting, but only partly correct, to see the past half-century of health reform as bookended by two Democratic moments of power and activism—1965 and 2010. In both years, Democrats controlled the House, the Senate, and the White House—leading, in this interpretation, to Johnson's Medicare and Medicaid, and to Obama's Affordable Care Act. Such a view of history, however appealing, ignores the reality of intervening Republican administrations in the story of big government. The real lesson of the past 50 years, then, is that the logic of expansion often defies party ideology. Republican administrations had come to appreciate that the diverse stakeholders in these programs (doctors, dialysis companies, pharmaceutical companies, hospitals, nursing homes, the elderly, and so on) are important constituencies for the party. This fact, a byproduct of the long history of these programs, ensures that these programs will endure and grow.

As these four examples—from ESRD to the prescription drug benefit—illustrate, demographic trends, economic pressures, and electoral calculations have made expansion an ever-recurring reality. Nevertheless, not all expansions are driven by the same calculation; and some types of expansion—for instance, coverage for ESRD—stand out as unique.[44] At crucial junctures in the history of Medicare and Medicaid, the pressing needs of particular recipients (dialysis patients, the elderly, children in poverty) were turned into politically potent appeals, reframing political discourse despite powerful calls for retrenchment. Finally, expansion has also been driven by political expediency. For governors in the states, for representatives in Congress, and for presidents, politics often has trumped ideology, especially in the face of impending elections. These factors (the demography of aging and childhood infirmity; their enduring potency as political concerns; and how elected officials responded to them amid electoral concerns) explain why the so-called "era of big government" decried by conservatives and eulogized by Clinton in 1994 remains very much alive and thriving in the realm of healthcare policy. The true political and economic beneficiaries of expansion have become numerous.

If rhetoric about big government has often withered in the face of governing at the national level, then so too at the state level have the realities of governance shaped unlikely Medicaid expansions. One need only consider the case of Arizona in 2013 and 2014. The state was the last in the nation to implement Medicaid, doing so in 1982—17 years after its passage. In 2013 its Republican governor, Jan Brewer, staunchly opposed the ACA; the state of Arizona was one of the 25 states that filed suit against the ACA. But once the Supreme Court ruled in favor of Obama's signature legislation, Brewer pivoted. Arizona then became the twenty-fourth state to sign onto ACA expansion.[45] Calls of traitor and "communist" greeted her, but she held firm—insisting that the federal money provided by the law was too good for the state to pass up.[46] Brewer wielded a powerful tool to get her way; she vetoed five bills until her Republican colleagues went along with the Medicaid expansion—which she characterized as "Medicaid restoration."[47]

Looking past the rhetoric, Brewer was joining a handful of Republican governors (including neighbors in New Mexico and Nevada) in endorsing the ACA's Medicaid expansion. The fight, in her view, was not about ideology and big government anymore; it was about budgets and bottom lines, and the realities of governance. "Medicaid has been here forever...," she said in one interview. "This [Obamacare] is a tiny little piece. We have a responsibility.... Other states ought to be following Arizona's lead and deliver good service at the most reasonable cost."[48] With support of Democrats and some Republicans, Arizona agreed to accept Medicaid expansion and begin receiving $1.6 billion from the federal government over the next three years; hospitals in Brewer's state would spend fewer dollars on uncompensated emergency room care. As Brewer noted, rejecting the law would mean that Arizona taxpayers would be subsidizing health care for other states. Brewer's actions are not the exception in the history of Medicare and Medicaid expansion; her case is the rule.

To be fair to politicians, this big-government doublespeak with regard to social programs is widely shared by the media and the general public. The gap between rhetoric and action (between anti-big government rhetoric running alongside support for expanding individual programs) has been observed elsewhere—often with invectives like "traitor" hurled at the breach. But as one observer noted, "When pollsters ask questions about specific government measures, it turns out that the public overwhelmingly supports virtually every aspect of big government, unless the named beneficiaries are blatant ne'er-do-wells (and sometimes even if they are)."[49] (For more on Medicare, Medicaid, and public opinion, see Chapter 11 by Andrea Louise Campbell in this volume.) In the end, we must look beyond rhetoric and discourse alone to understand what drives policy.[50]

After five decades of Medicare and Medicaid expansion, the surprising durability of these programs under both Democratic and Republican stewardship speaks to a complex relationship between Americans of all political persuasions and their big government. One observation by Ben Wattenberg in the 1980s about Social Security sheds light on another way to understand the forces shaping expansion. His observations equally apply to Medicare's appeal, and more tangentially to Medicaid. Quoting an unnamed person, Wattenberg observed that the need for government and the criticism of it were, in fact, two sides of the same coin:

> We [elderly people] don't like to take money from our kids. We don't want to be a burden. They don't like giving us money either. We all get angry at each other if we do it that way. So we all sign a political contract to deal with what anthropologists could call the "intergenerational transfer of wealth." The young people give money to the government. I get money from the government. That way we can both get mad at the government and keep on loving each other.[51]

Medicare's popularity no doubt follows a similar intergenerational logic; Medicaid involves government in different transfers of wealth and responsibility for those less fortunate, making government a third party in what many people regard as a fraught exchange—giving support directly to those in need. The anecdote captures nicely how it is that, decade after decade, the era of big government did not end, and why government could be both heatedly reviled yet also deeply valued; it remains, in short, a vital force buffering our most important and difficult relationships, regardless of party or ideology.

NOTES

1. On the anti-big government theme (a concept lumping opposition to large institutions, taxes, red tape, and waste) in the Ford 1976 campaign, see David Miles,
   "Political Experience and Anti-Big Government: The Making and Breaking of
   Themes in Gerald Ford's 1976 Presidential Campaign," *Michigan Historical Review*
   23 (Spring 1997): 105–122.
2. Ronald Reagan, inauguration address, January 21, 1981, Youtube video posted by
   C-SPAN on January 14, 2009, www.youtube.com/watch?v=hpPt7xGx4Xo.
3. Newman, 1972.
4. Richard Lyons, "Nixon's Health Care Plan Proposes Employers Pay $2.5-Billion
   More a Year," *New York Times*, February 19, 1971, 1.
5. David Zarefsky, "Presidential Rhetoric and the Power of Definition," *Presidential
   Studies Quarterly* 34 (September 2004): 607–619, quote on 615.
6. Alonzo Plough, *Borrowed Time: Artificial Organs and the Politics of Extending Lives*
   (Philadelphia: Temple University Press, 1986).
7. Howard Rusk, "Aid to Kidney Patients," *New York Times*, June 2, 1968, 90.
8. Marian Gornick, "Ten Years of Medicare: Impact on the Covered Population,"
   *Social Security Bulletin* 39 (July 1, 1976): 4.
9. "Ultimately," as Richard Rettig has argued, "the ESRD entitlement was added to
   Medicare because the moral cost of failing to provide lifesaving care was deemed
   to be greater than the financial cost of doing so."
10. Richard D. Lyons, "Concern Rising over Costs of Kidney Dialysis Program,"
    *New York Times*, April 28, 1978, A16.
11. Lyons, "Concern Rising."
12. On the cost-containment challenge in dialysis, and how the experience with
    ESRD lay the groundwork for later cost-containment strategies in Medicare,
    see James H. Maxwell and Harvey M. Sapolsky, "The First DRG: Lessons from
    the End Stage Renal Disease Program for the Prospective Payment System,"
    *Inquiry* 24 (Spring 1987): 57–67. Patricia McCormack has argued that "since
    1972, the government has been paying Renal dialysis for patients with kidney
    failure. Now there are profit-making renal dialysis centers where the charges
    add up to $24,000 a year for a patient. In a nonprofit setting the charge is
    much less—$8800. Yet the government, which is trying to contain healthcare
    costs, pays the higher bill with no public questioning of the cost." Patricia
    McCormack, "The Rising Cost of American Hospital Care," *Boston Globe*,
    April 8, 1978, 48. By 1988, the tables turned on home dialysis—now seen as
    more expensive, with costs said to be $2 billion a year. Martin Tolchin, "U.S. to
    Reduce Its Payments for Home Kidney Dialysis," *New York Times*, November
    30, 1988, A20.
13. M. Keith Weikel and Nancy A. LeaMond, "A Decade of Medicaid," *Public Health
    Reports* 91 (July–August 1976): 303–308.
14. Frank J. Thompson, *Medicaid Politics: Federalism, Policy Durability, and Health
    Reform* (Washington, DC: Georgetown University Press, 2012).
15. Quoted in Dan Wood, "Presidential Rhetoric and Economic Leadership,"
    *Presidential Studies Quarterly* 34 (September 2004): 573–606, quote on 595.

16. As Marilyn Moon has written, "It is one thing to gradually introduce income-related premiums for Medicare and quite another to have the first step be an $800 maximum premium tied to a benefit with an actuarial value of $250." Marilyn Moon, "The Rise and Fall of the Medicare Catastrophic Coverage Act," *National Tax Journal* 43 (September 1990): 380.
17. See Marmor, *Politics of Medicare*, 110–113.
18. Jessica S. Banthin and Thomas M. Selden, "The ABCs of Children's Health Care: How the Medicaid Expansions Affected Access, Burdens, and Coverage between 1987 and 1996," *Inquiry* (Summer 2003): 133–145, citing R. M. Weinick and A. C. Monheit, "Children's Health Insurance Coverage and Family Structure, 1977–1996," *Medical Care Research and Review* 56 (1999): 55–73.
19. Banthin and Selden, "ABCs of Children's Health Care."
20. Lisa C. Dubay and Genevieve M. Kenney, "The Effects of Medicaid Expansions on Insurance Coverage of Children," *The Future of Children* 6 (Spring 1996): 153.
21. L. Christopher Plein, "Activism in an Age of Restraint: The Resiliency of Administrative Structure in Implementing the State Children's Health Insurance Program," *Journal of Health and Human Services Administration* 27 (Fall 2004): 210.
22. Debra Street, "Maintaining the Status Quo: The Impact of Old-Age Interest Groups on the Medicare Catastrophic Coverage Act of 1988," *Social Problems* 40 (November 1993): 435.
23. Beth C. Fuchs and John F. Hoadley, "Reflections from Inside the Beltway: How Congress and the President Grapple with Health Policy," *PS* 20 (Spring 1987): 212–220.
24. Moon, "Rise and Fall," 371.
25. Hugh Heclo, "The Mixed Legacies of Ronald Reagan," *Presidential Studies Quarterly* 38 (December 2008): 555–574, quote on 560. See also Thomas R. Oliver, Philip R. Lee, and Helene L. Lipton, "A Political History of Medicare and Prescription Drug Coverage," *Milbank Quarterly* 82 (2004): 283–354, quote on 325.
26. Theodore R. Marmor, "The Politics of National Health Insurance: Analysis and Prescription," *Policy Analysis* 3 (Winter 1977): 25–41.
27. Richard Meckel, *Save the Babies: American Public Health Reform and the Prevention of Infant Mortality, 1850–1929* (Baltimore, MD: Johns Hopkins University Press, 1990); David Oshinsky, *Polio: An American Story* (New York: Oxford University Press, 2005).
28. Jerry Gray, "Through Senate Alchemy, Tobacco Is Turned into Gold for Children's Health," *New York Times*, August 11, 1997, A12.
29. Alison Mitchell, "Stung by Defeats in '94, Clinton Regrouped and Co-opted G.O.P. Strategies," *New York Times*, November 7, 1996, B8.
30. Katherine Schwartz, "Medicare Expansions 35 Years Later," *Inquiry* 35 (Spring 1998): 6–8.
31. Senator Edward Kennedy, in *Congressional Record: Proceedings and Debates of the 105th Congress, First Session* (May 21, 1997), 9152.
32. Cindy Mann, Diane Rowland, and Rachel Garfield, "Historical Overview of Children's Health Coverage," *The Future of Children* 13 (Spring 2003): 30–53.

33. See, for instance, John Hood, "Spoiled Rotten," *National Review* 50 (April 20, 1998): 39. As Hood commented in the conservative *National Review*, the expansion would allow states to "fund relatively free-market conservative ideas such as vouchers, tax credits, and Medical Savings Accounts." What states did, however, was more pragmatic and less ideological—they used the federal funds to support expansions of their Medicaid programs or to create or expand separate state-run health-insurance programs.

34. Jonathan Cohn, "True Colors," *New Republic*, July 12, 1999, 15–16.

35. Timothy Stoltzfus Jost, "Governing Medicare," *Administrative Law Review* 51 (Winter 1991): 81.

36. Mann, Rowland, and Garfield, "Historical Overview," 37.

37. Lawrence D. Brown and Michael S. Sparer, "Poor Program's Progress: The Unanticipated Politics of Medicaid Policy," *Health Affairs* 22 (2003): 41.

38. Michael D. Tanner, *Leviathan and the Right: How Big Government Conservatism Brought Down the Republican Revolution* (Washington, DC: Cato Institute, 2007). Bruce Bartlett, *Impostor: How George W. Bush Bankrupted America and Betrayed the Reagan Legacy* (New York: Doubleday, 2006). See also Tim Conlan and John Dinan, "Federalism, the Bush Administration, and the Transformation of American Conservatism," *Publius* 37 (Summer 2007): 279–303.

39. Calvin Woodward, "Election 2000 Tab—The Presidency—Seventeen Questions," *Yakima [WA] Herald Republic*, October 25, 2000, 1.

40. Robin Toner, "Bush, Like Clinton, Learns Perils of Health Policy," *New York Times*, February 2, 2003, 21.

41. Toner, "Bush, Like Clinton."

42. Toner, "Bush, Like Clinton."

43. "Bush's Medicare Gamble," [editorial], *Wall Street Journal*, June 23, 2003, A13.

44. John K. Ingelhart, "Health Policy Report: The American Health Care System, Medicare," *New England Journal of Medicine* 327 (November 12, 1992): 1467–1472. As Ingelhart has written, "Medicare's end-stage renal disease program is unique; it is the only instance in which a diagnosis provides the basis for Medicare benefits for persons of all ages."

45. Cindy Carcamo, "Arizona Gov. Jan Brewer Pushes Through Obama's Medicaid Expansion," *Los Angeles Times*, June 14, 2013, http://articles.latimes.com/2013/jun/14/nation/la-na-nn-ff-jan-brewer-arizona-medicaid-20130613.

46. Amanda Crawford, "Arizona's Brewer Labeled 'Traitor' as She Pushes Medicaid," *Bloomberg News*, May 23, 2013, http://www.bloomberg.com/news/2013-05-24/arizona-s-brewer-labeled-traitor-as-she-pushes-medicaid.html.

47. Website of the Office of the Governor, State of Arizona, http://www.azgovernor.gov/Medicaid.asp.

48. "Arizona Governor Staking Legacy on Medicaid," Interview with Governor Jan Brewer, 12 News Sunday Square-Off, May 19, 2013, http://www.usatoday.com/story/news/politics/2013/05/19/arizona-jan-brewer-medicaid-legacy/2324781/.

49. See, for example, Robert Higgs, "The Era of Big Government Is Not Over," *The Good Society* 9 (1999): 97–100, quote on 98. See also Richard A. Harris, "The Era of Big Government Lives," *Polity* 30 (Autumn 1997): 87–192.

50. See Jacob Hacker, "Privatizing Risk Without Privatizing the Welfare State: The Hidden Politics of Social Policy Retrenchment in the United States," *American Political Science Review* 98 (May 2004): 243–260.

51. Ben Wattenberg, *The Good News Is the Bad News Is Wrong* (New York: Simon and Schuster, 1984).

# 13

# THE MISSING PIECE
## *MEDICARE, MEDICAID, AND LONG-TERM CARE*

JUDITH FEDER

The US social insurance system that developed over the past half-century is missing a piece: protection against the unpredictable and potentially catastrophic risk of needing personal help with the basic tasks of daily life (like bathing, eating, and toileting), known as long-term care. The gap in protection reflects an explicit policy choice made when Medicaid and Medicare legislation was first crafted. In 1965, Medicaid assumed responsibility for the relatively long-standing welfare function of providing service to impoverished people of all ages unable to manage on their own. Today, Medicaid serves as the nation's long-term care safety net, financing care at home as well as in nursing homes for people who are poor or who exhaust their resources purchasing health or long-term care. By contrast, the 1965 statute explicitly prohibited Medicare from covering "custodial care," ignoring the fact that many medical conditions create long-term care needs. With the exception of some short-lived lapses, Medicare rules have restricted the program's benefits to avoid financing long-term care, even as it has paid long-term care providers, often excessively, for medically related "post-acute" services.

The results are predictable—failure to provide adequate insurance protection for people who need long-term care despite substantial, and growing, public costs. Reflecting Medicaid's welfare orientation, its spending is aggressively managed. Access to long-term care varies enormously across state programs and, in general, falls short of demonstrable need. Families accordingly bear enormous responsibility for caregiving at substantial physical and economic cost. And, as Jill Quadagno has discussed in Chapter 5 of this volume, impoverishment remains a condition for receipt of essential public services. By contrast, Medicare's far less constrained payments to long-term care providers—albeit primarily for short-term, post-acute care—have fueled growth in expenditures without actually covering long-term care.

Ironically, the overlap between the two programs in the people they serve, and the providers they pay, mislead policymakers and the public about the nation's actual long-term care investment. The result appears to be a policy paradox: rising spending on long-term care providers while, at the same time, underspending for long-term care. Misperceptions feed policy and political preoccupation with overspending, when the real problem in long-term care financing—today and, even more so, in the future—is underspending that leaves most Americans uninsured and underserved.

The paradoxical combination of substantial expenditures and limited coverage creates a political challenge: how to effectively finance long-term care for a growing elderly population, as well as for people with disabilities of working age (who make up over 40 percent of the roughly 12 million adults who currently need care). This chapter will analyze the policy decisions that have led to this position, what it means for people who need costly care, and the politics that will determine whether we eliminate, rather than perpetuate, this gaping hole in social insurance protection in the future.

THE TWO PROGRAMS AND HOW THEY GREW

Like the history of healthcare spending, the history of long-term care spending (and other spending on long-term care providers) reflects considerable growth with little planning. A distinct difference, however, is that Medicaid, a means-tested entitlement, is a major purchaser of, and states are the primary policymakers for, long-term care. States' willingness to use market and regulatory power to limit both spending on and access to long-term care differs markedly from the federal government's cautious approach to containing Medicare costs (see Uwe Reinhardt's Chapter 9 in this volume). Although Medicaid is generally an entitlement, states indirectly and directly limit access to long-term care service by paying low rates, controlling the supply of nursing home beds, and establishing waiting lists for care at home. By contrast, even when constrained, Medicare payments to some of the same providers—albeit for short-term, post-acute care—have supported excessive spending on post-acute care that has called Medicare's overall efficiency into question.

Medicaid did not initiate the federal role in financing nursing home care.[1] Support for welfare recipients in private nursing homes began with the establishment of Old Age Assistance in the 1935 Social Security Act; it expanded over the 30 years leading up to Medicaid's enactment. Just five years before Medicaid's passage, the Kerr-Mills legislation gave nursing home care a substantial boost by adopting open-ended federal matching payments to states and extending eligibility beyond people officially deemed poor to the "medically needy."

Medicaid absorbed, raised, and rapidly extended that federal commitment to all states, and both policy and business entrepreneurs aggressively responded to the newly available federal funds. An early review of program experience found that "Medicaid alone was disbursing more money on nursing homes in 1971 than had been spent in the entire industry five years earlier."[2] By consistently providing about half its revenues and contributing support for an even larger share of patients, Medicaid policy essentially built the nation's nursing home industry.

But from early days to the present, Medicaid policy toward long-term care has been a struggle. Early access expansion not only rapidly escalated spending, it also supported scandalously inadequate care and engendered egregious financial shenanigans. Legislative and administrative responses to this officially recognized "public policy failure" reflected conflicting policy goals and political pressures.[3] Federal law and state administration repeatedly promoted participation and access at the expense of quality enforcement, as policymakers responded to demands from states and providers, as well as from consumers seeking care. Not until 1986 did Congress establish detailed quality standards for nursing home care, significantly reducing, though by no means eliminating, quality concerns.[4]

On payment, federal initiatives requiring states to tie nursing home payment to costs, ostensibly to promote quality, were superseded by state efforts to constrain spending, whether by limiting the rates they paid or by directly limiting the supply of nursing home beds. Over the 1980s and 1990s, some states developed sophisticated reimbursement mechanisms designed to promote both quality and appropriate access. But the persistence of the bed shortage, which had itself been created by state policies, not only impeded the closure of substandard facilities (since patients had nowhere else to go) but also enabled nursing homes to favor profitable over unprofitable patients, including private-pay patients over Medicaid patients.[5]

The overwhelming dominance of nursing homes as long-term care providers began to shift in the mid-1980s. People able to fund their own care began to use care in less institutional settings, like assisted-living facilities, and Medicaid too began expanding options for long-term care outside the nursing home.[6] But states exercised both caution and control in their coverage of home and community-based services (HCBS). Unlike coverage of nursing home care, which the original Medicaid statute requires, coverage of care at home or in home-like settings in the community is optional. Until the 1990s, states offered very little coverage for long-term care outside institutions. Their willingness to expand these services has been largely limited to waivers from federal Medicaid requirements that require "budget neutrality"—spending no more than the program would spend without the new services. States have generally attempted to meet this requirement, and control their own spending, by limiting the numbers of people they serve.[7] Despite arguments that home care is less costly than nursing home care, states have been consistently skeptical that they could actually replace one type of service with another. So far, states have only been able to expand HCBS without increasing costs by aggressively restricting access to nursing home care and by limiting both access to and level of benefits in the community.[8]

But even by relying heavily on waiver programs that capped enrollment, states increased their investment in HCBS from 10 percent of Medicaid long-term care spending in 1988 to 28 percent in 1999.[9] A Supreme Court decision in that year, *Olmstead v L. C.*, constrained, but did not eliminate, states' use of waiting lists for home and community-based services.[10] Although waiting lists persist,[11] spending on home and community-based care has grown substantially since then, rising to 45 percent of total Medicaid long-term care spending in 2011.[12] But that average masks considerable variation, both across populations (66 percent for people with developmental disabilities, 36 percent for older people and people with physical disabilities) and across states: half the states direct more than 70 percent of their long-term spending for older people and people with physical disabilities to nursing home and other institutional services.[13] A comparison across states showed that people at home needing long-term care were more likely to go without services—risking falls; being unable to bathe, eat, or dress; or soiling themselves—in states with more limited coverage.[14]

States vary widely in supporting long-term care services for their residents—and not just with respect to home and community-based services. In 2009, the five states with the highest Medicaid spending levels spent, on average, six times as much as did the five lowest-spending states (and more than twice the level in the median state). An analysis of 2007 showed that half the states reached just over a third of low-income adults needing long-term care. The five states with the most extensive coverage reached almost two-thirds of their populations; the five states with the most restricted coverage reached only 20 percent.[15]

Medicare's approach to long-term care has a different history. Its policy reflects its designers' efforts to fend off the political charge that insurance could turn hospitals into warehouses for frail elderly people, at full public expense. To prevent such an outcome, the statute not only prohibited coverage for custodial or long-term care; it also created a new kind of post-hospital benefit intended to facilitate hospital discharge: post-acute skilled nursing and rehabilitative services, to be provided in a nursing home or at home. When the envisioned medically oriented nursing homes failed to emerge, standards were waived, terms of participation amended, and Medicare became a provider of care in the same nursing home industry that grew to serve Medicaid patients.[16]

After an initial surge in claims and spending, administrators acted swiftly to restore a limited benefit—strictly administering, or retroactively applying, coverage restrictions.[17] As a result, until the 1990s, Medicare spending on post-acute care remained relatively modest. Access to nursing homes for the relatively small number of Medicare-covered post-acute patients depended on the facilities that sprang up to serve Medicaid long-term care patients. In 1977, Medicaid provided 50 percent of nursing home industry revenues (and contributed to payment for 60 percent of residents). Medicare provided only 2 percent. Nursing homes demonstrated their considerable ability to select among patients. And Medicare patients—who were more costly, administratively burdensome, and therefore less profitable than Medicaid patients—were primarily attractive to relatively well-staffed homes for whom Medicare admissions were the entry point for longer-term stays paid for with private funds.[18]

Home health agencies, by contrast, developed primarily to serve Medicare patients. Congress grew that industry with 1980 legislation that loosened the benefit's tie to prior hospitalization and extended participation to for-profit agencies in states without licensure requirements. For a brief period spending grew in response. But aggressive application of coverage restrictions quickly reined in home health, along with nursing home spending. Tight controls limited a significant increase in spending, even when Medicare's adoption of the hospital prospective payment dramatically shortened hospital lengths of stay.[19]

Near the end of the decade, however, the courts upended the program's "arbitrary" restrictions on both nursing home and home health coverage. The resultant loosening of restrictions, exacerbated by disinvestment in claims oversight, led to dramatic escalation of Medicare spending on post-acute care.[20] From 1988 to 1996, Medicare spending on nursing home care increased from $0.9 billion to $11.7 billion; home health spending grew from $1.9 to $17.2 billion (more than three times the growth rate for the rest of the program).[21]

Over that period, the proportion of Medicare beneficiaries using nursing home or home health benefits, respectively, roughly doubled. The proportion of nursing home residents paid for by Medicare grew from 2 percent to 13 percent.[22] Medicare payments per day also increased, as nursing homes—for whom daily rates for routine nursing services had been capped—provided more uncapped and unregulated non-routine or ancillary services (like physical or occupational therapy). Much of the home health spending increase was also driven by increased use, especially the receipt of home health aide visits by people with long-term care needs. Although most Medicare beneficiaries with long-term care needs were not receiving benefits, analysts concluded that the Medicare home health benefit had moved beyond its post-acute focus into at least some long-term care to patients needing both.[23]

Congress responded to the expansion of post-acute benefits with legislation requiring the Health Care Financing Administration (the precursor to CMS) to alter its payment methods—specifically, to shift from a retrospective to a prospective payment method, as Medicare had done for hospitals in 1984. The intent was to replace the incentive of the cost-based reimbursement model with one that promoted efficiency (see Uwe Reinhardt's Chapter 9 in this volume). The shift did get Medicare home health spending out of long-term care, but it did not contain post-acute spending growth.

Medicare spending on nursing homes and home health care grew twice as fast as the rest of the program between 2006 and 2011, increasing post-acute care's share of overall (traditional Medicare) spending from 12.9 percent in 2001 to 15 percent in 2011. Medicare profit margins for nursing homes and home health agencies have been consistently high (at about 19 percent, on average, in 2010) relative to other Medicare providers. Setting payment rates in advance and allowing providers to keep amounts not spent have not increased overall efficiency. Nursing homes have taken advantage of the remaining cost-based elements of the payment system to boost per diem payments. And home health agencies have responded to powerful profit incentives by identifying more people to serve (apparently fraudulently, in some parts of the country), selecting favorably priced patients, and skimping on care.[24]

The enactment of the ACA has stimulated initiatives for Medicare payment reform, and post-acute care has been identified as a prime target for achieving better value for the dollar. A recent Institute of Medicine study determined that geographic variation in post-acute care (provided overwhelmingly but not solely by nursing homes and home health agencies) explains 40 percent of the overall geographic variation in per capita Medicare spending. This pattern fuels challenges to the program's overall efficiency. Although proposals to reduce what is widely perceived as excessive spending abound, not all take advantage of lessons from past experience that teach us that profit incentives pose potential risks to patient care—particularly when, as is the case for long-term care, quality measures and enforcement are lacking.[25]

In 2012, the nation spent an estimated $219.9 billion on long-term care. Medicaid paid the lion's share (61 percent or $134 billion), with long-term care recipients and their families paying about half the rest directly out of pocket. (A mix of public and private insurance—some similar to Medicare's post-acute care rather then actual long-term care—accounts for the rest.)[26] Current constraints on service levels and variations in states' future burdens and fiscal capacity call into question the likelihood that the current system of shared federal-state financing will be adequate to meet the needs of the nation's growing elderly population.[27]

Complicating the political challenge is the fact that not all analysts measure the current and future costs of long-term care spending in the same way. In 2013, the Congressional Budget Office issued a report assessing the impact of the growth in the nation's elderly population on public spending for long-term care.[28] Despite explicit recognition that Medicare's coverage generally focuses on short-term post-acute care rather than long-term care, the analysis simply added Medicare spending on home health and nursing homes to Medicaid's long-term care spending to measure public expenditures on "long-term care" for elderly people. The result was to approximately double actual long-term care spending, both currently and in future projections.

CBO attributed its decision to explicitly ignore differences in coverage between the two programs to the overlap of beneficiaries, providers, and—in some cases—services. But the gross exaggeration of public investment that comes from combining spending on these very different programs skews policy and political concerns about the future. Specifically, this distortion of actual public investment in long-term care reinforces political attacks on the "sustainability" of entitlement programs, while obscuring the inadequacy and inequity of public financing mechanisms for people who need long-term care.

## The Absence of Insurance for Long-term Care

Without insurance, the people who need care, and their families, bear the risk of extensive long-term care.[29] The bulk of long-term care is today provided not by public programs, but by families. Roughly 80 percent of the 11 million with long-term care needs living at home or in the community do not receive any paid services, relying solely on family and friends to provide it.[30] For many people, that may be as it should be—families doing what families do. But the health and economic costs of caregiving can be substantial.[31]

Perhaps even more important, families cannot always provide the full amount or type of care that is needed, nor can they necessarily provide it consistently over a long period of time. When paid care is necessary, its costs can far exceed most families' resources. In 2012, personal assistance at home averaged $21 an hour, or almost $22,000 annually for 20 hours a week of assistance. Adult daycare center services cost an average of $70 per day, or about $18,000 annually for five days of service per week. Assisted living services averaged $42,600 annually for a basic package of services. For people who need the extensive assistance provided by nursing homes, the average annual cost was $81,000 for a semi-private room, but costs varied widely among markets and exceeded $100,000 a year in many of the country's most expensive areas.[32]

The mismatch between the costs of these services and the resources of the people who need them is dramatic. Fewer than a third of people age 65 and over have incomes equal to or greater than four times the federal poverty level[33]—or about $44,000 for an individual age 65 or older, or $56,000 for an older couple in 2013.[34] Most people clearly cannot afford the expenses of institutional or intensive home care.

Although, in theory, savings can help fill the gap between income and service costs, in practice, savings are inadequate to the task. Most older people lack sufficient assets to finance extensive care needs. In 2013, half of the population over age 65 living in the community had savings of less than $73,000—less than the cost of a year in a nursing home.[35] Unfortunately, many people in their fifties and early sixties are not accumulating sufficient resources to cover their basic living expenses in retirement, let alone to finance potential long-term care needs. Working-age people who find themselves in need of long-term care often have not yet had the opportunity to accumulate the savings that might help pay for long-term care costs.

In contrast to health insurance, private insurance for long-term care has never really gotten off the ground and—in recent years—several insurance companies have given up on trying to market a successful product.[36] Only about 7 million people are estimated to currently hold any type of private long-term care insurance,[37] and most purchasers have relatively high incomes. The available long-term care insurance policies offer limited and uncertain benefits—raising questions about the wisdom of purchasing. Policies limit benefits in dollar terms to keep premiums affordable, but can therefore leave policyholders with insufficient protection when they most need care. Moreover, these policies have often lacked the premium stability that can assure purchasers of their ability to continue payments, a necessary condition for receiving benefits if and when the need arises.

It is not surprising, then, that people turn to Medicaid when they need long-term care. To qualify for Medicaid protection, individuals must either have low income and savings to begin with, or must exhaust the resources they have in purchasing medical and long-term care. Given the high cost of service, Medicaid support is critical to ensuring that people have access to care. But Medicaid limits the availability of care at home, where most people prefer to stay, and recipients of Medicaid benefits in nursing homes are required to spend all of their income on their nursing home care (subject to limits for people with spouses at home), except for a small monthly "personal needs allowance" of $30 to $60 in most states. Medicaid's availability is of enormous value to middle-class people who need care and otherwise lack the means to pay for it (see Chapter 5 by Jill Quadagno in this volume). But unlike insurance that protects people against financially catastrophic risks, Medicaid protection becomes available only after catastrophe strikes.[38]

Policymakers frequently overlook the unpredictable, catastrophic nature of the need for extensive long-term care. The unpredictability is obvious for people under the age of 65, only 2 percent of whom experience long-term care needs. Despite the fact that younger people with disabilities account for 5 million of the 12 million people now receiving care, public debate tends to focus overwhelmingly on older people. Evidence that 70 percent of people now turning age 65 will need some long-term care before they die is frequently cited as an argument for personal responsibility and financial planning. But the same research also demonstrated the variability of long-term care needs among people over age 65. Analysis showed that while 30 percent of older people are likely to die without needing any long-term care, 20 percent are likely to require more than two years of care. Just over 40 percent of older people are predicted to incur no care costs at all, but expenses for the costliest 5 percent are estimated in the hundreds of thousands of dollars.[39]

From a policy perspective, the logic of an insurance approach to spreading long-term care's catastrophic risk is patently obvious. But creating that policy requires political action. And that action has not been forthcoming.

## THE ABSENCE OF POLITICAL WILL

Unfortunately, political and policy logic have never been in sync when it comes to long-term care. Over the last 25 years, policymakers have attempted to remedy the gaps in Americans' health insurance, while utterly failing to address the almost total absence of long-term care insurance protection. Efforts to improve that protection have had little impact, and currently, both policy and politics focus on limiting existing benefits, rather than on establishing social insurance for long-term care.

The failed Medicare Catastrophic Coverage Act (MCCA), as discussed in several chapters of this volume, is primarily remembered for its repeal in 1989, which ended the new benefits the amendments had brought: a cap on out-of-pocket spending, coverage for prescription drugs, and elimination of the prior hospitalization requirement for Medicare coverage of post-acute nursing home care.[40] Two pieces of the law relevant to long-term care, however, survived intact: an easing of spend-down requirements to preserve some income and assets for community-dwelling spouses of Medicaid nursing home beneficiaries; and the establishment of the Pepper Commission (formally known as the Bipartisan Commission on Comprehensive Health and Long-term Care Coverage, but more familiarly after its congressional champion and initial chair, Claude Pepper). When Pepper died a few months after the commission's authorization, Senator John D. Rockefeller IV became the chair.

For Pepper, who had wanted a universal home and community-based services program, the Commission was, at best, a consolation prize. But once in existence, the Commission engaged both Democratic and Republican health leaders in Congress in deliberations on long-term care as well as healthcare policy. Eleven of the Commission's 15 members (which included three presidential appointees, in addition to members of Congress) explicitly supported enactment of a new, limited, social insurance benefit for long-term care, plus a new floor of protection against impoverishment for all nursing home users. By contrast, the Commission barely (8–7) endorsed an employer-based health insurance expansion—specifically a "pay-or-play" requirement that employers either provide health insurance or contribute to a public program that would serve their employees as well as non-workers. Two congressional Democrats joined all the congressional Republicans in voting against the recommendations to expand health insurance coverage.

At the time, Senator Rockefeller attributed members' broad endorsement of long-term care coverage—as opposed to their objection to universal health insurance—to their perceptions of political benefits and risks. On long-term care, he argued, the gains were substantial and the risks small: most Americans were uninsured; no entrenched private insurance system would be threatened; older Americans and their families were a powerful constituency; and providers would see more and better-paying patients. The opposite was true for reforming health insurance. Most Americans had insurance and were afraid of losing it; insurers and other stakeholders were well entrenched and were opposed to public intervention; the "uninsured" were not politically organized; and providers saw the prospect of less, not more, generous payment.[41]

Rockefeller's observations proved more prescient for opposition to expanding health insurance coverage than they did for support of social insurance for long-term care. In the years following the Commission's report, Congress actively considered health reform legislation that had much in common with the Commission recommendations. The Clinton health reform proposals, which were resoundingly rejected by Congress, actually included a substantial, albeit capped, universal public home care program. But throughout the contentious 1993–1994 health reform debate, the long-term care piece appeared and disappeared on the legislative landscape without attracting much political notice.[42]

When Congress picked up the problem of enacting health insurance coverage for the 15 percent of Americans without it 20 years later, it once again turned to the issue of long-term care. Given the lack of interest from both members of the public and most politicians, the law's inclusion of long-term care provisions, in the form of the Community Living Assistance and Supportive Services (CLASS) program, might be considered miraculous. Championed by Senator Edward Kennedy, whose committed staff ably and, for the most part, quietly maneuvered it through the legislative process even when he could no longer participate, CLASS established limited and voluntary public insurance for long-term care. Its benefits were constrained to fit its premium-generated financing—both benefits and premiums would be largely left to the administration to define. But the Obama administration, skeptical not only of the fiscal wisdom but also the fiscal viability of the new program, quickly abandoned its implementation and soon after acquiesced in its repeal.

The budget legislation that repealed CLASS called for a new commission to address long-term care financing—this time as a consolation prize to Senator Rockefeller, by now a long-term champion of long-term care. But, unlike the Pepper Commission, this commission lacked both congressional membership and, with few exceptions, congressional support. Its majority decided to punt on financing—presenting alternative approaches (tax credits for private insurance vs. social insurance) but offering no recommendations. Five members issued a minority report calling for tax-financed social insurance—whether comprehensive or limited—as essential to fulfilling the commission's charge and assuring meaningful access to affordable long-term care.[43] But aside from generating a modest revival of a long-standing conversation about private versus public insurance for long-term care, the commission had no impact.

In recent years, a preoccupation with the federal deficit has elevated concerns about the federal deficit to the top of the political agenda. Long-term care spending gets attention primarily as a budget issue (witness, for example, the above-mentioned CBO report that mischaracterizes Medicare payments to long-term care providers as spending on long-term care, thereby exaggerating long-term care spending). As in the budget debates of the mid-1990s, conservatives have suggested that Medicaid's open-ended federal financing be replaced with a block grant, with a substantial reduction of federal funds. And, as in the 1990s, those who push back against such so-called "entitlement reforms" argue that cutting funding and ending the entitlement would force frail elderly patients out of nursing homes.[44]

During the 1990s, however, this debate took place against the backdrop of a soaring economy. Economic growth, accompanied by tax increases, replaced budget deficits with a budget surplus. And entitlement reform—specifically, Medicare reform—morphed from spending reductions to benefit expansions. Prescription drug coverage, not long-term care, took center stage—perhaps because virtually all beneficiaries take medicine, while only some will need costly long-term care. The political conflict surrounding enactment of the Medicare Modernization Act of 2003 centered on the question of whether insurance benefits should be publicly or privately managed, not over the benefits themselves. (With George W. Bush as president and the House under Republican control, private management won.) No mention was made of long-term care.

Today, with a weak economy, and with even many Democrats in favor of limited public investment, such a shift is unlikely. The Obama administration's primary long-term care initiative illustrates the point.[45] As one of many ACA initiatives designed to promote better care at lower cost, the administration has launched demonstrations to consolidate Medicare and Medicaid for "dual eligibles"—beneficiaries who receive both—primarily in the form of managed care plans under state contracts. Both programs pay for services in nursing home and at home, albeit for different purposes, under different rules, and at different payment rates. Consolidation aims to overcome current incentives to shift costs from one program to another as providers aim to maximize revenues. Moreover, it allows plans to redistribute spending from expensive, preventable hospitalizations—a phenomenon particularly prevalent among dual eligibles—to primary and long-term care, both of which are currently underfunded.

Although consistent with other ACA initiatives to improve care and reduce costs through coordination, the dual eligible demonstrations differ in two fundamental respects. First, these demonstrations are initiated and operated by state Medicaid programs, not the federal Medicare program—despite the fact that the federal government finances 80 percent of dual eligibles' combined health and long-term care spending. The demonstrations turn governors' long-standing displeasure with financing Medicare beneficiaries' long-term care on its head. Rather than shifting dual eligibles' long-term care financing from state Medicaid programs to Medicare, as the nation's governors have long advocated, this policy shifts Medicare dollars to state Medicaid programs, potentially reducing their costs (or replacing their spending). The approach represents a "second best" solution to states preoccupied with resource constraints.

Second, these dual eligible demonstrations reduce Medicare and Medicaid payments from the outset, in contrast to most other Medicare delivery reforms that only yield public savings (which are "shared" with providers) if and when savings actually occur. These demonstrations pay health plans willing to serve dual eligibles a lower fixed rate (or capitation) per enrollee than what each program would be otherwise projected to spend and allow managed-care plans to keep any savings—or bear any excess costs—that actually result. Plans' inexperience with frail elderly and disabled beneficiaries needing a lot of care raises concern about the wisdom of this approach—perhaps contributing to the slower-than-expected rate at which they have been implemented. Nevertheless, the design of these demonstrations illustrates that, when it comes to long-term care, the policy priority is to reduce, not expand, federal financing.

## Overcoming the Medicare-Medicaid Legacy to Socially Insure Long-Term Care

Political pressure to shrink federal spending—or, more broadly, to shrink the role of government—clearly hampers political will to add the long-term care piece to the nation's social insurance. With politics challenging even existing social insurance commitments, mustering political support to extend its protections is obviously a challenge.[46] But a legacy from Medicare and Medicaid that unfortunately combines overspending with under-protection heightens the challenge. That we need a larger investment to secure meaningful insurance protection is hard—and unpleasant—for policymakers and the public to accept.

As baby boomers become caregivers and then care recipients, political leaders may come to demand better access to affordable quality care on their behalf, and possibly even gain support for the additional revenues required to finance it. If baby boomers mobilize, they will have allies in their children, who will face the financial challenges of caring for their parents while raising their own families; younger people with disabilities, who regard support for independent living as a civil right; and unions, who regard decent pay in decent jobs as a worker's right. The combination has significant potential political influence.

But success in achieving social insurance for long-term care will depend on a fundamental change in its perception. Unless the public and policymakers come to see the need for long-term care as the kind of unpredictable, catastrophic risk that individuals and families cannot be left to bear by themselves—that is, as a shared, not just a personal, responsibility—action is unlikely. Leaving care primarily in the hands of family members and underpaid workers virtually guarantees its inadequacy. Good care simply does not come on the cheap.

Achieving expanded financing for long-term care may require a fundamental change in social insurance. Decades of experience with provider-driven spending increases have made policymakers understandably reluctant to enact a new blank check. More than two decades ago, the Pepper Commission and then the Clinton administration proposal reflected these concerns by limiting benefits and, in the latter case, capping federal funds—creating the odd concept of a "capped entitlement." The CLASS design evidences even more reluctance to make open-ended commitments.[47]

Efforts to manage public spending are legitimate—indeed, they are long overdue. Other industrialized nations, who are far ahead of the United States in the aging of their populations, are reworking their social insurance models to balance spending constraints with equitable, adequate, and assured protection for long-term care.[48] But not every "innovation" will achieve that balance, and we know from experience that the United States is unlikely to follow other nations' paths. The barrier to an effective American path is, however, political, not technical. That knowledge should help its advocates chart a realistic strategy to achieve it.

## NOTES

1. For the history of Medicaid policy toward long-term care, see David Barton Smith, *Reinventing Care: Assisted Living in New York City* (Nashville, TN: Vanderbilt University Press, 2003); Robert Stevens and Rosemary Stevens, *Welfare Medicine in America* (New Brunswick, NJ: Transaction Publishers, 2003); and Bruce Vladeck, *Unloving Care* (New York: Basic Books, 1980). For a recent synthesis and update, see Sidney D. Watson, "From Almshouses to Nursing Homes and Community Care: Lessons from Medicaid's History," *Georgia State University Law Review* 26, no. 3 (2010): 937–969.
2. Stevens and Stevens, *Welfare Medicine in America*, 139.
3. "Nursing Home Care in the United States: Failure in Public Policy," Report of the Subcommittee on Long-Term Care of the Senate Special Committee on Aging, quoted in Vladeck, *Unloving Care*, 59.
4. Catherine Hawes et al., "The RAI and the Politics of Long-Term Care: The Convergence of Science and Politics in U.S. Nursing Home Policy," in *Implementing the Resident Assessment Instrument*, Milbank Memorial Fund Electronic Reports, May 2003, http://www.milbank.org/uploads/documents/interRAI/030222interRAI.html#usfn4.
   On current compliance issues, see Center for Medicare Advocacy, "Federal Nursing Home Enforcement System Is Not Punitive: Setting the Record Straight Again," http://www.medicareadvocacy.org/federal-nursing-home-enforcement-system-is-not-punitive-setting-the-record-straight-again/.
5. On nursing home payment, regulation, and the shortage of beds, see Vladeck, *Unloving Care*; William Scanlon, "A Theory of the Nursing Home Market," *Inquiry* 17 (1980): 25–41; Judith Feder and William Scanlon, "Regulating the Supply of Beds in Nursing Homes," *Milbank Quarterly* 58, no. 1 (1980): 54–88; Josh Wiener

and David Stevenson, "Repeal of the Boren Amendment: Implications for Quality of Care in Nursing Homes" (Washington, DC: The Urban Institute, 1998), http://www.urban.org/publications/308020.html.

6. Christine Bishop, "Where Are the Missing Elders?" *Health Affairs* 18, no. 4 (1999): 146–155, doi:10.1377/hlthaff.18.4.146; David Grabowski et al., "Assisted Living Expansion and the Market for Nursing Home Care," *Health Services Research* 47, no. 6 (2012): 2296–2315, December 2012, doi:10.1111/j.1475-6773.2012.01425.x.

7. "Understanding Medicaid Home and Community Services: A Primer," Office of the Assistant Secretary for Planning and Evaluation, US Department of Health and Human Services [HHS], October 2000.

8. For a review of the literature, see Pam Doty, "Cost Effectiveness of Home and Community-Based Long-Term Care Services," Office of Disability, Aging, and Long-Term Care Policy, HHS, June 2000, http://aspe.hhs.gov/daltcp/reports/2000/costeff.htm. For a more recent view and a longer-term perspective, see H. Stephen Kaye, Mitchell LaPlante, and Charlene Harrington, "Do Noninstitutional Long-Term Care Services Reduce Medicaid Spending," *Health Affairs*, 28, no. 1 (2009): 262–272, doi:10.1377/hlthaff.28.1.262.

9. HHS, "Understanding Medicaid Home and Community Services," p. 8.

10. Sara Rosenbaum, "The Olmstead Decision: Implications for Medicaid," Kaiser Family Foundation, March 2000, http://kff.org/medicaid/issue-brief/the-olmstead-decision-implications-for-medicaid/.

11. Kaiser Family Foundation, "Waiting List for Medicaid Section 1915 (c) Waivers," 2010, http://kff.org/health-reform/state-indicator/waiting-lists-for-hcbs-waivers-2010/; Terence Ng, "HCBS Waiver Wait List Estimates 2012," September 10, 2013, http://nasuad.org/documentation/HCBS_2013/Presentations/9.11%2010.00-11.15%20Roosevelt.pdf.

12. Terence Ng et al., "Medicaid Home and Community-Based Services: 2010 Data Update," Kaiser Commission on Medicaid and the Uninsured, March 2013, http://kff.org/medicaid/report/medicaid-home-and-community-based-service-programs/.

13. Judy Feder and Harriet Komisar, "The Importance of Federal Financing to the Nation's Long-Term Care Safety Net," Georgetown University and The Scan Foundation, February 2012, http://www.thescanfoundation.org/sites/thescan-foundation.org/files/Georgetown_Importance_Federal_Financing_LTC_2.pdf.

14. Harriet Komisar, Judith Feder, Judith Kasper, "Unmet Long-Term Care Needs: An Analysis of Medicare-Medicaid Dual Eligibles," *Inquiry* 42, no. 2 (2005): 171–182.

15. Feder and Komisar, "The Importance of Federal Financing."

16. Vladeck, *Unloving Care.*

17. Vladeck, *Unloving Care.*

18. Judith Feder and William Scanlon, "The Underused Benefit: Medicare's Coverage of Nursing Home Care," *Milbank Quarterly, Health and Society* 60, no. 4 (1982): 604–632.

19. William J. Scanlon, "Medicare Post-Acute Care," Testimony before the Committee on Finance, US Senate, April 1997, http://www.gao.gov/assets/110/106821.

pdf. See also "Medicare's Post-Acute Care Benefit," Office of Disability, Aging, and Long-Term Care Policy, HHS, January 1999, http://aspe.hhs.gov/daltcp/reports/1999/mpacb.pdf.

20. Scanlon, "Medicare Post-Acute Care."

21. Scanlon, "Medicare Post Acute Care," and HHS, "Medicare's Post-Acute Care Benefit."

22. Bishop, "Where Are the Missing Elders?"

23. Scanlon, "Medicare Post-Acute Care"; and Harriet Komisar and Judith Feder, *The Balanced Budget Act of 1997: Effects on Medicare's Home Health Benefit and Beneficiaries Who Need Long-Term Care*, The Commonwealth Fund, February 1998, http://www.commonwealthfund.org/~/media/files/publications/fund-report/1997/dec/the-balanced-budget-act-of-1997--effects-on-medicares-home-health-benefit-and-beneficiaries-who-need/komisar_bba-pdf.pdf.

24. This discussion reflects the author's summary of findings by the Medicare Payment Advisory Commission (MedPAC), as presented in Kaiser Family Foundation, *Policy Options to Sustain Medicare for the Future*, January 2013.

25. Judith Feder, "Bundle with Care—Rethinking Medicare Payment for Post-Acute Care Services," *New England Journal of Medicine* 369 (August 1, 2013): 400–401, doi:10.1056/NEJMp1302730.

26. Carol O'Shaughnessey, "National Spending for Long-Term Care Services and Support (LTSS) 2012," National Health Policy Forum, March 27, 2014, http://www.nhpf.org/library/the-basics/Basics_LTSS_03-27-14.pdf.

27. Feder and Komisar, "The Importance of Federal Financing."

28. Congressional Budget Office, "Rising Demand for Long-Term Services and Supports for Elderly People," June 2013, http://www.cbo.gov/publication/44363.

29. This section draws heavily on Feder and Komisar, "The Importance of Federal Financing," with data updated as noted.

30. This estimate of the long-term care population comes from Stephen Kaye's analysis of the 2012 National Health Interview Survey, 2010 Census, and 2010 Nursing Home Data Compendium, presented in testimony to the Long-Term Care Commission, September 17, 2013. The estimate of family caregiving relies on Kaye's analysis of the 2007 National Health Interview Survey and 2004 National Nursing Home Survey, presented in Feder and Komisar, "The Importance of Federal Financing."

31. Lynn Feinberg et al., "Valuing the Invaluable 2011 Update: The Growing Contribution and Costs of Family Caregiving" (Washington, DC: AARP Public Policy Institute, June 2011), http://assets.aarp.org/rgcenter/ppi/ltc/i51-caregiving.pdf; and Susan Reinhard, Carol Levine, and Sarah Samas, "Home Alone: Family Caregivers Providing Complex Care," AARP and United Hospital Fund, October 2012, http://www.aarp.org/home-family/caregiving/info-10-2012/home-alone-family-caregivers-providing-complex-chronic-care.html.

32. Prices are from the MetLife Mature Market Institute, *Market Survey of Long-Term Care Costs: The 2012 MetLife Market Survey of Nursing Home, Assisted Living, Adult Day Services, and Home Care Costs*, November 2012. Retrieved on March 24, 2014 from https://www.metlife.com/mmi/research/2012-market-survey-long-term-care-costs.html#keyfindings.

33. Zachary Levinson et al., "A State-by-State Snapshot of Poverty among Seniors," Kaiser Family Foundation, May 20, 2013, http://kff.org/medicare/issue-brief/a-state-by-state-snapshot-of-poverty-among-seniors/.

34. US Census Bureau, Poverty Thresholds 2013, https://www.census.gov/hhes/www/poverty/data/threshld/.

35. Gretchen Jacobson et al., "Income and Assets of Medicare Beneficiaries 2013–2030," Kaiser Family Foundation, January 2014, http://kff.org/medicare/issue-brief/income-and-assets-of-medicare-beneficiaries-2013-2030/.

36. For a recent assessment of the long-term care insurance market, its limitations, and suggestions to improve it, see Richard Frank, Mark Cohen, and Neale Mahoney, "Making Progress: Expanding Risk Protection for Long-Term Services and Supports Through Private Long-Term Care Insurance," The Scan Foundation, March 2013, http://www.thescanfoundation.org/sites/thescanfoundation.org/files/tsf_ltc-financing_private-options_frank_3-20-13.pdf.

37. Frank, Cohen and Mahoney, "Making Progress."

38. Some critics have argued that people "transfer," rather than exhaust, their assets to qualify for Medicaid, allowing even well-to-do people to qualify for Medicaid benefits. But evidence shows the following realities: (1) few older adults have the income or wealth that would warrant such transfer; (2) people in poor health are more likely to conserve than to exhaust assets; (3) for the elderly population as a whole, the transfers that do occur are typically modest (less than $2,000); and (4) transfers associated with establishing eligibility are not significant contributors to Medicaid costs. Feder and Komisar, "The Importance of Federal Financing."

39. Peter Kemper, Harriet Komisar, Lisa Alecxih, "Long-Term Care over an Uncertain Future: What Can Current Retirees Expect?" Inquiry 42, no. 4 (Winter 2005–2006): 335–350.

40. Jonathan Oberlander, The Political Life of Medicare (Chicago: University of Chicago Press, 2003).

41. Senator John D. Rockefeller IV, "The Pepper Commission Report on Comprehensive Health Care," New England Journal of Medicine 323 (October 4, 1990): 105–107, doi:10.1056/NEJM199010043231429.

42. Joshua Wiener et al., "What Happened to Long-Term Care in the Health Reform Debate 1993–1994?" Milbank Quarterly 79, no. 2 (2001): 207–252.

43. "A Comprehensive Approach to Long-Term Services and Supports," Alternative Report of the Long-Term Care Commission, September 23, 2013, https://georgetown.app.box.com/s/h6ri85lam79vt58bma3e.

44. Edwin Park and Matt Broaddus, "Ryan Medicaid Block Grant Proposal Would Cut Medicaid by One-Third by 2022 and More after That," Center for Budget and Policy Priorities, March 27, 2012, http://www.cbpp.org/files/3-27-12health.pdf; Frank J. Thompson, Medicaid Politics: Federalism, Policy Durability and Health Reform (Washington, DC: Georgetown University Press, 2012).

45. Judy Feder et al., "Refocusing Responsibility for Dual Eligibles: Why Medicare Should Take the Lead," Urban Institute, October 2011, http://www.urban.org/UploadedPDF/412418-Refocusing-Responsibility-For-Dual-Eligibles.pdf.

46. On budget politics and Medicare, see Oberlander, *Political Life of Medicare*; on Medicaid, see Thompson, *Medicaid Politics*.

47. For a review of policy proposals on long-term care financing, see Alice M. Rivlin and Joshua M. Wiener, *Who Will Pay?* (Washington, DC: The Brookings Institution Press, 1988); *Report of the U.S. Bipartisan Commission on Comprehensive Health Care* [The Pepper Commission] (Washington, DC: GPO, 1990), http://www.allhealth.org/publications/Uninsured/Pepper_Commission_Final_Report_Executive_Summary_72.pdf; Joshua Wiener, Laura Illston, and Raymond Hanley, eds., *Sharing the Burden: Public and Private Strategies for Long-Term Care Insurance* (Washington, DC: The Brookings Institution Press, 1994); Judith Feder, Harriet Komisar, and Robert Friedland, "Long-Term Care Financing Options for the Future," Georgetown University, June 2007, http://hpi.georgetown.edu/ltc/papers.html; William Galston, "Live Long and Pay for It: America's Real Long-Term Care Crisis," *The Atlantic*, September 12, 2012, http://www.theatlantic.com/business/archive/2012/09/live-long-and-pay-for-it-americas-real-long-term-cost-crisis/262247/; Majority and Minority Reports of the Congressional Long-Term Care Commission, September 2013, http://mccourt.georgetown.edu/mspp-professor-issues-alternative-report.

48. Jose-Luis Fernandez et al., "How Can European States Design Efficient, Equitable and Sustainable Funding Systems for Long-Term Care for Older People?" World Health Organization, Policy Brief No. 11, 2009, http://www.euro.who.int/__data/assets/pdf_file/0011/64955/E92561.pdf.

# 14

# FROM SERVANT TO MASTER TO PARTNER?

## MEDICARE, COST CONTROL, AND THE FUTURE OF AMERICAN HEALTH CARE

JACOB S. HACKER

The TV ad warned, "$700 billion cut from Medicare for seniors," as grainy images of distressed older Americans passed across the screen.[1] Such ads are a staple of election campaigns in Florida, the state with the oldest population in the nation. And so it was no surprise that they dominated the airwaves during the 2014 midterm election. The surprise was who sponsored them: the Republican Party. After all, most Republicans opposed Medicare in 1965, and the party has been repeatedly battered since then for even hinting at program cuts. Yet here was the GOP accusing President Barack Obama and congressional Democrats of trashing Medicare to fund the Affordable Care Act (ACA), the biggest expansion of publicly guaranteed insurance since the creation of Medicare itself. It was as if Obama had been transformed into former GOP House Speaker Newt Gingrich, who infamously suggested that Medicare would "wither on the vine" if his party had its way.[2]

Since the roiling debate over the ACA in 2009 and 2010, Republicans have successfully positioned themselves as Medicare's protectors—the last line of defense against nefarious Democratic plans, real or imagined, to gut the program to aid the poor and uninsured. Perhaps the most successful attack concerned "death panels," a minor provision allowing Medicare to fund end-of-life counseling that became, in extreme portrayals, a federal plan for euthanizing America's aged. Though fabricated, the charge stuck: more than a third of Americans older than 65 said they believed that the ACA would "allow a government panel to make decisions about end-of-life care for people on Medicare."[3] Perhaps worse for Democrats, fully half said the law—which expanded Medicare's prescription drug coverage and expressly prohibited cuts in Medicare benefits as a way of slowing spending—would reduce benefits that were previously provided to all people on Medicare.[4] In the 2010 midterm elections, older Americans favored Republicans by a 21-point margin after essentially splitting their vote between the parties four years prior. Almost a quarter of the voters who gave the House of Representatives back to the GOP were over 65, a demographic share that won't be reached in the United States (where roughly 13 percent of people are over 65) until at least 2050.[5]

This reversal—and the backlash that contributed to it—opens the door to a new era in Medicare's history. It is an era that contains perils as well as opportunities: for the Democratic Party, for the Medicare program, and above all for the goal of medical cost-containment. Over the 50 years of Medicare's operation, as this chapter will trace, the program has undergone an epochal transformation. From a "servant" of the medical industry, Medicare has moved, step by step, toward a very different role: a "master" of medical costs, exercising the kind of broad powers over prices, practices, and performance deployed by public authorities in other rich nations. When it comes to serious cost control, as the debate over the ACA made clear, the scale, purchasing power, and established infrastructure of Medicare now make it the only game in town. Yet, as that debate also revealed, it is a dangerous game. Excessive reliance on Medicare as the engine of national cost control could foster a political backlash inimical not only to cost-containment but also the successful implementation and expansion of the ACA. Indeed, the belief that the ACA threatens Medicare has become a powerful new barrier to the program's assumption of greater and more effective purchasing power.

In the famous words of Joseph Heller in *Catch-22*, "Just because you're paranoid doesn't mean they aren't after you." Older Americans are certainly paranoid about Medicare, but they aren't responding entirely to wisps of GOP fantasy. The ACA *does* rely heavily on reducing the growth of Medicare spending—not merely to fund benefits for the uninsured but to make American health care fiscally sustainable overall. For all the talk about innovative ways of "bending the cost curve" during the ACA debate, federal policymakers consistently focused on the one lever they have used again and again over the last generation: Medicare. Born as a passive purchaser that fueled medical inflation, Medicare has become an increasingly assertive buyer. As discussed by Uwe Reinhardt in Chapter 9 of this volume, the program has pioneered some of the most consequential developments in provider reimbursement, from diagnosis-related groups (DRGs) that fix hospital payments according to a patient's initial diagnosis, to the resource-based relative value scale (RBRVS) that links physician payments to skill, resource intensity, and effort. Though hardly unambiguous successes, these reforms have reduced the growth of Medicare spending per patient to a level significantly below the private-sector standard, and it has held the prices paid by Medicare to much lower and more consistent levels as well.

Today, however, reformers are asking Medicare to do something new—to become the vehicle for system-wide cost control. And this presents a Catch-22 of its own. Medicare's success to date has rested as much on supportive political conditions as capable policy levers. Tight federal budgets impelled policymakers to strengthen Medicare's capacity for cost restraint. But these policy moves were made palatable by politically dividing the providers of care from those who received it, by restraining prices while preserving benefits. Explicitly harnessing Medicare as a means to reduce spending across the board threatens to undo this jujitsu balance, creating increasingly stark conflicts between Medicare's role as a guarantor of health security for the aged and its role as a restrainer of health costs for all Americans. This the Catch-22: the more policymakers lean on Medicare to do what they could not do during the 2009 debate—directly confront the healthcare industry to reduce costs and improve care—the more they threaten the political foundations of both Medicare and the ACA.[6]

Perhaps this dilemma will lessen. If the modest medical inflation of recent years continues, Medicare's finances may improve so much that GOP attacks become hard to sustain (since 2009, the date at which the Part A trust fund is expected to be exhausted has increased by 13 years). Slowed spending growth would also give policymakers the breathing room to move gradually toward stronger cost-control. Yet in today's polarized politics, the ACA can't and won't follow Medicare's post-1965 trajectory, in which bipartisan coalitions, leaning heavily on technical analyses of payments and processes, gradually tightened the spending screws. Even if medical inflation remains muted—a big *if* given the historical trajectory of US spending—the political foundations for such coalitions simply do not exist. Nor should one underestimate the capacity of committed politicians to sustain distorted images of policy realities. If Medicare is to escape its Catch-22, neither cosmetic changes nor better talking points will be enough. Instead, efforts at medical spending restraint will need to move beyond its confines, so that cost control becomes increasingly separate from the operation of a defined program for the aged and disabled. Medicare, in short, needs to become a *partner* in the process of system-wide cost control, not the sole agent. Whether Medicare makes this leap depends on how well reformers learn the lessons from its remarkable transformation thus far.

## Medicare as Servant

Medicare is distinctive in cross-national perspective. No other affluent democracy began national insurance coverage with the aged. Nor does any other act so passively with regard to health coverage and spending for kids and working-age adults. These two exceptional characteristics are linked. The struggles that preceded Medicare resulted in a program both limited in scope and largely hands-off when it came to costs. Most nations conceded price-setting to providers at the outset, but because they created publicly overseen insurance plans covering most citizens, they had *latent* capacity to restrain rising expenditures across the board.[7] Medicare had some hidden capacities, it turned out. But it would not extend its reach—and hence its scope for direct control of costs—beyond the aged and disabled.

What was a bane for cost control, however, was a boon for political entrenchment. Medicare virtually created the modern senior lobby, and its single insurance pool and close association with Social Security encouraged a sense of shared fate and common interest among its members.[8] With a highly engaged beneficiary population, the program quickly became politically entrenched, as Paul Starr discusses in Chapter 16. But this engagement also created serious barriers to cost control. In a system of diffuse insurance pools, Medicare was the one big payer. While this gave it leverage, it also created a cohesive enrollee lobby that limited cost control to certain relatively limited forms of price regulation for providers accepting Medicare. The effects of Medicare on medical reimbursement more broadly had to come mainly through the diffusion of Medicare practices into private insurance plans.

In its early years, however, diffusion went the other way.[9] The private insurance market—dominated by provider-friendly Blue Cross and Blue Shield plans—paid doctors "usual and customary" rates, and so, therefore, did Medicare. The problem was that these rates were neither standard nor stable. Doctors and hospitals charged Medicare whatever they felt they could, with the predictable result of skyrocketing costs. Medicare's backers and administrators largely saw this as the price to pay for establishing the program, and they hoped that an established program would become the basis for insuring other segments of the population, such as children. Needless to say, this hope was not borne out. Runaway costs gelled an elite perception of the program as costly and inefficient, while proposals for expanded coverage went down in flames.

By the early 1980s, however, a rapprochement of sorts had emerged. Conservatives conceded that Medicare was impregnable; a core public program would exist, even if private plans might come to assume a larger role within it. Many in the political center, meanwhile, came to believe that Medicare was not a realistic foundation for expanding insurance. They focused instead on expanding Medicare's step-sibling, Medicaid, while pursuing various (invariably failed) strategies for increasing private coverage. The big programmatic fights over Medicare had ended—at least for a time.

Instead, policymakers enacted a series of rationalizing reforms to rein in Medicare's spending growth without challenging its fundamental premises or core benefits. Cast as technical fixes, carefully calibrated to focus the pain on providers rather than patients, these adjustments transformed Medicare from an inflationary emulator of the private sector into an increasingly efficient pioneer of payment innovations. In each case, the changes resulted from bipartisan deals brokered by Republican presidents and the leadership of Democratic congresses. And in each case, after some fixes and fights, the changes stuck.

More important, they largely worked. From the fastest-growing part of the health system in the 1970s, Medicare soon became the slowest, and its edge grew over time. Figure 14.1 compares per-person spending growth for the same set of benefits between Medicare and private plans between 1969 and 2012. Medicare's strong comparative performance is all the more remarkable because over this period its beneficiaries were growing older as life expectancy of the aged increased. In addition, Medicare out-performed the private sector despite the adoption by private plans of many of its payment modalities, including, most notably, the DRG approach to paying hospitals.

There was one notable exception to this story of structural stasis alongside purchasing leadership: at the insistence of Republicans, Congress and the executive branch pursued regulatory changes that increased the role of private insurance plans within the program. The original rationale for incorporating private plans rested on the assumption that tightly managed health maintenance organizations (HMOs) could deliver better outcomes at a lower cost. For a variety of reasons, however, the expanding role of private plans *increased*, not lowered, Medicare spending—by almost $300 billion

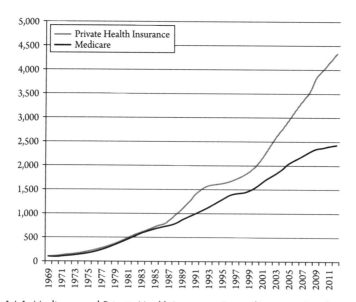

FIGURE 14.1 Medicare and Private Health Insurance Expenditures per Enrollee, 1969–2012 (1969 = 100).

Source: https://www.cms.gov/Research-Statistics-Data-and-Systems/Statistics-Trends-and-Reports/ NationalHealthExpendData/Downloads/tables.pdf, Table 21

between 1985 and 2012, according to a recent calculation.[10] For starters, most of the plans that enrolled Medicare beneficiaries were *not* tightly managed HMOs, but were looser plan models (including, remarkably given the original rationale, plans that used the same payment approach as Medicare). What's more, under the reforms, any savings won by private plans had to be funneled back into broader benefits rather than lower premiums. Indeed, Medicare beneficiaries in these plans came to expect these broader benefits and, in turn, to oppose efforts, such as those contained in the ACA, to reduce the implicit and explicit subsidies for generous private plans.

Even more important, Medicare reimbursed private plans using a formula that based payments on the average cost of Medicare beneficiaries, but the plans generally enrolled healthier, lower-cost beneficiaries. Though Congress repeatedly changed the payment formula in an effort to more accurately capture the risk of plan subscribers, plans in turn became adept at gaming these "risk scores," sometimes through outright fraud. From 2008 to 2013, plans received more than $70 billion in "improper" payments, according to the Centers for Medicare and Medicaid Services—most of them increased charges due to mischaracterization, or lack of documentation, of patients' actual risk. Over this period, risk scores rose roughly twice as fast within private plans as within traditional Medicare, a disparity that can only be explained by the aggressive inflation of risk scores.[11] In the fictional town of Lake Wobegon described by the humorist Garrison Keillor, "all the children are above average." In Medicare private plans, it seemed, all the old people were sicker than average.

Finally, Medicare beneficiaries enrolled in generous private plans were not the only ones who wanted them subsidized. Republicans who thought that Medicare should be replaced with a federal voucher for private coverage (sometimes called "premium support") also sought to encourage the plans to remain in the program to create the case for this more privatized approach. In this sense, the expansion of private plans, though not highly partisan on the surface, signaled the re-emergence of the long-dormant partisan schism over Medicare's basic structure.

The expansion of Medicare to include prescription drugs in 2003 bore the mark of this increasing polarization. After Republicans gained control of both Congress and the White House, they pushed for this traditionally Democratic goal to improve their standing with seniors and to head off Democratic plans for a prescription drug benefit within Medicare. Rather

than the simple option of incorporating drug coverage into Medicare's benefit package, the new benefit would be handled by private plans—either
existing comprehensive plans of the sort Medicare already paid or new
stand-alone plans just for drug coverage. A moment's reflection on Medicare's
history—or the experience of other rich nations, all of which have much
lower drug costs—would suggest that dividing responsibility for coverage
among many new plans would reduce the chance of bargaining down prescription prices. But that was precisely the point. The pharmaceutical industry and providers wanted a benefit design that did as much as possible to put
money in their pockets and as little as possible to hold down prices.

It was a pattern that would repeat itself during the battle over the
Affordable Care Act, with major potential consequences for Medicare's
future.

## The Contentious Beginnings of a New Era

The struggle over the ACA in 2009 brought to the fore the two dominant
features of Medicare's post-1965 development: Medicare's growing role as
the one big purchaser in American health care, and the continuing resistance of Medicare beneficiaries to reforms that might impose visible losses
on them. For the first time, however, these two realities directly conflicted
with each other. Given the political and budgetary constraints, reformers
could have cost control through Medicare or they could have the support, or
at least acquiescence, of the aged. They could not have both.

The conflict reflected the political resistance to cost control *outside*
Medicare. As in 2003, providers and insurers sought support without
restraint. Americans should be required to have private insurance, they
argued, but neither federal nor state governments should be able to exercise
control over spending or compete directly with private plans. Shore up a
crumbling market, in other words, but don't restrict that market's size.[12]

Politicians had good reason to pay attention to these demands. Health
reform went down in flames under President Bill Clinton in 1993 in significant part because of the energized resistance of insurers, drug companies, and medical providers. This time around, companies lobbying on
healthcare spent $1.2 billion in 2009 alone, with over 1,700 companies and
organizations hiring roughly 4,525 lobbyists—eight for each member of
Congress—to press their case on the issue.[13] Not surprisingly, the money

was mostly on the side of the medical industry. For example, the pro-reform group Health Care for America Now! spent less than $300,000 on four lobbyists in 2009. By comparison, Pharmaceutical Manufacturers and Research of America, the advocacy arm of the drug industry, employed 186 lobbyists and spent over $26 million.[14]

In 2009, unlike in 2003, federal policymakers could not so blithely ignore the total bill. For one, Democrats had reinstated so-called pay-as-you-go rules that required that all new spending be financed through new revenues or lower spending elsewhere. Expanded coverage had to be paid for. For another, the long-term viability of any health reform rested on reducing the rate of growth of American health spending. If costs continued to climb as they had in the past, not only would consumers and corporations be impoverished, so too would federal and state governments.

And so it was that the unstoppable force of cost control ran headlong into the immovable object of Medicare's unified constituency. In the resulting collision, all the hopes (and fears) surrounding "bending the cost curve" fell onto Medicare. Talk of death panels, bureaucratic rationing, and Medicare as a fiscal piñata were wrong in almost every respect but one: Medicare was indeed being harnessed for system-wide cost control.

Consider the official numbers from Congress's budgetary watchdog, the Congressional Budget Office. According to CBO estimates, expanded coverage for the uninsured through Medicaid and state-based insurance "exchanges" would cost around a trillion dollars over 10 years. That amount would be financed in two primary ways—actually more than financed, since the law was projected to reduce the federal deficit. The first was new taxes of around $500 billion. (Most of these also concerned Medicare: the ACA broadened and increased the program's dedicated payroll tax.) The second, and far more controversial, source of financing was a roughly $700 billion reduction in projected Medicare spending. These cuts, in turn, consisted of three roughly equal sources: reduced payments to private plans, reduced payments to hospitals, and a series of smaller tweaks, such as lower payments to home health providers.[15]

Put another way, virtually all of the "scorable" savings in the ACA—that is, savings the CBO was willing to forecast—came from reductions in the projected growth of Medicare. For good reason, the CBO looked skeptically on the claims of the law's defenders that huge efficiencies would come from competition among health plans, expanded preventive care, and new health plan models with fancy acronyms (such as ACOs, or account-able care organizations—networks of providers that are supposed to work together to deliver better care). The CBO wanted to see strategies of spending restraint that had worked in the past. The cuts in Medicare payments to plans and providers fit the bill.

The law also created an Independent Payment Advisory Board (IPAB) for the program that would be quite different from the largely toothless payment advisory commission the program has long had. IPAB would be required to put forth cost-containment proposals whenever recent and projected Medicare spending rose faster than a predetermined rate. More important, these recommendations would go into effect automatically *unless Congress voted otherwise.* In an age of gridlock, such votes were unlikely to succeed.

Whether IPAB ever gets off the ground remains very much in doubt. The medical industry hates it, and a majority in Congress would probably repeal it immediately if they had a chance (indeed, they have already voted to cut the funding for its creation). To supporters of stricter cost control, IPAB's potential currently looks weak, given that spending has been far below the specified target and given that slated—but perpetually postponed—reductions in physician payment levels make future growth rates look rosier than they actually will be. (CBO is required to assume that Congress will let these reductions go into effect even though it has voted to block them again and again.) To make IPAB's mandate harder still, Republicans in Congress will do everything they can to block nominations to the board. Yet if IPAB survives, it could become the foundation for more sustained and aggressive efforts to control Medicare costs. Moreover, the incentive to use Medicare to cut federal spending growth will remain, whether or not IPAB survives.

None of the ACA cuts to Medicare reduced benefits directly. Again, the law *expanded* prescription drug benefits, as well as Medicare coverage of no-cost preventive care. Going forward, the ACA explicitly forbids IPAB from considering benefit cuts in its efforts to slow spending. In keeping with history, Medicare would use its purchasing power to hold down prices. This time, however, it would be holding down prices to improve American health care—not just the sustainability or performance of Medicare. That was a fateful difference: no matter how many new benefits for seniors or assurances that benefits were sacrosanct were in the ACA, the reality was that Medicare would spend less than projected so that people outside Medicare would get more.

It did not take long, of course, for Republicans to discover the many benefits of pointing this reality out. Older Americans were once relatively reliable Democratic voters. For more than two decades, however, they have leaned Republican. They are less diverse racially than younger Americans, and a nontrivial share are dismayed by the country's ongoing demographic transformation. Older Americans also form the backbone of the Tea Party—a movement whose anti-government animus does not extend to programs for the aged, which adherents portray as wholly earned benefits, unlike alleged giveaways such as health coverage for the poor.

No matter that Republicans had long criticized both Medicare and Social Security programs as runaway "entitlements."[16] No matter that they would soon take for granted Medicare's reduced spending in their own budget proposals. Foolish consistency may not be the hobgoblin of little minds, but it is certainly the hobgoblin of savvy politicians. Attacking the ACA as a mortal threat to Medicare was political gold for Republican politicians: it hurt the popularity of reform, and it helped the popularity of the GOP with its most engaged voters.

In a sense, Medicare's designers did their job too well. They wished to create a strong constituency to protect against regression, thinking that additional steps forward were in the cards. But, as Mark Schlesinger argues in Chapter 7 of this volume, the structure of Medicare and the mobilization of the aged that it fostered meant that this constituency was acutely sensitive to benefit threats and deeply resistant to larger health reforms if they appeared to pose such threats. The ACA was almost tailor-made to provoke this threat-response. Its long-term success—in following Medicare's path toward entrenchment as well as in restraining costs—rests on whether reformers can overcome it.

## MEDICARE AS MASTER?

Since the financial crisis of 2008, health costs have done something unusual: they have stopped rising, or at least have stopped rising at the meteoric rates that have made the United States the highest-spending nation in the world. Initially, the slowdown could be attributed to the economic downturn, as families tightened their belts and workers lost coverage. But the slowdown has persisted even as the economy has (painfully and gradually) recovered. To be sure, employers and insurers have shifted more costs onto insured workers, jacking up premiums, deductibles, and copayments. But no changes of this sort have happened in Medicare, and Medicare has seen the greatest deceleration of any payer. From 2011 until 2014, the real growth of spending per beneficiary was essentially zero. In early 2014, it fell into negative territory.[17] As already noted, thanks to slowed growth (and the new taxes contained in the ACA), the date at which the Medicare trust fund begins to run a deficit has shifted more than a decade into the future.[18]

Yet no one should be sanguine about the continued restraint of Medicare costs, much less those of American health care as a whole. Even if Medicare spending per person remains stable, the share of the population on Medicare is growing quickly. Starved of bureaucratic capacity for years—fewer people work for Medicare today than did in 1980—the program is also administratively taxed.[19] Moreover, the ACA's mechanisms for cost control are politically vulnerable. A unified Republican government could reverse them overnight, though Republicans would have to say how they would make up the difference (something that no GOP budget plan so far has done; all of them have instead assumed the ACA's level of restraint).[20] Though Medicare can continue to ratchet down payments to providers, savings from further-reaching reforms of the delivery of care are likely to prove more distant and elusive. And there is no guarantee that even successful reforms adopted within Medicare will diffuse into the private sector. Providers have become increasingly consolidated and, with their substantial market power, are demanding higher rates. In some markets, they receive payments that are double the rate of Medicare payments. Some exclusive hospitals charge five to seven times as much.

Most important, however, Medicare and the ACA are likely to remain in an uneasy alliance so long as Republicans have strong incentives and capacities to mobilize beneficiaries of Medicare against perceived threats. To be sure, the strength of these attacks may lessen as it becomes clear that Medicare savings will not come from direct benefit cuts. But decades of research on public opinion and political behavior do not foster great confidence that experience alone will turn the tide.[21] If end-of-life counseling can become death panels, the possibilities for creative distortion are pretty expansive. So long as Medicare remains in the vulnerable position of restraining its beneficiaries' expenditures to increase those of Medicaid patients and the previously uninsured, the ACA and its cost-containment strategies will rest on shaky foundations.

Thus policymakers of the future face a twin challenge: how to simultaneously strengthen Medicare's tools of cost control and shift the strategy of system-wide control away from the near-exclusive reliance on Medicare. Doing so will require tackling the underlying source of both rising Medicare spending and America's exorbitant healthcare costs: the lack of broad price restraint in American health financing.

## THE HEALTHCARE RENT IS TOO DAMN HIGH!

During one of the 2012 Republican presidential debates, an unexpected contestant shared the stage with Mitt Romney and other top contenders. His name was Jimmy McMillan, a former male stripper running under the banner of the Rent Is Too Damn High Party. (Perhaps recognizing how few Republican voters are renters, the candidate known for his odd facial hair and Jiminy-Cricket-style white gloves changed the slogan for the campaign to "The Deficit Is Too Damn High!") Given that McMillan comes from New York City, one can understand why he chose to focus on housing costs. But if there is one form of rent that is really too damn high, it is the exorbitant amount that Americans pay for health care. In the lingo of economics, a "rent" is excess payment made to market actors because of their political or economic power. The rents in health care consist of enormously wasteful levels of spending that result from policies tilted toward the medical industry within a market marked by vast imbalances of information and influence between patients and providers.

That's the bad news. The good news is that getting control of these costs would provide a major boost to the US economy—directly because health costs are a major threat to the economic security of workers and their families, and indirectly because they are the biggest threat to America's long-term fiscal outlook. Without "rent control" in health care, public and private budgets will be crushed under the ever-growing burden of medical costs.

The United States spends vastly more than other rich nations on medical care—almost twice as much per person as the next most profligate nation, Switzerland, and about $700 billion more overall in 2006 than predicted by our per capita income.[22] The main reason for this higher spending is not greater utilization of care: Americans visit doctors less often and spend less time in the hospital after treatment, they are younger on average, and there are fewer doctors and hospital beds per capita than is the norm among rich nations.[23]

Instead, the main reason we spend so much more is that our healthcare prices are so much higher than those found in other rich nations. In 2012, a routine office visit cost $30 in Canada and France—and an average of $95 in the United States. The total hospital and physician cost of bypass surgery was $26,432 in New Zealand, $17,729 in Switzerland—and an average of $73,420 in the United States. The cost of hip replacement was $11,187 in the Netherlands, $11,889 in the United Kingdom—and an average of $40,364 in the United States. And these are just the averages. At the 95th percentile (that is, the price just below the top 5 percent of prices), that office visit runs $175, that bypass costs $150,515, and that hip replacement costs $87,987.[24] Prices are not just extraordinarily high in the United States, in other words; they are extraordinarily variable as well.

High prices equal high incomes for providers, drug companies, medical device manufacturers, and other industry players. They do not, alas, equal better health outcomes. Whether analysts are comparing across nations or across regions of the United States, they typically find little or no link between prices and quality.[25] Despite all the excess spending in the United States, Americans live shorter lives, experience poorer overall health than citizens of most other rich nations, and die from preventable causes at higher rates.[26] The quality of American health care is not the sole, or even the primary, reason for this poor performance. But at the very least, we are not getting good value for our money.

These cost differences add up. If American expenditures had risen at the rate of Swiss expenditures between 1980 and 2010, we would have spent $15 trillion less on health care overall. Even in the jaded world of health costs, that is a lot of money (enough, for example, to send more than 175,000 kids to a four-year college).[27] Looking forward, America's long-term deficit problem is basically a healthcare-spending problem. Take out Medicare and Medicaid, and the federal budget is more or less balanced as far as the eye can see.[28] Ever-escalating health spending means not just less disposable income for workers and their families, but also less budgetary scope to upgrade non-health benefits or to invest in education, infrastructure, technology, and other critical sources of future growth. No healthcare cost-containment, no American Dream.

Fortunately, effective public and private efforts to control costs could make an enormous difference. Other countries restrain spending better than we do for a simple reason: they create countervailing power to push back against all the industry players seeking higher incomes. These strategies do not require a "single payer," where the government acts as a public insurer for basic services. The Swiss, for instance, purchase private insurance—but the government closely regulates the insurance industry and the prices charged by providers. In other nations, the state oversees negotiations between providers and insurance funds. But no rich nation besides the United States leaves cost control to decentralized negotiations between private insurers and providers—negotiations in which increasingly consolidated and politically mobilized providers almost invariably hold the upper hand.

We do not need international experience to demonstrate this point. Medicare, as we have seen, has controlled costs better than private insurers precisely because it has some measure of countervailing power. Yet, as we have also seen, Medicare's power is limited in many ways. Not only does it cover only the elderly and disabled, but the medical-industrial complex has also managed to limit Medicare's countervailing power in myriad ways. Take Medicare's highly passive model of pharmaceutical insurance. Because Medicare does not have the power or capacity for drug price negotiation, companies have been able to charge exorbitant prices. Lipitor, a cholesterol drug used by many beneficiaries, costs roughly $100 a month in the United States—and $6 in New Zealand. The nasal medication Nasonex runs $108 a month for Medicare beneficiaries—and $29 in Canada. On most dimensions, Canada and New Zealand are as market-oriented as the United States.[29] They just don't allow manufacturers with limited-duration monopolies (thanks to patent protections) to charge whatever a distorted market will bear.

## WHITHER MEDICARE?

Faced with the reality of runaway prices, many on the Right blame patients' lack of "skin in the game." They insist that shifting more risk and costs onto patients—especially Medicare beneficiaries—will increase their incentive to shop around and bargain for better prices.[30] But health care is not a normal market. The asymmetry of information between providers and patients is huge. Shopping around, especially at the time of treatment, is often prohibitively difficult ("Wait, don't pull out my rupturing appendix; I want to see what the place down the street charges!"). High-tech care simply cannot be financed without insurance, but insurance rightly protects the most costly patients whose expenses account for the vast bulk of our overall spending. (The costliest 10 percent of Medicare beneficiaries account for more than 60 percent of spending.)[31] They cannot have skin in the game unless we allow them to lose all their skin.

Transforming Medicare's guaranteed benefits into a fixed voucher makes sense only if we pretend that the health costs borne by individuals are fundamentally different from those borne by the federal government. Simply shifting costs from the federal government to patients will not control them for all the reasons just mentioned—and may even cause costs to rise by reducing the pressure on federal policymakers to improve Medicare's efficiency. That is a poor bargain for today's older Americans. It is an even worse bargain for younger generations, who are facing greater insecurity in the workforce today and will be required to face greater insecurity in retirement, too.

If shifting costs and risks isn't the solution, what is? Real spending control—as opposed to measures that just shift spending around—depends on sustained restraint on the actual costs of care. And the only proven way to achieve that restraint is through active purchasing by public authorities who either buy care directly or establish rules that set prices for multiple purchasers. This could be achieved through a variety of strategies. Medicare could be expanded to include younger Americans—for example, 55 to 64-year-olds and children under age 10, with coverage gradually extended to all age groups. Or the so-called exchanges through which Americans can buy regulated and subsidized private insurance under the ACA could include a "public option" (that is, a public insurance plan that pays rates based on those of Medicare), allowing younger Americans without secure workplace coverage to have the same kind of choices that older Americans have. Or "all-payer" rates could be established at the state or federal level to create standard prices across all insurers that pay doctors and hospitals on a fee-for-service basis.

All of these strategies would involve breaking open the demographic silos of our present inefficient system and fostering countervailing power on the purchasing side of health care. Rather than move Medicare toward the private model of multiple plans and limited coverage, these approaches would do just the opposite: they would augment the Medicare model of concentrated bargaining power and move it outside Medicare to encompass younger Americans. This would not only allow the public sector to better control costs, but would also create pressures on private insurers to adopt public innovations in cost control and care management. More important, it would reduce the current tension between Medicare and the ACA created by the law's heavy reliance on slowing Medicare spending to finance new coverage for the non-elderly.

## LEARNING FROM THE PAST

The problem, of course, is the politics. But the politics of system-wide cost control is arguably no less fraught than the politics of shifting ever more expenses onto Medicare beneficiaries, a constituency not exactly known for its quiescence.[32] Medicare's history suggests that policymakers will sometimes do the right thing—when they exhaust all other alternatives. Caught between the rock of rising costs and the hard place of imposing losses on Medicare beneficiaries, politicians of both parties chose again and again to augment Medicare's capacity to hold down prices.

The ACA is much more complex than Medicare, of course. It relies on private plans and on state Medicaid programs and health exchanges, rather than a relatively simple national program. Nor are its main beneficiaries anywhere near as politically engaged or powerful as America's aged. Nonetheless, if the basic aspects of the ACA became substantially entrenched—as they are likely to if Democrats hold the White House after President Obama—fiscal imperatives will likely take center stage, as they did in the debate over Medicare, encouraging political leaders to push back against provider demands for blank-check reimbursement.

The prospects for bipartisan deals in response to these imperatives are much less certain. The contemporary GOP differs dramatically from the Republican Party of Ronald Reagan and the George H. W. Bush. By every measure, the Republican Party has moved substantially to the right, and at a faster pace than the Democratic Party has moved left.[33] With the Tea Party fielding primary challengers and the most conservative elements of the business community spending hundreds of millions to push an anti-government agenda, the kinds of bipartisan deals that elevated Medicare's capacity for cost control are much harder to envision. Serious forward movement may therefore depend on splits within the GOP coalition—and the strengthening of moderate forces more generally, including within the business community. Needless to say, these outcomes are by no means guaranteed.

Money also matters more in American politics than it did a generation ago, and the medical industry has learned how to use that money to significant effect. Consider the fate of the ACA's cuts in Medicare payments to private plans. Private health plans lost the battle in 2010, but they may yet win the war. In 2013, the ACA was supposed to cut Medicare's payments to private plans by 2 percent; instead, lawmakers of both parties stepped in to pressure CMS to reverse the cuts. In the end, CMS *increased* them by 3 percent. As one industry consultant boasted, the reversal was a "direct reflection of muscle this program has obtained. It's now nearly 30 percent of the [Medicare] program and that gives it a lot of juice."[34] The 10 largest insurers that market private plans to Medicare beneficiaries (in terms of enrollment of people within the program) had more than 140 lobbyists working for them. Yet insurers are not content to rely exclusively on inside-the-Beltway strategies. They have also created the Coalition for Medicare Choices, a classic "astroturf" organization designed to rile up older Americans to ensure that private plans continue to be overpaid. The architect of Medicare, Wilbur Cohen, liked to say that successful social policy was 1 percent inspiration and 99 percent implementation. That may be true, but it's also the case that implementation is when the self-interested, the resourceful, and the organized often have the upper hand.

Still, advocates of more effective policies have won battles in the past, and they could do so yet again. The key will be recognizing the two big lessons of Medicare's increasingly successful strategy for restraining costs: cost control requires countervailing power, and politics cannot be an afterthought. Indeed, cost control depends at least as much on getting the politics right as it does on getting the policies right.

For now, the primary political imperative must be reducing the perceived conflict between strengthening Medicare and providing all Americans with affordable coverage. Unless we give up on cost control—and failure here really is not an option—this will require political coalitions strong and broad enough to win victories against well-resourced and politically savvy industry players. It would be good if these coalitions crossed traditional political lines, uniting labor unions concerned about the security of benefits and business leaders worried about the bottom line, Democrats hoping to make coverage more available, and Republicans wishing to make government leaner. It would be even better if these coalitions included the tens of millions of Americans older than 65 who rely on America's most popular and successful health program.

NOTES

1. "NRCC Says Obamacare Cuts Money from Medicare and Seniors," *PoliticFact.com*, February 14, 2014, http://www.politifact.com/truth-o-meter/statements/2014/feb/14/national-republican-congressional-committee/nrcc-says-obamacare-cuts-money-medicare-and-senior/.

2. Gingrich's entire statement (made in 1995) was: "Now, we don't get rid of it in round one because we don't think that's politically smart, and we don't think that's the right way to go through a transition. But we believe it's going to wither on the vine." Quoted in Adam Clymer, "The Ad Campaign: Organized Labor Goes on the Offensive and the Republicans Cry Foul," *New York Times*, 20 July 1996, http://www.nytimes.com/1996/07/20/us/politics-ad-campaign-organized-labor-goes-offensive-republicans-cry-foul.html.

3. Elise Viebeck, "Poll: Four in 10 Believe in Obama Healthcare Law 'Death Panels,'" *The Hill*, September 26, 2012, http://thehill.com/policy/healthcare/258753-poll-four-in-10-believe-in-health-law-death-panels.

4. Viebeck, "Poll."

5. Byron Tau, "Seniors Fled Democrats in Midterm," *Politico*, November 7, 2010, http://www.politico.com/news/stories/1110/44802.html; "Mid-Term Voters: Older, Whiter, Righter," *The Economist*, May 17, 2014, http://www.economist.com/news/united-states/21602212-mid-term-electorate-year-will-be-white-america-was-1983-and-old-it.

6. For example, the "public option" (a reform idea that, full disclosure, I helped develop) would have created a Medicare-like public plan for Americans younger than 65, but this provision was killed during the legislative battle. See Jacob S. Hacker, "The Road to Somewhere: Why Health Reform Happened," *Perspectives on Politics* 8, no. 3 (2010): 861–876.

7. Theodore R. Marmor and David Thomas, "Doctors, Politics and Pay Disputes: 'Pressure Group Politics' Revisited," *British Journal of Political Science* 2, no. 4 (1972): 421–442.

8. Jonathan Oberlander, *The Political Life of Medicare* (Chicago: Chicago University Press, 2003), 45.

9. Jacob S. Hacker, *The Divided Welfare State: The Battle over Public and Private Social Benefits in the United States* (New York: Cambridge University Press), ch. 5.

10. Ida Hellander, Steffie Woolhandler, and David U. Himmelstein, "Medicare Overpayments to Private Plans, 1985–2012," *International Journal of Health Services* 43, no. 2 (2013): 305–319.

11. The CMS conclusions, released through a Freedom of Information Request, as well as the rate of growth in risk scores, are discussed in a three-part series by the Center for Public Integrity, available at http://www.publicintegrity.org/health/medicare/medicare-advantage-money-grab.

12. A discussion of these concessions can be found in Paul Starr, *Remedy and Reaction: The Peculiar American Struggle for Health Care Reform* (New Haven, CT: Yale University Press, 2011), 203–206.

13. Joe Eaton and M. B. Pell, "Lobbyists Swarm Capitol to Influence Health Reform," Center for Public Integrity, February 24, 2010, http://www.publicintegrity. org/2010/02/24/2725/lobbyists-swarm-capitol-influence-health-reform.

14. Data from Center for Responsive Politics, http://www.opensecrets.org/lobby/ (retrieved on June 12, 2014).

15. The most complete recent estimate of these savings was done by the CBO in 2012: CBO, "Letter to the Honorable John Boehner Providing an Estimate for H.R. 6079, the Repeal of Obamacare Act," July 24, 2012, http://www.cbo.gov/ publication/43471.

16. Theda Skocpol and Vanessa Williamson, *The Tea Party and the Remaking of Republican Conservatism* (New York: Oxford University Press, 2012).

17. Jason Furman and Matt Fiedler, "Alongside Expanded Coverage, Underlying Slow Growth in Health Costs Is Continuing," May 27, 2014, http://www. whitehouse.gov/blog/2014/05/27/alongside-expanded-coverage-underlying-slow-growth-health-costs-continuing.

18. Testimony of Paul Van de Water, Senior Fellow, Center on Budget and Policy Priorities, before the Committee on the Budget, US House of Representatives, January 26, 2011, http://budget.house.gov/uploadedfiles/vandewater012611. pdf.

19. Robert A. Berenson, John Holahan, and Stephen Zuckerman, "Can Medicare Be Preserved While Reducing the Deficit?" Urban Institute, March 2013, http:// www.urban.org/UploadedPDF/412759-Can-Medicare-Be-Preserved-While-Reducing-the-Deficit.pdf.

20. Couldn't Democrats simply filibuster such a move? Not if Republicans undid these provisions through the so-called reconciliation process through which the US federal budget is made. Reconciliation bills cannot be filibustered under Senate rules. Indeed, Democrats used the reconciliation process to pass the final healthcare legislation that combined separate House and Senate bills. To be sure, there are germaneness rules that limit the use of reconciliation, but changes in Medicare financing would surely pass the test.

21. For a good introduction to this research, see Larry Bartels, "The Irrational Electorate," *Wilson Quarterly* 32, no. 4 (Autumn 2008): 44–50.

22. Diana Farrell et al., "Accounting for the Cost of U.S. Health Care: A New Look at Why Americans Spend More," McKinsey & Company, December 2008, http://www.mckinsey.com/insights/health_systems_and_services/accounting_ for_the_cost_of_us_health_care.

23. Gerard F. Anderson et al., "It's the Prices, Stupid: Why the United States Is So Different from Other Countries," *Health Affairs* 22, no. 3 (2003): 89–105, doi:10.1377/hlthaff.22.3.89.

24. Ezra Klein, "21 Graphs That Show America's Health-Care Prices Are Ludicrous," *Washington Post* Wonkblog, March 23, 2013, http://www.washingtonpost.com/ blogs/wonkblog/wp/2013/03/26/21-graphs-that-show-americas-health-care-prices-are-ludicrous/.

25. Peter S. Hussey, Samuel Wertheimer, and Ateev Mehrotra, "The Association Between Health Care Quality and Cost: A Systematic Review," *Annals of Internal Medicine* 158, no. 1 (January 2013): 27–34.
26. Steven H. Woolf and Laudan Aron, eds., *U.S. Health in International Perspective: Shorter Lives, Poorer Health* (Washington, DC: National Academies Press, 2013), http://obssr.od.nih.gov/pdf/IOM%20Report.pdf.
27. David Blumenthal, "Controlling Cost Through Increasing Value: A View from the South," Keynote Address at the Canadian Association for Health Services and Policy annual conference, Vancouver, British Columbia, May 28, 2013, https://www.cahspr.ca/web/uploads/presentations/Keynote_David_Blumenthal.pdf.
28. Henry J. Aaron, "Budget Crisis, Entitlement Crisis, Health Care Financing Problem—Which Is It?" *Health Affairs* 26 (November 2007): 1622–1633, doi:10.1377/hlthaff.26.6.1622.
29. Diane Archer, "Strengthen Medicare: End Drug Company Price Setting," *Health Affairs* blog, May 28, 2013, http://healthaffairs.org/blog/2013/05/28/strengthen-medicare-end-drug-company-price-setting/.
30. The most prominent of such plans was introduced by Paul Ryan in 2011. The CBO concluded that it would require that a typical 65-year-old would pay 68 percent of the total cost of their coverage (premiums and all out-of-pocket costs) by 2030, compared with 25 percent under current law. For example, by 2030, under the plan, typical 65-year-olds would be required to pay 68 percent of the total cost of their coverage, which includes premiums, deductibles, and other out-of-pocket costs, according to CBO. CBO, *Long-Term Analysis of a Budget Proposal by Chairman Ryan* (Washington, DC: CBO, April 5, 2011), 22, http://www.cbo.gov/sites/default/files/cbofiles/ftpdocs/121xx/doc12128/04-05-ryan_letter.pdf.
31. Congressional Budget Office, *High-Cost Medicare Beneficiaries* (Washington, DC: CBO, 2005), 5, http://www.cbo.gov/sites/default/files/cbofiles/ftpdocs/63xx/doc6332/05-03-medispending.pdf.
32. Jacob S. Hacker, "Healthy Competition: The Why and How of 'Public-Plan Choice,'" *New England Journal of Medicine* 360 (2009): 2269–2271, doi:10.1056/NEJMp0903210.
33. Jacob S. Hacker and Paul Pierson, *Winner-Take-All Politics: How Washington Made the Rich Richer—And Turned Its Back on the Middle Class* (New York: Simon & Schuster, 2010), 264–266.
34. Fred Schulte, "Medicare Advantage Lobbying Machine Steamrolls Congress: Fear of Senior Voters Turns Critics into Champions," Center for Public Integrity, June 10, 2014, http://www.publicintegrity.org/2014/06/10/14881/medicare-advantage-lobbying-machine-steamrolls-congress. The remainder of this paragraph draws on the Center's report.

# PART V

# LOOKING AHEAD

That programs conceived amid the social turmoil of the 1960s have endured and have remained cornerstones of American social policy 50 years later requires that we look not only backward, to explain how and why they have withstood the test of time, but also forward. What can Medicare and Medicaid tell us about the future of the Affordable Care Act? How do compromises in the course of fashioning such legislation create and entrench some rights—giving Medicare beneficiaries, for example, a strong sense of entitlement? How do those legislative compromises give rise to features of law that even supporters may come to regret?

James Morone and Elisabeth Fauquert, in Chapter 15, look back to examine not only the origins of these programs, but also the ways in which Democratic administrations have gestured toward the social insurance ideal present at the inception of Medicare, only to embrace the market thinking that has become so prevalent in modern healthcare politics. They analyze the political tides bringing this neoliberal vision to bear, and speculate on what the next chapter might be in the rise and fall of social insurance. Paul Starr, in Chapter 16, looks both back and ahead, asking what makes a reform built to last? He analyzes the design of Medicare, Medicaid, and the Affordable Care Act as producing different kinds of entrenchment, and sees the ACA as at risk for becoming entrenched, but in a much-degraded form.

# 15

# MEDICARE IN AMERICAN POLITICAL HISTORY

## THE RISE AND FALL OF SOCIAL INSURANCE

JAMES MORONE AND ELISABETH FAUQUERT

After Harry Truman won his long-shot presidential election, he put national health insurance before Congress. Democrats had won majorities of 92 votes in the House and 12 in the Senate. Even so, the unlikely proposal provoked ferocious opposition—cries of socialism were especially effective as the Red scare began to engulf the nation. *Newsweek* summed up the conventional wisdom about his prospects: "No chance." In 1952, near the end of his term, Truman grudgingly agreed to a tactical retreat: win the national health plan for elders, show America how well it works, and then extend the program to the rest of the population.

Thirteen years later, President Lyndon Johnson signed Medicare (along with Medicaid) into law, sitting next to a beaming Harry Truman. As a program, Medicare became indispensable—one of the pillars of American social welfare policy. As a political strategy for winning national health insurance, it proved a bust. Medicare thrived but, if anything, it subverted the effort to expand healthcare coverage. Two questions dominate the analyses of Medicare and American politics. How and why did legislation win? And why did it fail to expand?

Scholars have been exploring these questions for decades. Medicare won in 1964 because a small cadre of health reformers kept the idea alive; because the second-largest Democratic landslide in presidential history burst the congressional stalemate; and because adroit leadership seized the moment and added physician care and Medicaid to the original proposal.[1] The program never expanded beyond elders because, once enacted, the policy changed the politics: Medicare's rising costs put expansion out of bounds; senior citizens organized to fight off any changes to "their" program; and pusillanimous Democrats lost their verve and focused on the easy fight to protect what they had already won.

Most of these accounts focus tightly on Medicare and the debates surrounding it. Here we zoom out to explore the political and economic frame of the debate. Placing Medicare in historical time offers a fresh perspective on why such an ambitious social policy was on hand in 1965, why the concept of social insurance vanished, and how it might fare in the future.

Four features of the waning New Deal era help explain the Medicare moment. A discordant Democratic coalition—very liberal and highly conservative—dominated American politics; though conservatives routinely blocked liberal reform, when conditions were right, they eased passage in ways that would not be possible once the parties sorted themselves by ideology. A highly egalitarian American political economy—the most equal since the Civil War—offered a plausible setting for ambitious universalism. Very low immigration rates lowered the temperature of the American culture wars. And, for a brief instant, the American racial divide looked tractable to a majority in both parties.

Then everything changed. The Democratic coalition shattered. The United States careened from its most egalitarian era to what may be its most gilded age. Immigration reform (signed just two months after Medicare) injected the high-temperature tribal politics of "us and them." Race once again fractured the society. The new dynamics fostered very different politics and made ambitious social policy increasingly implausible.

These two eras—the New Deal and the "gilded age"—produced very different ideas about national healthcare reform and the future of Medicare. Even Democratic presidents spoke in a different tongue. Social insurance segued into arguments about individual choice, efficiency, and maximizing returns.

Our purpose here is to look beyond healthcare politics and to place Medicare in the larger context of American political history. The first part of the chapter examines Medicare's passage. A second section underscores what made 1965 unique by contrasting it with the very different era that followed. After that, we suggest how the new political economy changed the politics of Medicare. Finally, we briefly speculate about what Medicare might look like after another 50 years.

## THE MEDICARE MOMENT

When Wilbur Mills strode to the House floor to preside over the final debate and passage of Medicare, he did so in the twilight of a New Deal dispensation that stretched back 30 years. There were few signs that this Congress—about to enact its most important social reform—would be the last of its kind. The Medicare program was perfectly fit to the times. Consider four features of the political economy that facilitated universal social insurance.

First, the Democratic Party dominated national politics. It had won seven of the last nine presidential elections, averaging a whopping 424 Electoral College votes compared to Republicans' 101. In Congress, the Republicans had managed only four years in control. The lopsided results, however, obscure the Democratic Party divide between Southern conservatives and Northern liberals.

The Southerners ferociously protected segregation, fought unions, and subverted most social reforms. Seniority rules and the South's pattern of re-electing its members (until they retired or died) meant that conservative Southerners dominated both chambers. In 1938, President Franklin Roosevelt grew so frustrated that he campaigned against right-wing Democrats like Senator Walter George of Georgia—who easily beat the president's candidate in the primary. When Harry Truman proposed his national health insurance, there sat the implacable Walter George, chairing the Senate Finance Committee. The only way the administration could get around George—who would have buried the bill in committee—was to strip all financial provisions out of the proposal. The media of the day wrote Truman's bill off as a non-starter partially because it included no funding mechanisms.

On the other side of the Democratic Party, Northern liberals crafted their social insurance proposals: Social Security expansion, national health insurance, robust labor protections, child welfare programs, and so on. Democratic presidents—Roosevelt, Truman, Kennedy, and Johnson—all fell, some more and some less, into this faction. Even though conservatives dominated Congress, being part of a permanent majority conferred advantages on the liberals. Their ideas and programs, articulated by the presidents, stayed fresh and remained on the agenda. The social insurance ideal was always present—albeit normally blocked.

The contemporary reading of the New Deal Democrats emphasizes how conservatives bedeviled the liberals. Ira Katznelson has described it as a coalition of Swedish welfare state and South African apartheid—dominated by the latter.[2] And there is much to that version of the story. It seems extraordinary, even now, that over a hundred legislators in the House and Senate would threaten Democratic presidents for even the mildest condemnations of lynching. How could some of the most respected political leaders in the United States raise such an uproar—launching long filibusters full of bluster and threats and cries of doom—at the prospect of black children playing in the same park as white ones?

The racial story is horrific. But the image of implacable opposites pressed together in the same party distorts the historical experience. Beyond race, the sides negotiated, accommodated, and log-rolled—adjusting to the issue and the political alignment of the moment. Southerners, in particular, were committed to Congress as an institution. Yes, they routinely frustrated health reformers. But Democrats on both the Left and the Right were members of the same party, with overlapping ideas and goals. (Walter George may have vexed both Roosevelt and Truman on social issues, but they found him to be indispensable on foreign policy.) As we shall see, being part of a majority coalition kept the liberals' agenda in play, offered them incremental gains, and gave them occasional opportunities for breakthrough.

A second distinctive feature of the Medicare moment was equality. The Johnson administration operated during a deeply egalitarian era. Table 15.1 ranks nations on their level of economic equality (based on the Ginni index) in 1970. Note how the United States fits between Japan and France. Although social scientists did not appreciate it at the time, the United States was part of a league of wealthy, European nations: It fell a bit (about 12 percent) behind such northern egalitarians as Denmark, Germany, and Canada.

TABLE 15.1  Inequality, 1970 (Ginni Coefficient)

| | |
|---|---|
| United Kingdom | 24.3 |
| Denmark | 31 |
| Germany | 31.3 |
| Canada | 31.6 |
| Sweden | 31.6 |
| Japan | 34.1 |
| **United States** | **35.8** |
| France | 36.2 |
| Brazil | 56 |
| Mexico | 58.3 |

Note: A completely equal society would come
in at 0. An entirely unequal society would be at 1
(We've multiplied the index by 100 to simplify).

In the 1960s, it would not have made any sense to compare the United States to, say, Brazil or Mexico, which were deeply inegalitarian societies.

A program like Medicare—collective, universal, and compulsory—reflected the American political economy of the era. The logic of social insurance rests on a faith in equal treatment. And that fits a nation that values—and practices—economic equality.

Of course, this relative equality emerged from three decades of Democratic politics. Democratic rule had produced high tax rates on the wealthy, strong unions, a rising minimum wage, and government regulations on business, finance, and even the media (the FCC required radio and television stations to offer equal air time to each political position). Postwar economic expansion facilitated this consensus. So too, perhaps, had the shared experience of war.

The Medicare moment was unusual for a third reason: more than 95 percent of the American population had been born in the United States. Immigration had defined nineteenth-century century America, but by 1965, had been tightly restricted for 40 years. When President Kennedy visited Ireland in 1963, he stood in a pub and lamented that his hosts could not move to the United States as his great-grandparents had done. In retrospect, the lowest immigration rates in a century carried important political consequences.

High immigration generally fosters contentious debates about wealth, poverty, and social welfare. It complicates communitarian sentiment and the effort to win social insurance. Immigration offers the raw material for American culture wars. By 1965, that hot, messy cultural matter had all but vanished in the United States.

Finally, consider race. No issue reverberates through American history like race. The issue divided (and would soon wreck) the Democratic Party. However, 1963–1964 saw a flash of optimism, along with the terrible violence meted out to the civil rights protesters in the South. The great March on Washington, in August 1963, might well have been, as *New York Times* columnist Anthony Lewis put it, "a national high water mark in…sweetness, patience, and mass decency." The following year, the Civil Rights Act faced a Senate filibuster that lasted from March 9 to June 10. But when the cloture vote was finally called, 27 (out of 33) Republican Senators joined 45 Democrats to break the Southern filibuster. For a brief moment, it might have seemed that most of America—across party, across regions—had finally united to deal with the South's racial intransigence. Public approval of the *Brown v. Board of Education* ruling striking down segregated schools had risen from 55 percent (right after the decision) to 87 percent (in April 1964). Foreign observers like Gunnar Myrdal began to speculate that Americans had finally—finally!—faced up to their original sin.[3]

This was a rare moment in American race politics: 72 Senators went on record suggesting that America's race problem lay in oppressive laws and discriminatory practices. In Chapter 2 in this volume, David Barton Smith suggests that the Civil Rights Act facilitated—and perhaps even enabled—Medicare's passage. A long historical view reinforces the point: for a brief season the American race binary—the inexorable otherness of African Americans—seemed to slip into abeyance. Deep divisions over race, class, and ethnicity imperil the kinds of solidarity that make universal social insurance plausible. Medicare's moment occurred when many Americans clung to the hope that their country was on the verge of bridging the deepest division of all.

The visions of solidarity did not last long. The very night he signed the Civil Rights Act, on July 2, 1964, President Johnson turned to his advisor, Bill Moyers, and said, "I think we just delivered the South to the Republican Party for a long time to come."[4] Two weeks later a race riot—also known, ominously, as an urban insurrection—burst out in Harlem. And two weeks after President Johnson signed Medicare into law, in July 1965, the largest riot of all engulfed Watts, Los Angeles. The American racial saga had taken a terrifying and violent turn. The racial "us and them" was back with a vengeance. The cities would burn for four sweltering summers; by the time the fires had died down, late in 1968, the New Deal Democratic era was gone.

Fifty years give new perspective to the historical conditions under which Medicare passed. American society was relatively egalitarian—dramatically so, compared to the eras that came before and after. While the race politics were more ferocious than usual, the racial divisions were less so; for a brief period, both political leaders and public opinion turned optimistic. In addition, low immigration meant less cultural backlash. All these conditions fostered a universal social policy like Medicare. The design of the program fit the times.

In historical perspective, the behavior of the Congressional Democrats is even more striking. Liberals and conservatives—bound together in the same Democratic Party—behaved in ways that are unimaginable today, when liberals and conservatives inhabit different parties. Consider some of the political twists and turns in the road to passage.

Soon after assuming the presidency in November 1963, President Johnson began pushing for Medicare. Wilbur Mills, the chair of the House Ways and Means Committee, had blocked the plan before and, in the summer of 1964, he blocked it again. The House passed only an increase in Social Security benefits; the Senate also voted for the Social Security increase but added Medicare to the legislation. When the package went to the conference committee, to reconcile the differences between House and Senate versions, Wilbur Mills made a startling proposal: drop Medicare and crank up the Social Security increase to 7 percent. That would require a large increase in the payroll tax—effectively blocking Medicare for the foreseeable future. The idea had originally come from Senator Russell Long, a Democrat from Louisiana, and was supported by Senator George Smathers, a Democrat from Florida. Both were on the conference committee. A trio of savvy Southern conservatives—Mills, Long, and Smathers—had outmaneuvered President Johnson. Yet each would dramatically shift sides and would eventually play a role in winning the reform.

When Mills called for a vote, he was stunned to find the conference committee deadlocked. Long and Smathers, who had long opposed Medicare, now voted down the entire package and saved the program for the next Congress. When reporters asked Senator Smathers why he had switched, he said cheekily, "Lyndon [Johnson] told me to."[5]

Six weeks later, a Democratic landslide appeared to make Medicare's passage inevitable. Now it was Wilbur Mills's turn to flip. In the famous, often retold story, he led the Ways and Means Committee through its paces and, at the last moment, in secret collaboration with Johnson, pulled his legendary coup and combined three competing bills. At the time, Mills's switch seemed like savvy politics as usual—he maximized his own influence by transforming the program he had long blocked. But from the perspective of our own era, where such flipping is hard to imagine, we can see how unusual—how fluid—the Democratic alliance could be.

In brief, the Democratic era took a divided party—a situation that reformers found deeply frustrating—and saw its members negotiate and accommodate each other in ways that liberals and conservatives could not do today. Medicare was one of the last great efforts of the long Democratic era. Beginning with the next election, everything would change.

## A New Gilded Age Shifts the Policy Frame

Every dimension described in the previous section changed following the Medicare moment. A radical new context would incubate an entirely different vision of healthcare reform. Republicans, who had always been skeptical of social insurance, designed an alternative. Slowly, Democrats adopted the new ideas.

The Eighty-Ninth Congress (1965–1966), which passed Medicare, was the last hurrah for the New Deal coalition. Putting aside the anomalous post-Watergate (1976) election, consider the dismal string of Electoral College scores attained by Democratic presidential candidates across the next 24 years: 191 (1968), 17 (1972), 49 (1980), 13 (1984), and 111 (1988). Republicans could count on many states through this entire period (California, for example); but not a single state stayed in the Democratic column—not one—between 1968 and 1992. Put another way, Democrats strung up the worst electoral run since the people started voting directly for the president in 1828. The comparable change in Congress took a generation, as Southern states continued to return their Democrats to their seats until they retired—at which point most Southern states and districts went red.

Figure 15.1 illustrates just how bad things got by mapping the Dukakis vote in 1988. Of course, Dukakis lost in a landslide, but his campaign team might have taken some solace in a bit of historical perspective: this was the second-best Democratic effort over these five presidential elections.

Policy analysts normally ascribe the election results to individual failure: Hubert Humphrey was tied to an unpopular administration, George McGovern was a hopeless candidate, Jimmy Carter was inept, Walter Mondale too liberal, and Dukakis most of the above. However, a series of defeats this large suggests some underlying problem. What might that have been? One phenomenon leaps from the electoral record: white people stopped voting for Democrats. To be sure, the results are skewed by the Southern vote, but they held, more weakly, for the entire country. And the white vote remains Republican to this day. Over the last nine presidential elections (from the election of Ronald Reagan in 1980 to Barack Obama in 2012), the Democrats averaged 39 percent of the white vote—exactly what Obama won in 2012. President Johnson had been more prophetic than he could have dreamed on the night he signed the Civil Rights Act.

Scholars have since gone back and questioned the Democrats' original Medicare strategy. Presidential advisers thought they were following the original Truman blueprint. "Medicare was the first step," recalled a health policy advisor to Senator Edward Kennedy, "and the next step was coming."[6]

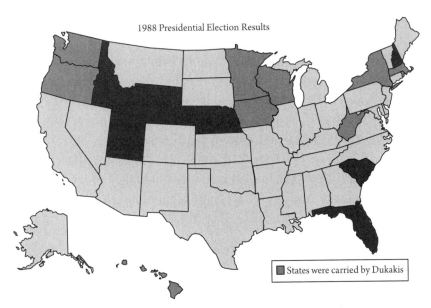

FIGURE 15.1 Still Looking for the New Democratic Coalition: The Republican landslide of 1988.
Source: *The American Presidency Project*, University of California, Santa Barbara.

Why did they fail? The analysis ought to begin, not with the program itself, but with the radical new electoral setting. Not even the most pessimistic Democratic Cassandra could have imagined the kind of electoral wilderness awaiting them. And regardless of Medicare's flaws in program design or implementation, any serious effort to build on it—any serious expansion on the social insurance model—was very unlikely from a party that was averaging 74 electoral votes per election. Reforms would have to await the construction of a new Democratic presidential coalition. That coalition, as we will see, finally became visible in 2000, when, for the first time in 36 years (again, putting aside the 1976 Watergate election), a Democratic candidate managed to win a majority of the popular vote. After decades of Republican dominance, notions about health reform—what was needed, what was possible—had profoundly changed.

This new electoral alignment had formidable political consequences for the political economy. Washington rolled back the New Deal policies. Republicans (eventually with Democratic support) deregulated business, finance, and the media; squeezed unions; slashed taxes; reduced welfare; and resisted redistribution at every turn. The policies helped produce new levels of inequality. Table 15.2 offers one measure of the consequences: a stunning rise in inequality—far greater than most other industrialized (and many developing) nations.

In effect, the United States dropped entirely out of the Western European equality league. Rather than lagging slightly behind the Western European democracies in equality, it has come to reflect the wealth distribution of the largest Latin American nations—closer to Mexico or Brazil than it is to Germany, France, or Canada. In fact, the United States is nearer to the least egalitarian nation on record (Lesotho) than it is to the most (Sweden).

Table 15.2 explodes a lazy myth: that globalization has unleashed rampant inequality everywhere. On the contrary, six of the cases in this sample have seen rising *equality*. And only Great Britain underwent a spike in inequality comparable to the American case. Since Britain started as a far more egalitarian society, and its rates of inequality have leveled out in recent years, it now finds itself almost exactly where the United States was in 1970—at the rear of the rich industrial nations, right between France and Japan.

Inequality on the new American scale powerfully subverts social insurance. It becomes far less plausible to argue for programs that put all citizens in together. On the contrary, recent health policy—from Democrats

TABLE 15.2  Economic Inequality

| Country | Index (2005–2011) | Change (from 1970) |
| --- | --- | --- |
| Sweden | 23 | –8.6 |
| Denmark | 24.8 | –6.2 |
| Germany | 27 | –4.3 |
| Canada | 32.1 | +.7 |
| France | 32.7 | –3.5 |
| Great Britain | 34 | +10 |
| Japan | 37.6 | –3.5 |
| **United States** | **45** | **+9.2** |
| Mexico | 48.3 | –10 |
| Brazil | 51.9 | –4.1 |
| Lesotho | 63.1 | (n/a) |

Source: Central Intelligence Agency, World Factbook: https://www.cia.gov/library/publications/the-world-factbook/rankorder/2172rank.html.

as much as Republicans—rests on the assumptions of individualism, markets, and choice. A nation with 160 billionaires (there were 32 before the New Deal and 16 during the Medicare moment, all in current dollars) is far less likely to put all citizens in a compulsory program where everyone gets more or less the same rights. The idea does not fit a culture where people are always scrambling from coach to business to first class—with private jets the prize for real winners.

Analysts who focus too tightly on health policy miss this critical frame: the United States is now a society with yawning gaps between rich and poor. Different classes segregate themselves from one another in almost every possible way. The health policy conversation reflects the larger political economy.

At the same time, the nation is split by cultural divides over race and immigration. By 1968, white liberal optimism about race had vanished. The urban insurrections—or riots—had racked the inner cities for four years. Richard Nixon found a way to mobilize racial fears without saying the word "black" in public: "law and order." After screening a campaign ad, Nixon exulted to his staff: that "hits it right on the nose. It's all about law and order and the damn Negro and Puerto Rican groups out there." In 1968, only a single Southern state (Texas) remained in the Democrats' column in the presidential election—the Deep South went for the segregationist George Wallace before turning Republican. The border states went straight into the Republican column.[7]

White racial fears grew more intense—and more white voters fled the Democrats—when the Supreme Court unanimously accepted school busing to achieve racial integration. The busing strategy took a volatile turn in 1973 when the courts applied it first to Denver and then to other cities outside the Jim Crow South. Suddenly, white Northerners discovered that they had a race problem, too. Busing may have been a plausible policy for confronting 300 years of racial apartheid, but it created deep divisions in American politics and culture.

The imagery of race politics took another powerful turn when the media discovered a new American scourge: the underclass. *Time* magazine luridly introduced this latest racial trope in 1977. "Behind the [ghetto's] crumbling walls lives a large group of people who are more intractable, more socially alien and more hostile than almost anyone had imagined. They are the unreachables: The American underclass." Here was the source of crime, violence, drug abuse, and family decay. And the pictures delivered the punch line: these alien, hostile, intractable people were—black.[8] The response would be the wars on crime and drugs. President Ronald Reagan put real muscle into the effort. The result, now vivid after three decades of crime fighting, is a policy so racially skewed that many analysts tag it "the New Jim Crow." Black Americans are six times more likely to be incarcerated than white Americans.

A new era of immigration compounded racial divisions. Just two months after signing Medicare into law, President Lyndon Johnson signed the Hart-Cellar Act, removing the immigration quotas that had existed since the 1920s. The idea provoked little debate or controversy at the time. The limits on Asians or Eastern Europeans seemed like just another form of racism—and one that could be righted without unleashing the racial furies. The legislation passed with large bipartisan majorities (although some Southerners voted no). Supporters insisted that this would not have undesirable consequences—like changing the nation's ethnic composition or, as LBJ put it, "flooding" the cities with foreigners.

This time, LBJ was entirely wrong. The legal change permitted the second largest period of immigration in American history. Today, more than one in eight American residents was born abroad. Like every immigrant generation, the newcomers inject new ethnicities, races, religions, ideas, foods, entertainments, sins, and physical types into the national mix. The arrival of immigrants that began in the late 1960s changed the cultural debate and touches every social issue because social policy always turns, in part, on the image of the beneficiary. Recall that it was President Barack Obama's pledge that the Affordable Care Act (ACA) would not benefit undocumented aliens that made Representative Joe Wilson shout, "You lie!"[9]

The idea behind Truman's national health insurance rested on a simple notion: everyone goes into the same program, each is treated (more or less) alike. The idea draws from a sense of solidarity: we all get sick, we all need help. The idea's power diminished as the United States changed. There are, of course, divisions in every society, but American divisions grew fiercer after the 1960s—indeed, many Americans blamed the Great Society programs for aggravating crime, welfare, the decline of cities, drug abuse, and family breakdown. And note how every one of these problems emits a little racial jolt.

Inequality made social insurance—with its premium on treating all citizens equally—a far more difficult sell. The new images of a racialized "us and them" further divided the society, and the Republican Party now led a conservative coalition that dominated Washington for three decades. Together, all these trends made an egalitarian, compulsory program like Medicare far less likely. An entirely different approach offered a far better fit for the era.

## NEOLIBERALISM RISING

Three years after Medicare went into effect, President Richard Nixon sounded the alarm: "We face a massive crisis . . . and unless action is taken . . . within the next two to three years, we will have a breakdown of our medical system." Medicare was so expensive, he explained, that it threatened to crash American medicine. In fact, healthcare costs had been rising for 15 years; Medicare quickened the inflation (by a factor of two) and made the rise visible and politically charged by placing the burden on the federal government. The crisis became a permanent fixture of healthcare reform. The Truman vision—rights, social justice, help, equality—gave way to four decades (and counting) of the plumbing metaphor: fix the broken system.[10]

What might solve the crisis? Over time, a bundle of reforms emerged that reflected the values of a fractious, highly unequal society self-consciously committed to hard capitalism: markets, competition, choice, and the search for profits.

In the early 1970s, two visions of health reform briefly squared off. When Ted Kennedy, the lion of social insurance, considered supporting Richard Nixon's health plan, union leaders dourly gathered in his office and backed him off the idea. But as the Republican landslides began to pile up and the unions declined, the debate evaporated. The neoliberal model became the dominant approach to health reform in Washington.

President Ronald Reagan introduced the new thinking. Over the ardent objection of almost his entire Cabinet, Reagan introduced a plan to expand Medicare to cover catastrophic costs (in 1987). The final package, negotiated with fiscally conservative Democrats, broke with the universalism that had marked Medicare. Seniors would pay for their own benefits. Liberal Democrats immediately decried the new thinking. Why should seniors bear the full cost of the program? Conservatives despised the new entitlement; wealthier seniors were furious about having to cover the bulk of the costs. With enemies on both Left and Right, Reagan's catastrophic program would be struck down in a little more than a year. The underlying principle, however, remained: groups and individuals were responsible for funding their own care. The "departure from the social insurance principles," as Congressman Henry Waxman described it, would prove permanent.[11]

Seven years later, in 1994, the Republicans captured both the House and the Senate (for the first time in 40 years), and the full market model came clearly into view. Republican reformers scoffed at the old Medicare—a dinosaur of federal authority, centralized regulation, compulsion, and one-size-fits-all. Instead, they promised to "modernize" Medicare, by which they meant, establish it firmly on market principles. The federal government would simply subsidize beneficiaries who could then shop for private insurance. People would leave the old program for the modern market alternative, predicted House speaker Newt Gingrich, leaving traditional Medicare to "wither on the vine."[12]

Medicare beneficiaries, however, proved stubborn; they clung to their old program despite regular efforts to nudge them into modernity. For example, President George W. Bush made reforming Medicare one of the centerpieces of his domestic agenda. In his inimitable way, he announced that the old defenders of the status quo would not cow him: "Medicare is—they usually call it in the political lexicon, 'Mediscare'. . . . That doesn't deter me, however, from making sure the system works." Then he got down to substance: "Why shouldn't we say, 'Let's give seniors choices.'"[13] The Medicare Modernization Act was originally designed to permit beneficiaries to choose among different private health plans for their Medicare benefits; if they wanted, say, prescription drug coverage, they could choose a plan that offered it. After running into stubborn opposition—even many Republicans refused to remake a popular program—the administration proposed using prescription drugs as a modernization carrot: seniors who left traditional Medicare and selected a private plan would get prescription drug care. By the time the reform had worked its way through Congress, the reform left traditional Medicare alone and introduced prescription coverage for all beneficiaries, but required them to select the benefits from private insurance plans in the marketplace. This fell far short of what the administration had hoped to attain. Still, for the first time, competition among private insurance companies was grafted onto one part of Medicare. The old social insurance model may have survived, but Republicans believed that their market plans were inevitable: old Medicare was a program out of time, out of step with the new American political economy.

Still, it was the Democratic leaders, even more than the Republicans, who demonstrated the potential scope and power of neoliberal thinking. During the New Deal, Democrats had championed the social insurance model over Republican opposition. Now Republicans pushed a model much more congenial to their anti-governmental values. Every Democratic administration in this period, from Jimmy Carter and Bill Clinton to Barack Obama, gestured to social insurance before embracing market thinking. While the Democratic base clung to Truman's vision—Medicare for all—Washington shucked it aside as romantic illusion. Even when Washington Congressman Jim McDermott rounded up over one hundred Democrats to sign on to Medicare for all in 1993, many of his signatories were quick to tell anyone who asked that they intended the petition as a mere bargaining chip to wring concessions from the marketeers.[14]

Indeed, the two most audacious pro-market reforms came from Democrats. President Bill Clinton, elected with just 43 percent of the popular vote (in a three-way race) dismissed his experienced healthcare advisors six weeks after the election and brought in a business consultant to rethink health reform from the ground up. The Clinton plan famously offered universal coverage through managed competition. Private companies—elaborately overseen by neutral arbiters—would compete for the people's healthcare business. Carefully managed competition would discipline American health care. Here was a Democratic version of modernization: coverage would be nearly universal, and careful oversight would limit market excess. But beneath these values lay a deeper reality: the flight from social insurance was close to complete.

President Barak Obama's Affordable Care Act—despite the furious opposition it encountered from the Right—offers another Democratic version of the Republican idea. Originally designed by the conservative Heritage Foundation, a previous version of the act had been sponsored by Republicans Robert Dole and John Chaffee as a rejoinder to the more expansive Clinton reform; a very similar version had been legislated by a Republican governor (and future presidential candidate) in Massachusetts.[15] Organized insurance marketplaces established in each state formed the centerpiece of the plan. The logic of the reform: send each citizen out to shop for health insurance, many of them with federal subsidies. Conservatives thinkers quietly champion the ACA's marketplaces as the mechanism by which they can finally modernize Medicare. Why not let the program's beneficiaries shop for their healthcare coverage, just like everyone else?[16]

Many Democrats, including the president, reached for a sliver of the old model by proposing a "public option." Citizens could voluntarily opt into something akin to social insurance: one large, Medicare-style plan for all who chose it. After a vociferous attack, the Democrats could not muster the final handful of votes to get beyond a Senate filibuster. House Speaker Nancy Pelosi caught the spirit of the times when she tried to rebrand (one might say modernize) the "public option" as "the consumer option." We can map the evolution of health reform from social insurance to neoliberalism more precisely by tracing presidential rhetoric. One of us, Elisabeth Fauquert, has examined over 1,200 presidential addresses devoted to health care.[17] She delineated two rhetorical paradigms and noted the words and phrases evocative of each paradigm, and coded the frequency that presidents referred to one or the other. For instance, words like "birthright," "compassionate," "deserve," "fairness," "protection," and "rights" code as *social insurance paradigm.* "Choice," "consumer," "empower," "individual," "market," "taxpayer," and "responsibility" code as *neoliberal perspective.* Figure 15.2 lays out the extent to which presidents relied on one or the other vision. The upshot reflects a sharp rise in the market vision among Republicans—but even more strikingly so among Democrats.[18]

When Truman's bills were before Congress, the social insurance perspective dominated his rhetoric (80 percent in 1947). Likewise, as Medicare passed, Johnson invoked social insurance 55 percent (1964) and 65 percent (1965) of the time. After that, the neoliberal pattern grows dominant. As Congress debated healthcare reforms, neoliberal speech took up over 65 percent (Clinton, 1994), and later 89 percent (Bush, in 2003). That trend continued unabated during the Obama administration.

In short, the change in rhetoric—in ideas and purpose—reflects the changing content of healthcare reform. Whether the subject is fixing Medicare (as in the Bush years) or expanding healthcare coverage (Clinton, Obama), the American way of thinking—and talking—about health care has changed. We have suggested that those changes, in turn, reflect the larger American political economy.

Health analysts often pore over the structure and politics of Medicare—its organization, its compromised implementation, the tactics of its supporters—to explain why Medicare never worked as a stepping-stone to national health insurance. Those microanalyses yield far more complete explanations when we place them in the context of American political history. The shift in party politics, the radical rise of inequality, and the evolution of cultural conflict all undermined social insurance and advantaged neoliberalism.

## MEDICARE: THE NEXT 50 YEARS

If the past decades help explain the rise of the neoliberal paradigm, what might the future hold? What will Medicare look like at its hundredth anniversary? One social trend in particular is worth noting. The Republican Party has remained 87 percent white for more than a decade, with scarcely any variation; the Democratic Party, in contrast, is now 55 percent white, a number that declines with every election.[19]

This matters because, as Figure 15.3 quite dramatically shows, the number of voters who consider themselves white is steadily falling. When Ronald Reagan clobbered Jimmy Carter, the electorate self-reported itself as 88 percent white; by the 2012 election, that number had fallen to 72 percent. Long

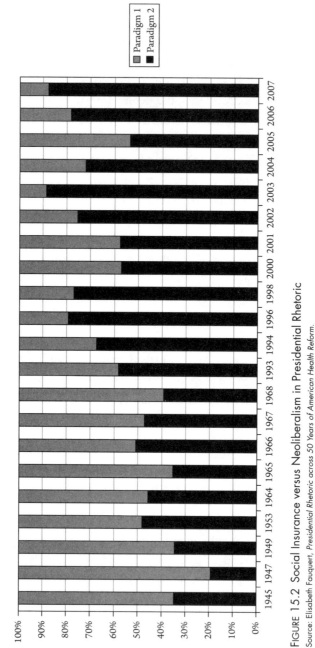

FIGURE 15.2 Social Insurance versus Neoliberalism in Presidential Rhetoric

Source: Elisabeth Fauquert, *Presidential Rhetoric across 50 Years of American Health Reform.*

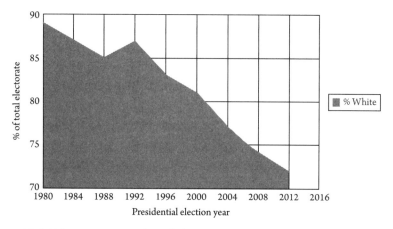

FIGURE 15.3 White Vote in Presidential Elections, 1980–2012.
Source: Chris Cilizza and Jon Cohen, *Washington Post* polling, November 8, 2012.

before Medicare's hundredth birthday, white Americans will make up less than half the voters—indeed, less than half the population.

How will that affect the larger political frame? Of course we cannot say, but demographic change surely suggests the possibility of another major shift in political coalitions. In the late 1960s, a sudden shift in politics—driven to a considerable extent by race—helped flip the paradigm of health-care reform. A comparable sea change, again driven by race, may lie ahead.

Of course, demography is not destiny. Political change requires leadership and vision. That's the hidden story in this history of two paradigms. After President Truman's legislation failed, a group of reformers—led by Truman himself—kept the social insurance vision alive. They took every opportunity to demand Medicare. Even President Dwight Eisenhower warned his fellow Republicans that they would lose the debate unless they came up with an alternative. By the 1980s, the leadership and vision had passed to the Republicans. Now, even Democrats proposed variations of their rivals' plans. In each era, the larger political economy bolstered the rising view. But it always took adroit leaders to convert the spirit of the times into a concrete reform. The larger political trends we have discussed here only enable, they never determine.

The political tides are always turning. After wandering in the electoral wilderness, Democratic presidential candidates have won the popular vote in five out of the six most recent elections—and they will continue to do so by ever-larger margins until the Republicans find a way to reach more than

11 percent of nonwhite voters. But electoral changes will have no effect on Medicare, health policy, or social insurance without leaders who envision new possibilities and articulate a different way. What may be most striking, as Democrats bid to reassert control of American politics, is the almost complete absence of serious thinking about how to adopt the social insurance model to a new era. Until that happens, neoliberalism—or modernization—will remain the dominant paradigm for Medicare and American healthcare reform.

NOTES

1. The classic account, written just six years after passage, is Theodore Marmor, *The Politics of Medicare* (London: Routledge and K. Paul, 1970). For updates, see Jonathan Oberlander, *The Political Life of Medicare* (Chicago: University of Chicago Press, 2003); and David Blumenthal and James Morone, *The Heart of Power: Health and Politics in the Oval Office* (Berkeley: University of California Press, 2009).

2. Ira Katznelson, *Fear Itself* (New York: Liverwright, 2013).

3. James Morone, *The Democratic Wish: Private Power and American Democracy* (New Haven, CT: Yale University Press, 1998), ch. 7; Anthony Lewis quoted at 213; Gallup poll reported in Julie Ray, "Reflections on the Trouble in Little Rock, Part II," *Gallup* March 4, 2003, http://www.gallup.com/poll/7900/Reflections-Trouble-Little-Rock-Part.aspx.

4. Todd S. Purdham, *An Idea Whose Time Has Come: Two Presidents, Two Parties, and the Battle for the Civil Rights Act of 1964* (New York: Henry Holt, 2014), 325.

5. The story is told in Richard Harris, *A Sacred Trust* (Baltimore, MD: Penguin Books, 1966), 171–173; Marmor, *Politics of Medicare*, 42–43; Blumenthal and Morone, *Heart of Power*, 183–185.

6. Lawrence Jacobs, "The Implementation and Evolution of Medicare: The Distributional Effects of 'Positive' Policy Feedbacks," in *Remaking America*, ed. Joe Soss, Jacob Hacker, and Suzanne Mettler (New York: Russell Sage, 2010), 88–89. Senate staffer Stan Jones, interviewed by David Blumenthal and James Morone, August 6, 2007.

7. Nixon quoted in Philip Kinker and Rogers Smith, *The Unsteady March: The Rise and Decline of Racial Equality in America* (Chicago: University of Chicago Press, 1999), 292.

8. Michael Katz, *Improving Poor People: The Welfare State, The Underclass, and Urban Schools as History* (Princeton, NJ: Princeton University Press, 1995), 63–64.

9. Barack Obama, "Address Before a Joint Session of the Congress on Health Care Reform," September 9, 2009. Available online by Gerhard Peters and John T. Woolley, *The American Presidency Project*, http://www.presidency.ucsb.edu/ws/?pid=86592.

10. Robert Hackey, *Cries of Crisis: Rethinking the Health Care Debate* (Reno: University of Nevada Press, 2012).

11. Blumenthal and Morone, *Heart of Power*, ch. 8, quoted at 315.
12. Jonathan Oberlander, "Medicare: The Great Transformation," in *Health Politics and Society*, ed. James Morone, Theodor Litman, and Leonard Robins (Stamford, CT: Cengage Learning, 2008), 310–327, Gingrich quoted at 320.
13. George W. Bush: "Remarks at Truman High School in Independence, Missouri," August 21, 2001. Available online by Gerhard Peters and John T. Woolley, *The American Presidency Project*, http://www.presidency.ucsb.edu/ws/?pid=62637.
14. Interviews by one of the authors, February–March 1993.
15. Jill Quadagno, "Right Wing Conspiracy? Socialist Plot? The Origins of the Affordable Care Act," *Journal of Health Politics, Policy and Law* 39 (December 2013): 35–56.
16. Douglas Holz-Eakin and Avik Roy, "The Future of Free Market Health Care," *Reuters*, February 20, 2013, http://blogs.reuters.com/great-debate/2013/02/20/the-future-of-free-market-healthcare/.
17. The graph was obtained with the following methodology (and the precious help of Victor Perron). For a given speech, a score is obtained by adding the occurrences of each of the words belonging to the set list of a given paradigm (1 or 2), divided by the total number of words in the analyzed text. A relative score for each of the two paradigms is therefore determined for each text under scrutiny. For a given year, the relative score for a paradigm is obtained by the sum of the scores obtained for each text analyzed, divided by the total number of analyzed texts that year. Thus, for each year, we calculated the percentages with the following formula: percent 1 = score 1 / (score 1 + score 2). Score 1 is obtained by dividing the words of paradigm 1 and score 2 by those of paradigm 2. This representation enables us to chart the relative presence of the terms of paradigm 1 compared to those of paradigm 2 in the texts of a same year.
18. Elisabeth Fauquert, "La rhétorique présidentielle sur les réformes de santé: cas d'étude sur l'adoption du *Patient Protection and Affordable Care Act*," Ph.D. to be defended in 2015.
19. "Partisan Divide Reaches New High," Pew Research Center, 2012 Values Survey. http://www.people-press.org/values/.

# 16

# BUILT TO LAST?

## POLICY ENTRENCHMENT AND REGRET IN MEDICARE, MEDICAID, AND THE AFFORDABLE CARE ACT

PAUL STARR

Laws generally qualify as historic achievements only if they last. But even laws that prove durable and popular often have lasting unhappy effects that must be reckoned with. This has been the case with the legislation that established Medicare and Medicaid in 1965. It gave millions of Americans legal rights to health care that have survived political challenges for half a century, while it entrenched features of policy that have contributed to the healthcare system's high costs and persistent inequities. That mixed experience suggests two questions about the Affordable Care Act (ACA): Will the expanded rights under the ACA become as entrenched as those created in 1965? And does the law risk entrenching new features of health policy that many of its supporters may come to regret?

By "entrench," I mean establish in such a way as to make policies and institutions exceptionally hard to undo or roll back. Entrenchment refers not to permanence but to mechanisms that resist or limit change. The origin of those mechanisms may lie in the strategic choices of political parties and their leaders or the unintended consequences of their actions, or some combination of the two. A good example of strategic entrenchment is writing a rule or principle into a constitution in order to make it hard to alter. Constitutional entrenchment pre-commits opposed parties to observe the same rules of the game. At the other extreme are measures adopted as temporary expedients or compromises that nonetheless become entrenched, or locked in, as a result of self-reinforcing economic and political effects. Over time, institutions and policies may also come to be so taken for granted that they seem the natural and inevitable way of doing things preventing alternatives even from being considered.

Such mechanisms preserve policies after those who instituted them have lost power. The test of entrenchment typically comes when an opposition party takes office; a policy has become entrenched to the extent that it survives transfers of power. In addition, the party that introduced a policy may also become dissatisfied with the results or may have introduced it as a first step toward a larger goal, only to find that the initial policy now stands in its way. In such cases, entrenchment turns into a "policy trap" by constraining or even subverting the larger substantive goals of its own initiators.

Entrenchment itself is neither good nor bad. Constitutionally entrenched rights and rules are necessary for a well-functioning democracy, whereas entrenched power and privilege may undermine democratic values. Entrenchment also does not necessarily depend on whether a policy is optimal or just. Policies that are inefficient or inequitable may generate self-reinforcing effects that make them highly resistant to change. Regret is always a risk when legislative bargains and even sought-after policies ("watch what you wish for") have the potential to become locked in.

With these considerations in mind, we can conceive of the developmental path of legislated reforms as lying along a spectrum of possibilities:

1. *Entrenchment and extension*: Policies may not only become entrenched but also serve as the foundation for additional measures that achieve more fully the substantive values of their originators. The most successful policies are extended in various dimensions, adapted to changing circumstances, and used as models for change in other areas.

2. *Walled-in entrenchment*: Policies may become entrenched, though only in a limited form. Such policies may become vulnerable to the kind

of erosion that Jacob Hacker calls "drift," when circumstances change and policies do not.[1]

3. *Degraded entrenchment*: An initial policy developed for one set of aims may become entrenched in a way that undermines important substantive values of its originators. In an extreme case, a measure gets turned into a vehicle for entirely different ends.

4. *Disentrenchment*: Policies may get repealed when they are overturned by their opponents, superseded by their original supporters, or abandoned on all sides.

The first of these possibilities, entrenchment and extension, represents the ideal case for most reformers. The second, walled-in entrenchment, has an ambiguous significance as a limited achievement, while the third—degraded entrenchment—is unambiguously a policy trap. Disentrenchment implies a policy failure unless the lessons of defeat prove to be instrumental for later success.

In the history of American social policy, Social Security is the paradigmatic example of successful reform: the program is highly entrenched and has been progressively extended in several dimensions (covered population, scale and scope of benefits). The Democrats who campaigned and voted for Medicare and Medicaid had the experience of Social Security in mind, and those who pressed for the ACA saw that legislation as a counterpart to both Social Security and Medicare. But despite the political appeal of these historical analogies, Medicare has not traveled the same path as Social Security, and the ACA seems even less likely to do so.

In a recent book, *Remedy and Reaction*, I argue that, by adopting a series of measures in the mid-twentieth century, the United States ensnared itself in a policy trap in health care. Those measures—including the tax exclusion of employer health insurance contributions, separate programs for veterans and other groups, and Medicare and Medicaid—skewed the allocation of national resources both *toward* health care and *within* health care, raising costs to much higher levels than in the other advanced economies and leaving millions of uninsured and underinsured in financial insecurity and with inferior access to care.

Despite intensifying problems through the late twentieth century, the healthcare system became exceptionally hard to change for four reasons: (1) it satisfied a majority of the public, including the best-organized groups; (2) it enriched the healthcare industry; (3) it obscured costs from many of those who ultimately bore them; and (4) it conveyed a moral rationale that those who enjoyed good protection (employees, veterans, seniors) had earned it, in contrast to less deserving groups who had not earned it and consequently did not deserve equal treatment. These effects ultimately did not prevent the enactment of the ACA in 2010, but they severely constrained its reach.[2] Hence the same questions hover over the ACA as over Medicare and Medicaid: Can the limitations and deficiencies of reform be repaired while the gains are entrenched? Or might the gains prove ephemeral, while other provisions are entrenched in a way that degrades and subverts the aims of reform?

### Entrenchment and Regret in Medicare and Medicaid

Medicare and Medicaid bear a distinctive time stamp from their enactment that subsequent generations have found difficult to erase or write over. In this respect, they are not unusual. The ideas, leadership, and conditions prevailing at the time of a policy's enactment often give a specific form and structure to resulting institutions, which may then generate "feedback" effects that obstruct further change. If the ideas, leadership, and circumstances at enactment had been different, other institutions might have become just as entrenched.

The institutional structures created by the 1965 Medicare and Medicaid legislation are downright peculiar. None of the other major democracies has either a separate, national health program for seniors or a mixed, federal-state program for categorical groups among the poor. To be sure, specific historical causes help explain why Congress in 1965 crafted a program of this kind. The sequence and timing of social-insurance programs were critical. The United States was already distinctive in having first adopted a national, compulsory, old-age insurance system without also instituting health insurance. That legacy created both an institutional base oriented to seniors and a skittishness among liberals and centrists about challenging the medical profession and other interest groups in health care.

After the defeat of national health insurance under Truman, the program executives in Social Security came up with the idea of adding hospital insurance as a benefit for the retired. Attaching a hospital benefit to the old-age program had obvious advantages in legitimacy, and it took on a political life of its own. As it turned out, Lyndon Johnson's landslide brought in majorities in both houses of Congress, which made it possible to enact more than a hospital benefit for the retired, but the standing promise to seniors defined the central concerns of the national agenda in health care.

The timing of the 1965 legislation also influenced its framework in other ways. One method of legitimating policy is through mimetic isomorphism—that is, adopting institutional structures that copy accepted forms. Many of the features of Medicare, such as the split between hospital and physician coverage as well as the payment provisions, matched the familiar structures of Blue Cross and Blue Shield. Medicaid fit into a previously developed structure for federal subsidies of medical care linked to state and local welfare programs. These examples illustrate how prior institutional forms in the United States shaped the elements of Medicare and Medicaid that departed from international patterns. But the particular combination was cobbled together in political bargaining; with different ideas and leadership, the results might have been different.

A key ideational influence on the bill was the theory of change that liberal policymakers of the Johnson era derived from the experience of Social Security. The basic premise was that compromises at the start of a program need not be consequential in the long run. Just as many of the original limitations of Social Security had been overcome through incremental measures, so, too, would Medicare's initial deficiencies be gradually overcome. Reversible errors, irreversible achievements—such was the theory of reform. This comforting set of expectations encouraged liberal politicians and policymakers to go along with concessions to interest groups on the assumption that they would be able to build on the Medicare-Medicaid legislation and correct the flaws while entrenching the gains.

That theory of change, however, turned out to be mistaken in critical respects. In Medicare, unlike Social Security, compromise inhibited program expansion. The spectacular cost increases that resulted from concessions on payment provisions (see Chapter 9 by Uwe Reinhardt in this volume) convinced many people that the United States could not afford universal health coverage on a social-insurance basis. Limiting Medicare to the aged also inhibited wider eligibility as seniors came to regard the program as exclusively for them. In addition, the design of Medicare reinforced the belief that, rather than being obligations of the community, access to health care and protection against its costs were benefits that needed to be earned. To be sure, Congress passed Medicaid at the same time, but in doing so it created a lower tier of coverage linked to welfare, institutionalizing inequalities in access to care and helping to wall in Medicare. In coming years, Congress would not open Medicare to other groups, except for the addition of the disabled and end-stage renal disease patients in 1972. Extensions of federally subsidized coverage ultimately came through Medicaid and private insurance, two systems that liberals originally hoped to supersede.

Compromise has been the mother of complexity in health care. The 1965 legislation gave rise to four systems for paying for seniors' medical care, each one based on different principles: Medicare Parts A and B, private Medigap plans to make up for the limited Medicare benefit package, and Medicaid for low-income seniors and those who spend down their assets. (When Congress later added Parts C and D, it based them on still different principles.) It is a measure of the gratuitous complexity of American health policy that the system for seniors, with its multiple methods of payment, is seen as a model of simplicity.

Many other original features of the originating legislation, such as the basic duality between Medicare and Medicaid, have survived intact for half a century and seem likely to remain entrenched for a long time to come. Congress did tighten Medicare's payment provisions in the 1980s and 1990s, but such measures have necessarily had their limits because reducing rates below other payers could impair seniors' access to care. (Lower payment levels relative to private insurance also increase provider opposition to expanding Medicare eligibility.) Depending on how tax expenditures are counted, the government pays for about half the costs of all healthcare—yet without the control over costs that more comprehensive regulatory systems give other countries. And this contradiction between budgetary exposure and budgetary control is at the root of the institutional instability of Medicare, as well as other federal health programs.

As a result, it would be a mistake to regard Medicare as being as well entrenched as Social Security. The two programs have much in common in their design and support, but the differences are crucial. (The following analysis may be contrasted with the chapters by Mark Peterson and others in this volume that see public opinion as a primary cause of policy, rather than being, in significant respects, produced by it.)

Both Social Security and Medicare benefit from the original, strategic choice to use an earmarked tax that would give workers a strong sense of entitlement. At the time that Social Security was enacted, Franklin D. Roosevelt was convinced that despite its regressive incidence, the payroll tax would entrench the program. As he famously told an aide, "With those taxes in there, no damn politician can ever scrap my social security program. Those taxes aren't a matter of economics, they're straight politics."[3] Although Medicare is partly financed from general revenues, the use of payroll taxes to pay for Part A has helped to create the belief among Medicare beneficiaries that they have paid for their coverage, and no "damn politician" should dare tamper with it.

In addition, the layering of Medicare on top of Social Security has contributed to the formation of an exceptionally powerful and well-organized beneficiary interest group (see Chapter 7 by Mark Schlesinger in this volume). The structure of the programs has helped to solve seniors' collective-action problems; for example, AARP derives its financing from the sale of Medigap coverage and other services.[4] Organizations representing other beneficiary populations do not have comparable bases for financing their activities.

The two programs have also become entrenched because of the adaptive responses of individuals and families. As one of several conditions making policies hard to reverse, Hacker points to "long-lived commitments" to beneficiaries on which they premise "crucial life and organizational decisions."[5] Social Security and Medicare have induced crucial life decisions about retirement and expectations about financial relationships between parents and children. The support for Social Security and Medicare comes not only from their current beneficiaries, but also from working adults who look forward to both their own benefits and not needing to support their retired parents. These effects contribute to the support for the programs registered in public opinion surveys (see Chapter 11 by Andrea Louise Campbell in this volume).

Social Security, however, is more deeply entrenched than Medicare for two distinct reasons, both related to budgetary concerns. First, the long-term fiscal problems in Social Security are manageable, whereas those facing Medicare are much more challenging and periodically provide a rationale for radically restructuring the program. Second, and more decisively, the costs of switching to privatized alternatives are much higher in Social Security than in Medicare. As a result of amendments adopted in 1939, which put Social Security on a pay-as-you-go basis, conservative proposals to privatize Social Security face a "double-payment problem": If current workers put their Social Security payments into their own individual accounts, what will be the source of funds to pay current benefits? Unless the federal government has a budget surplus, it would have to borrow the money, raise taxes, or cut benefits. When President George W. Bush proposed private accounts in 2005, projected budget deficits were already high, and the proposal collapsed in the face of overwhelming opposition.

But while high switching costs have blocked the privatization of Social Security, they have not prevented conservatives from introducing and promoting private Medicare Advantage plans. The plans do not save Medicare money; on the contrary, Medicare's costs would be lower if the beneficiaries stayed in the traditional program.[6] Nonetheless, Republicans have been able to enact favorable payment rules for the private plans, which have attracted about one-third of Medicare enrollees, partly by providing additional benefits out of Medicare's overpayments. The position of the plans is now entrenched; even after the ACA's changes in payment rules, their enrollment continued to grow. To be sure, enrollees can still switch back into public Medicare, but conservatives have created a mechanism for private-plan enrollment that may at some point allow them to privatize the entire program.

For the first 30 years after the 1965 legislation, there seemed to be no chance that the rights established under it would be repealed. But when Republicans under Newt Gingrich's leadership gained control of Congress in 1995, they began to call for changes that would limit federal commitments to a defined contribution for Medicare beneficiaries' coverage and a flat block grant to state Medicaid programs, neither of which would be tied to a measure of medical inflation. That was also true of the 2011 Ryan budget approved by Republican members of the House. In 2012, the Republican Party platform explicitly called for converting Medicare from a defined-benefit to a defined-contribution system.[7]

The significance of that change is fundamental. At the time of the first Ryan budget, Democrats accused Republicans of voting to "end Medicare"—or to "end Medicare as we know it"—an accusation that PolitiFact labeled the "lie of the year" in 2011.[8] But converting Medicare to a defined-contribution system would be a form of disentitlement; it would shift risk to the enrollees and end rights established by the 1965 law. The mere maintenance of the name "Medicare" does not signify that its protections would continue. The bill that some Republicans preferred in 1965—the "Bettercare" plan of Representative John Byrnes—would also have provided federal contributions for enrollment in private insurance. A half-century later, congressional Republicans have returned to the alternative to Medicare that at least some members of their party wanted from the beginning.

Between 2010 and 2014, the growth in Medicare's costs slowed considerably, and if that trend continues, it may weaken the budgetary justifications for privatization. But, whenever costs start rising quickly again, Republicans will have an alternative at the ready. If at that time they also have sufficient congressional majorities and control of the White House, they may well roll back the rights that Medicare and Medicaid established. What once looked locked in, no longer does.

## Entrenchment and the Potential for Regret in the ACA

For at least three reasons, the prospects for entrenchment of the ACA in coming years are more tenuous than they were for Medicare and Medicaid in the decades immediately after 1965.

First, as a result of the growing ideological distance between the parties, shifts in party control of the federal government are now more likely to result in substantial changes in national policy. In a generally partisan and polarized era, the ACA has been an especially partisan and polarizing issue—passed solely by Democrats and carried out over unrelenting opposition by Republicans, who have sought to stop the law in the courts, repeal it in Congress, and block its full implementation in the states. The ACA survived a critical challenge in the Supreme Court in 2012, when Chief Justice John Roberts, in an act of clemency, deemed the individual mandate constitutional under the taxing authority of Congress, but in that same decision the Court made the expansion of Medicaid optional for the states. As this book goes to press, the ACA faces another conservative legal challenge (*King v. Burwell*) that could severely undermine its goals—this time to the statutory basis of the affordability subsidies in the federal exchange. If Democrats had a congressional majority or the law were already entrenched, fixing the statutory language in question would be easy. The legal challenge to the subsidies in the federal exchange is a serious threat to the ACA only because the political position of the law remains precarious.

328 MEDICARE AND MEDICAID AT 50

Second, the uninsured and underinsured who benefit from the ACA have never been effectively organized. They do not have any coherence or stability as a group, and the ACA is unlikely to do for them what Social Security and Medicare have done in helping to constitute seniors as a powerful lobby. Seniors are the exception in the politics of the American welfare state. In *The Unheavenly Chorus*, Kay Schlozman, Sidney Verba, and Henry Brady survey interest-group representation at the national level and find that no group of beneficiaries of means-tested programs has effective representation in Washington.[9] To be sure, the ACA has increased coverage; in its first year of full implementation, the ACA reduced the number of uninsured by about 9.5 million, according to an estimate by the Commonwealth Fund.[10] But these numbers do not necessarily translate into political influence. The recipients of subsidized insurance in the exchanges and the newly added Medicaid beneficiaries are not likely to assemble themselves into an interest-group powerhouse.

Third, the ACA works in ways that have been, and will remain, mysterious to many people, in part because the federal government does not communicate directly with the people benefiting from the law. Although the ACA has resulted in rebates to many insurance subscribers, those rebates do not come with a letter from the president. Insurers do not inform their subscribers that they have Barack Obama to thank for closing loopholes in their coverage. Even the state insurance exchanges have separate names, obscuring their connection to the ACA. When bad things happen, however, both the insurance companies and state officials are happy to finger "Obamacare." In the public imagination, the Obama administration now "owns" every malfunction in health care, an impression that the administration seemed to confirm by botching the early rollout of Healthcare.gov. Despite improvements, the program labors under a cloud of doubt and in a fog of incomprehension.

As I suggested earlier, the key test of entrenchment comes when the opposition party gains control. Alternation in power sooner or later is the characteristic pattern in American politics, and in this case "sooner or later" may make all the difference. If Republicans had won both Congress and the White House in 2012, they would almost certainly have repealed the major provisions regarding Medicaid and the affordability subsidies, even while preserving some secondary aspects of the law, such as the extension of private coverage to young adults up to age 26 under their parents' policies.

Many of the law's supporters have assumed that once millions of people obtained coverage in 2014, Republicans would find it impossible to take it away. The Republican Party, however, has thus far shown no signs of accepting the ACA as a fait accompli. As a result of the obstacles that Republican state officials have thrown in the way of Medicaid expansion and exchange development, the ACA's major reforms will not yet be entrenched as of 2016. If the Supreme Court decides in *King v. Burwell* to overturn the subsidies in the federal exchange, the reform effort will likely collapse in many, if not most, of the red states. Even if the Court upholds the subsidies, the program will not yet be irreversible. The fate of the law will depend on the future of the Republican Party; at some point Republicans will win both the presidency and Congress, and when they do, the question will be what faction is in control. If the radical conservative wing dominates, Republicans could not only roll back the ACA but also convert Medicare into a defined-contribution system and cap federal spending for Medicaid. But if Republicans continue to lose the presidency, more centrist figures may gain influence, returning the United States to a more collaborative policy regime in health care.

Other potential sources of discontent with the ACA may increase pressure even among Democrats to renegotiate the law's provisions. As the penalties for failing to insure increase, so will anger among those who feel they cannot afford even the subsidized rates in the exchanges. The onset of the so-called Cadillac tax on high-cost health plans will exert intense pressure on employers to reduce the generosity of their coverage, and those affected are likely to seek political protection. Finally, if experience with Medicare Part D is any indication, enrollees in the exchanges will be highly sensitive to premiums, and plans with broader coverage at the gold and platinum levels may disappear.

Together, the Cadillac tax and the trends in the exchanges may produce a general degradation of the quality of insurance as more people are driven into plans with high cost-sharing and narrow networks. These and other developments may instill among many Democrats a sense of regret about the kind of health insurance that the ACA has helped to entrench. This is the possibility of degraded entrenchment that I referred to at the beginning of this chapter. Ironically, the model of insurance promoted by the ACA's insurance exchanges and the Cadillac tax could eventually find its principal support on the Right. Although conservatives lost their enthusiasm for the exchanges when Obama embraced them, they may again come to see in them a means of advancing a market-oriented design for health insurance. Support for the exchange model has switched hands once; a switch back to the Republicans would not be the strangest reversal in American politics. Such a turnabout would not necessarily bring stability to health policy. Rather than becoming entrenched, the ACA may just continue to be "in play" politically for a considerable time as a result of dissatisfaction among both parties and the public at large.

During most of the twentieth century, the dominant liberal narrative was a story of ascending rights. In T. H. Marshall's formulation, the democracies had seen a steady unfolding of civil, political, and social rights in a great march toward full and equal citizenship.[11] Although the United States did not constitutionally entrench social rights as European countries did, American liberals long believed that once Congress established such rights through legislation, they would become irreversible. When Congress enacted Medicare and Medicaid, America seemed to be irreversibly on its way to making health care a right.

But rather than realizing that hope, the last half-century has given us little reason to be confident that social rights are irreversible. "Entitlements" have become a pejorative; rights once taken for granted have to be fought for all over again. American health policy illustrates in a particularly sharp way the possibility that instead of entrenching rights, legislation may entrench power and privilege in ways that are ultimately destructive of liberal ends. That is not a counsel of despair. It is an honest reading of the historical record and a realistic warning about the difficult work ahead.

## NOTES

1. Jacob S. Hacker, "Policy Drift: The Hidden Politics of U.S. Welfare State Retrenchment," in *Beyond Continuity: Institutional Change in Advanced Political Economies*, ed. Wolfgang Streeck and Kathleen Thelen (Oxford: Oxford University Press, 2005), 40–82.
2. Paul Starr, *Remedy and Reaction: The Peculiar American Struggle over Health Care Reform*, rev. ed. (New Haven, CT: Yale University Press, 2013).
3. Luther Gulick, "Memorandum on Conference with FDR Concerning Social Security Taxation, Summer, 1941," http://www.ssa.gov/history/Gulick.html.
4. Frederick R. Lynch, *One Nation under AARP: The Fight over Medicare, Social Security and America's Future* (Berkeley: University of California Press, 2011).
5. Jacob S. Hacker, *The Divided Welfare State: The Battle over Public and Private Social Benefits in the United States* (New York: Cambridge University Press, 2002), 55.

6. Medicare Payment Advisory Commission, *Report to the Congress: Medicare Payment Policy* (Washington: MedPAC, 2014), 331, http://www.medpac.gov/documents/mar14_entirereport.pdf.

7. Republican National Committee, "2012 Republican Platform," 22, http://www.gop.com/wp-content/uploads/2012/08/2012GOPPlatform.pdf.

8. Bill Adair and Angie Drobnic Holan, "Lie of the Year 2011: 'Republicans Voted to End Medicare,'" *PolitiFact.com*, December 20, 2011, http://www.politifact.com/truth-o-meter/article/2011/dec/20/lie-year-democrats-claims-republicans-voted-end-me/.

9. Kay Lehman Schlozman, Sidney Verba, and Henry E. Brady, *The Unheavenly Chorus: Unequal Political Voice and the Broken Promise of American Democracy* (Princeton, NJ: Princeton University Press, 2012), 321–328.

10. S. R. Collins, P. W. Rasmussen, and M. M. Doty, "Gaining Ground: Americans' Health Insurance Coverage and Access to Care after the Affordable Care Act's First Open Enrollment Period," *The Commonwealth Fund*, July 2014, http://www.commonwealthfund.org/publications/issue-briefs/2014/jul/health-coverage-access-aca.

11. T. H. Marshall, *Citizenship and Social Class, and Other Essays* (New York: Cambridge University Press, 1950).

# CONCLUSION

## THE WORLD THAT MEDICARE AND MEDICAID MADE

ALAN B. COHEN, DAVID C. COLBY, KEITH A. WAILOO, AND
JULIAN E. ZELIZER

To speak of the world that Medicare and Medicaid made is not merely to speak about government's relationship to people who are elderly, disabled, and in poverty, but rather to discuss the ways in which these systems transformed American society more broadly. Medicare helped redefine the relationships and expectations between parents and children about responsibility and care, making government a source of security in their lives. Before 1965, older citizens were the face of poverty in America. Medicare changed that by helping to protect people over 65 (and after 1972, people with permanent disabilities and kidney failure) against the ravages of poverty and illness. Medicaid, too, changed the face of poverty, helping initially to ensure access to care for many people in poverty and with disabilities, and then, more recently, children and families above the poverty line. Both programs also blurred the lines between public and private. Though staunchly opposed by physicians at the time of passage, doctors and hospitals came to depend on the beneficiaries' benefits. Through this process, both programs stimulated the development of new private health sectors, such as the nursing home industry and the pharmaceutical and medical technology industries.

Political scientists use the term *policy feedback* to describe how policies create new politics, setting in motion new developments in the political environment, the electorate, and in society. Nowhere has this process been more evident than with Medicare and Medicaid. Broadly speaking, the beneficiaries of Medicare and Medicaid are also the hospitals, pharmaceutical companies, dialysis clinics, and physicians who treat Medicare and Medicaid patients—even as they bemoan the programs' at first generous but increasingly stingy fee schedules.[1] For some groups, these programs drove their growth. As W. Bruce Fye has noted, in the early days Medicare helped drive specialization by benefiting "procedurally oriented specialties like cardiology and cardiac surgery," feeding the field's costly technology-orientation.[2] By 1990, Medicare would pay these surgical specialists nearly $1 billion.[3] In a real sense, Medicare and Medicaid have contributed to a remaking of American society on multiple levels—from family relationships around health and economic security, to the financing of new institutions and specialization, to the development and growth of a "medical-industrial complex" that has become an economic engine of prosperity as well as a driver of escalating costs.

The complex web of political, economic, and moral commitments that sprang up around Medicare and Medicaid has not developed smoothly or without conflict. The problem of budgetary costs loomed large from the start. The programs' founders overcame the concerns of lawmakers like Wilbur Mills at first, but by 1970, critics, policymakers, politicians, and citizens were complaining loudly about rising costs. They wondered if America could afford to keep the social and moral commitments it had made in the Great Society era. By the twentieth anniversary in 1985, a new president, Ronald Reagan, had arrived in Washington with a stark vision of the federal government's role in the lives of Americans. No social welfare program was too sacrosanct to be cut; budget pressures loomed large; and the future of Medicare and Medicaid was imperiled. When Medicare and Medicaid reached 30, the struggle to control costs rose to new heights. For the first time ever in 1995, the programs faced Republican majorities in the House and Senate intent upon radically transforming them. Writing in 1995, James Tallon and Diane Rowland noted, "Medicaid is now at the center of a fiscal and philosophical tug-of-war between the federal and state governments over how responsibility is divided." At stake was whether the program would "continue as an entitlement program with federal funds matching state expenditures" or be completely converted to a block grant, giving states full latitude to build, shrink, or dismantle these commitments.[4] Medicare faced similar challenges with the push to privatize. At the time, Judith Feder commented, "It would be a bitter pill indeed, if, under the cloak of reform, we replaced Medicare's social insurance with a private insurance market filled with inequities, inefficiencies, and holes."[5]

But, even as Medicare and Medicaid were being transformed by the new political environment, the world that Medicare and Medicaid had created pushed back—shaping American politics in turn. Reformers now confronted the extraordinary difficulty of seriously retrenching or even substantially reforming these programs. As president, Ronald Reagan (who once criticized Medicare as "socialized medicine" and as a fundamental assault on American freedom and liberty in the early 1960s), faced fierce public support for the program; he, too, ultimately endorsed expansion of its benefits. Democratic President Bill Clinton espoused the idea that Medicare and Medicaid needed to be transformed by market-friendly reforms in order to be preserved. Barack Obama later embraced plans for saving Medicare (asking higher income beneficiaries to pay more), only to be accused by Republicans of harming Medicare beneficiaries with his Affordable Care Act (ACA) and its Medicaid expansion proposals. These political inversions and policy shifts highlight just how potent Medicare and Medicaid had become as political issues, and how embedded they were within the fabric of American politics.

Reform was difficult; but it was not impossible. In response to challenges to their structure in the 1980s and 1990s, Medicare and Medicaid policymakers chose to innovate, adapt, and change—incorporating many neoliberal market ideals into the liberal vision that had created them. But even before the Republican political ascendancy in the 1980s and 1990s, Medicare had innovated in cost containment by becoming the acknowledged leader in designing payment methods for hospitals and physicians that aimed to control costs. Private payers subsequently adopted the methods. Through these and other methods, liberals successfully fought proposals to block grant Medicaid and to shift costs to the states, accepting however the devolution of power from the federal government to the states in controlling costs, privatizing services, and shaping the future of health care for people below or near the poverty line. In this way, not only would Medicare and Medicaid survive, they would lay the foundation for program expansion in the 1990s and 2000s (adding children's health insurance, new prescription drug benefits for seniors, and so on). Such expansions would have been unimaginable in the early and mid 1980s.

The harsh reality of health care in the United States is that Medicare and Medicaid expansion could not stem the rising numbers of people who fell in the gaps—that is, those lacking access to private insurance and ineligible for both government programs, estimated at 48 million people in 2012.[6] The passage of the 2010 Affordable Care Act aimed to alleviate this situation through two mechanisms: (1) establishing new state-based health insurance exchanges (marketplaces) where individuals could purchase private insurance policies; and (2) the expansion of state Medicaid programs to include individuals whose incomes were below 138 percent of the federal poverty level. The Supreme Court's June 2012 ruling gave states the power to refuse to expand their Medicaid programs, and many states have exercised that right. These developments have blunted the impact of the ACA. Yet, as of December 2014, 27 states and the District of Columbia had opted to expand Medicaid eligibility,[7] and two Gallup polls revealed a sharp reduction in the uninsured rate nationwide. The sharpest reductions came in those states that had both expanded Medicaid and implemented their own insurance exchanges.[8]

Medicaid expansion now has become, improbably for many familiar with its origins, the principal means by which coverage of the uninsured will expand in the near future. This is a prospect that few, if any, of the program's architects would have envisioned in 1965.[9] Medicare (a true entitlement) was to be the model for future reforms, not Medicaid. Yet over time, Medicaid—ever in danger—ceased being merely a stigmatized poor person's program. As Michael Sparer and Lawrence Brown observed in 2003, its ambiguous boundaries had created room to innovate and grow; and the program had financed a growing constituency of "physicians, hospitals, community health centers, and public health clinics . . . [with] tangible interests not only in what Medicaid pays but also in whom it covers. . . ."[10] For Sparer and Brown, the lesson of the "poor program's" progress was that incremental approaches to reform (raise eligibility slowly, insure children, add families, etc.) actually work. Following this tangled path, by 2014, Medicaid had surpassed Medicare to become the largest health insurance program in the nation; with ACA expansions, it will continue to grow and evolve.

The expansion of health insurance coverage through Medicaid, of course, is a risky and vulnerable step. Medicare began as a quintessential entitlement, while Medicaid was not an entitlement in the same sense. The differences between Medicare's social insurance promise (supported by payroll taxes for hospital insurance) and Medicaid's weaker commitment (supported by general taxpayer funds) remain large. Medicaid became a weak legal entitlement over time, not through legislation but through judicial decisions establishing that eligibility by federal standards entitled an individual to Medicaid benefits. The scope and limits of the Medicaid obligation to US citizens has since become the topic of intense negotiations and arguments. In some conceptions (specifically legal and budgetary), Medicaid is considered an entitlement program by the federal government and the courts, as well as by policy analysts; but in political circles, the claim is highly contentious. The fact that its status is in dispute says much about its contested place in American health policy, and makes Medicaid expansion as the basis for future health reform a particularly precarious path to follow.

Looking back at the past half-century, what lessons can we carry into the future about this quintessentially American tale—a story of liberal ideals, conservative reactions, innovation, and tangled, often paradoxical, progress?

The authors in this volume suggest that we bear the following in mind as we move into the sixth decade of these programs. Contentious origins do not necessarily produce weak programs. Indeed, history shows that politically weak programs like Medicaid (however meagerly funded and politically contentious) still have the capacity to grow and to fulfill vital roles in society. The ACA, also born amid intense partisanship and intense cost cutting, may yet prove to be as resilient. We learn that even though much of the debate today might revolve around cost and cost containment, we should not lose sight of the fundamental realities and concerns that created them— the plight of families in poverty, the medical care needs of elderly people, and the essential moral questions of fairness and equality that created the need for these programs in the first place. We also learn that the design of Medicare and Medicaid has had lasting effects. Designed and implemented at a high point in the Civil Rights era, the law became a force for hospital desegregation and equality in health care. The architects of Medicare, however, did not anticipate that in the longer term, by enacting a program for older Americans in 1965, they effectively would remove that segment of the population from the battles to come over health care reform—creating a "what's in it for me" attitude among elderly beneficiaries that continues (and will continue) to impact reform efforts.

We learn that Medicare and Medicaid have remade values, relationships, and society far and wide, and that the courts continue to be a crucial force for defining the meaning of the entitlement and the limits of these programs. The entitlement question has been hotly contested over the past five decades. In contrast to Medicare, nowhere in the original Medicaid statute is there language granting beneficiaries access to the courts to protect their eligibility to services. The courts, however, exercised their own power—recognizing and continuing to debate this right of recipients.[11] Chief Justice Roberts, in another exercise of court power over the scope of Medicaid, ruled against the federal government's power to coerce states to expand Medicaid. In the decades ahead, shifts in balance of power in the courts, judicial appointments, and political philosophies about the respective roles of the federal versus state governments in people's lives will continue to shape Medicare and Medicaid. We must also consider that the social identities of beneficiaries of these programs will not remain static, but instead will be open to change—and that those changes will alter, and be altered by, the programs themselves.

Of course, the age of conservative retrenchment is still with us, and restraining the costs of these programs will create persistent challenges in the decades ahead. Pressure to cut the rate of growth in spending will remain intense. Faced with the challenge of rising costs, both Medicare and Medicaid have had to be inventive. Their supporters have had to fight hard to make sure that fundamental ideals were not harmed as the debate turned to privatization, shifting costs to beneficiaries, and block grant proposals. These battles continue today and will continue as long as deficits exist and state and federal budgets remain tight, and the struggle for inventive ways of controlling expenses that began with DRGs in the 1980s will also continue. Perhaps surprisingly, administrators of these programs have shown the capacity to be flexible and to innovate in hard times. Medicare, in fact, will continue to be a powerful vehicle for future cost containment. But too much reliance on Medicare to control the nation's healthcare costs could backfire, with negative effects for other reform efforts.

Despite all of the turmoil, those who support Medicare and Medicaid can take great satisfaction in the programs reaching 50, and may plan for its next decade. Throughout the half-century, the American public has supported the programs—and the freedom, independence, and fairness embodied by them—even as they have worried about the cost. Remarkably, even in the immediate wake of pitched battles over ending these programs, they have since expanded under both Democratic and Republican leadership in Washington, D.C. Yet, gaps in health protection continue to exist. Looking ahead, one new challenge will be filling the gap in coverage for more people needing long-term care. It remains to be seen if politicians (and the web of constituents now deeply connected through Medicare and Medicaid) can muster the will to act on this front.

The past cannot predict the future; but with the last 50 years as a guide, it is fair to say that the web of relationships created by Medicare and Medicaid, along with the related moral, social, and financial investments, has proven to be unusually durable. This fact alone will not ensure their future nor determine the next steps. Indeed, this web of relationships may even inhibit future reforms. However, for good or ill, these programs have remade American society, and it is likely that in families, in politics, in government, in the courts, in the medical and health professions, and in hospitals and nursing homes, their impact will be felt for many years to come.

## NOTES

1. As Rosemary and Robert Stevens commented in 1970, "the AMA opposed Kerr-Mills because it claimed that physicians already provided care to the elderly poor free of charge. . . . Thus when physicians became to be paid for their services under Kerr-Mills in 1960 and under Title XIX in 1965, they received a sudden and significant increase in their incomes, allegedly for services they were already donating." Rosemary Stevens and Robert Stevens, "Medicaid: Anatomy of a Dilemma," *Law and Contemporary Problems* 35 (Spring 1970): 409.
2. Asked about the impact of Medicare on cardiology in 1966, the former president of the American College of Cardiology, Charles Fisch, answered bluntly: "it made cardiologists rich, as simple as that." In W. Bruce Fye, *American Cardiology: The History of a Specialty and Its College* (Baltimore, MD: Johns Hopkins University Press, 226.
3. *Cardiovascular Specialists and the Economics of Medicine* (Bethesda, MD: American College of Cardiology, 1994), figure 9.1, p. 65. Cited in W. Bruce Fye, p. 227.
4. James R. Tallon, Jr., and Diane Rowland, "Federal Dollars and State Flexibility: The Debate over Medicaid's Future," *Inquiry* 32 (Fall 1995): 235–240. See also Jonathan Oberlander, *The Political Life of Medicare* (Chicago: University of Chicago Press, 2003)
5. Judith Feder, "Thoughts on the Future of Medicare," *Inquiry* (Winter 1995/96): 378.
6. http://www.census.gov/hhes/www/hlthins/data/incpovhlth/2012/highlights.html.

7. http://kff.org/health-reform/state-indicator/state-activity-around-expanding-medicaid-under-the-affordable-care-act/.

8. http://www.gallup.com/poll/172403/uninsured-rate-sinks-second-quarter.aspx; http://www.gallup.com/poll/174290/arkansas-kentucky-report-sharpest-drops-uninsured-rate.aspx.

9. As Rosemary and Robert Stevens wrote in 1970, "the Medicaid program is in constant danger of having the argument of costs used not to provide services more efficiently but to cut down the provision of services to those who need them most." Rosemary Stevens and Robert Stevens, "Medicaid: Anatomy of a Dilemma," *Law and Contemporary Problems* 35 (Spring 1970): 397.

10. Lawrence D. Brown and Michael S. Sparer, "Poor Progress: The Unanticipated Politics of Medicaid Policy," *Journal of Health Politics, Policy and Law* (2003) 22, no. 1: 41.

11. In addition to Chapter 6 by Sara Rosenbaum in this volume, see also Timothy Stoltzfus Jost, "The Tenuous Nature of the Medicaid Entitlement," *Health Affairs* 22 (2003): 145–153.

# LIST OF ABBREVIATIONS AND ACRONYMS

| | |
|---|---|
| ACA | Affordable Care Act of 2010 |
| ACO | Accountable Care Organization |
| AFDC | Aid to Families with Dependent Children |
| AFL-CIO | American Federation of Labor and Congress of Industrial Organizations |
| AMA | American Medical Association |
| AMPAC | American Medical Association Political Action Committee |
| CBO | Congressional Budget Office |
| CEA | Council of Economic Advisers |
| CLASS | Community Living Assistance Services and Supports Act (part of the ACA, repealed January 1, 2013) |
| CMS | Centers for Medicare and Medicaid Services |
| CNHI | Committee for National Health Insurance |
| CPR | Customary, prevailing, and reasonable |
| DRG(s) | Diagnosis-related group(s) |
| DSH | Disproportionate Share Hospital |
| EPSDT | Early and Periodic Screening, Diagnosis, and Treatment Program |
| ESRD | End-stage renal disease |
| FCC | Federal Communications Commission |
| FERPA | Federal Educational Rights and Privacy Act of 1974 |
| FPL | Federal poverty level |
| GDP | Gross domestic product |

| | |
|---|---|
| HCBS | Home and Community-Based Services |
| HEW | Department of Health, Education, and Welfare |
| HHS | Department of Health and Human Services |
| HIBAC | Health Insurance Benefits Advisory Council |
| HIFA | Health Insurance Flexibility and Accountability Demonstration Initiative |
| HMO | Health maintenance organization |
| ICF | Intermediate care facility |
| IPAB | Independent Payment Advisory Board |
| JCAH | Joint Commission on Accreditation of Hospitals |
| MAAC | Medical Assistance Advisory Council |
| MCCA | Medicare Catastrophic Coverage Act of 1988 |
| MCHR | Medical Committee for Human Rights |
| MFP | Money follows the person |
| MMA | Medicare Modernization Act of 2003 |
| NAACP | National Association for the Advancement of Colored People |
| NAACP-LDF | National Association for the Advancement of Colored People Legal Defense Fund |
| NCSC | National Council of Senior Citizens |
| NIH | National Institutes of Health |
| NMA | National Medical Association |
| OAA | Older Americans Act of 1965 |
| OACT | Office of the Actuary |
| OEHO | Office of Equal Health Opportunity |
| OEO | Office of Economic Opportunity |
| P4P | Pay-for-performance |
| PAC | Political action committee |
| PACE | Program of All-Inclusive Care for the Elderly |
| RBRCS | Resource-based relative cost schedule |
| RBRVS | Resource-based relative value scale |
| S-CHIP / CHIP | State Children's Health Insurance Program |
| SGR | Sustainable growth rate |
| SNF | Skilled nursing facility |
| SRS | Social and Rehabilitation Service |
| SSA | Social Security Administration |
| SSI | Supplemental Security Income |

| | |
|---|---|
| TANF | Temporary Assistance to Needy Families |
| UAW | United Automobile Workers |
| UCR | Usual, customary, and reasonable |
| VA | Veterans Health Administration |
| VPS | Volume performance standard |

# A FEW FACTS ABOUT
# MEDICARE AND MEDICAID

## The Medicare Program

The Medicare program, created under Title XVIII of the Social Security Amendments of 1965, today provides health insurance coverage as an *entitlement* for three groups of beneficiaries: adults aged 65 and older; younger adults with permanent disabilities who qualify for Supplemental Security Insurance; and individuals of any age who have end-stage renal disease.

The Medicare program is managed by the Centers for Medicare and Medicaid Services (CMS), an agency within the federal Department of Health and Human Services. The program contains four parts. Part A (Hospital Insurance) and Part B (Medical Insurance) were established with the enactment of Medicare in 1965. Part C (now called Medicare Advantage) was added under the Balanced Budget Act of 1997 and then was restructured under the Medicare Modernization Act (MMA) of 2003. Part D (Prescription Drug Coverage) was added by the MMA in 2003 but was not fully implemented until 2006.

Parts A and B constitute "traditional Medicare," whereas Part C represents Medicare "managed care" offered by private health plans. Beneficiaries may elect to enroll in Part C; otherwise, they receive traditional Medicare benefits. All beneficiaries, however, are eligible to enroll for Part D prescription drug benefits.

Of the 54 million Medicare beneficiaries in 2014, 30% (15.7 million) were enrolled in Medicare Advantage, while the majority of beneficiaries were in traditional Medicare. The number of beneficiaries enrolled in private plans almost tripled from 5.3 million to 15.7 million between 2004 and 2014.

**Part A: Hospital Insurance** covers services such as hospital care, post-hospitalization rehabilitative care in a skilled nursing facility, home health care, and hospice care. It is managed by CMS though private administrative contractors (e.g., Blue Cross plans) who perform actual administrative functions (e.g., processing of claims and payments). Part A is financed mostly through payroll taxes that are placed in the Hospital Insurance Trust Fund. Financial projections, based on demographic and actuarial trends, suggest that the Trust Fund eventually may be exhausted. Current estimates by the Congressional Budget Office indicate that the Fund should remain solvent until 2033.

**Part B: Medical Insurance** covers services (such as doctor visits, procedures, and lab tests) and supplies (such as oxygen therapy, wheelchairs, walkers, and other medical equipment) deemed medically necessary to treat a disease or condition and meeting accepted standards of medical practice. The Affordable Care Act of 2010 requires that preventive services also be covered. Part B is managed by CMS through private administrative contractors who handle claims and payments. It is financed through a combination of insurance premiums paid by beneficiaries ($104.90 per month in 2014) and general tax revenues collected by the federal government. Premium levels are set by Congress on an annual basis.

**Part C: Medicare Advantage** is the managed care alternative to traditional Medicare coverage. These plans are offered by private insurance companies according to specified rules set by CMS, but the plans are not required to match the benefits of traditional Medicare coverage. Part C is financed through a combination of payroll taxes and premiums paid by enrollees to managed care firms. Originally called the Medicare + Choice program when created under the Balanced Budget Act of 1997, Medicare Advantage was redesigned in 2003 to give beneficiaries a choice other than the traditional Medicare program.

**Part D: Prescription Drug Coverage** pays for pharmaceutical expenses of beneficiaries. Part D is managed by CMS through contractual arrangements with private companies that offer an array of alternative plans. It is financed through a combination of general tax revenues, monthly premiums paid by enrollees, and state contributions to drug costs. Monthly premiums vary by plan, with higher-income beneficiaries paying more.

Regardless of whether they opt for traditional Medicare coverage or Medicare Advantage, beneficiaries are responsible for paying some portion of their healthcare costs through a combination of deductibles, copayments, and coinsurance.

Although fairly comprehensive in scope, Medicare does not cover certain services, such as private rooms for hospital care, dental care, eye care, hearing aids, dentures, and cosmetic surgery. Many, if not most, beneficiaries, therefore, purchase **supplemental medical insurance** to cover gaps in Medicare coverage. These insurance policies (often called "Medi-gap" policies) are issued by private insurance firms and are paid out of pocket by beneficiaries.

Despite the fact that Medicare beneficiaries are primarily individuals aged 65 and older, the Medicare program does *not* cover long-term care in nursing homes. It does, however, cover skilled nursing services and other rehabilitative services, such as physical therapy, provided in the home that are required only intermittently and usually temporarily following an acute care episode such as a hospitalization.

Because of its considerable market power as a major payer of health care, Medicare is the de facto standard-setter for payment and procedure coding methods in the United States, with private insurance companies typically adopting Medicare payment methods, but generally paying for services at higher levels. The Medicare program pioneered prospective payment for hospitals and physicians in the 1980s and 1990s, and developed other innovative methods for paying other healthcare providers and facilities in more recent times. Medicare uses its market power to pay discounted rates to healthcare providers, thus keeping its costs lower than those of private insurers. However, the Medicare Modernization Act has prohibited the program from negotiating prescription drug price discounts for beneficiaries.

## THE MEDICAID PROGRAM

The Medicaid program, created under Title XIX of the Social Security Amendments of 1965, is a joint federal and state program that helps with medical costs for some people with limited income and resources. Initially, the program was designed to provide coverage for people who qualified for benefits under public assistance programs such as Old Age Assistance, Aid to Families with Dependent Children (AFDC), Aid to the Permanently and Totally Disabled, and Aid to the Blind. Over time, Medicaid has expanded to include other low-income and disabled individuals and offers benefits not normally covered by Medicare, such as skilled nursing home care and personal care services in the home.

To be eligible, individuals must have incomes that are at or below the federal poverty level, which, in 2014, was set at $11,670 for an individual and $23,850 for a family of four. Some states allow individuals with incomes exceeding the poverty level to receive coverage. Although the federal government sets general rules within which states operate, and also grants waivers allowing states to operate outside the rules, the Medicaid program is actually operated and managed by the states. Medicaid programs, therefore, vary substantially from state to state in terms of eligibility requirements, scope of coverage, and payment levels for healthcare providers. Historically, the federal government has covered 50%–70% of Medicaid's costs, depending on a formula related to the financial status of each state, with resource-poor states receiving higher federal subsidies. Medicaid expenditures, on average, account for nearly one-quarter of total state expenditures in many states, posing serious financial challenges for state budgets.

Although states always have had the option to offer Medicaid coverage to individuals with incomes above the federal poverty level, few opted to do so. The Affordable Care Act encourages states to expand Medicaid coverage to individuals with incomes at or above 138% of the federal poverty level by offering federal subsidies to cover the costs, but as of 2014, only about half of all states had elected to expand coverage.

Medicaid finances 43 percent of all spending on long-term care services and covers a range of services and supports, including those needed by people to live independently in the community, as well as services provided in institutions. PACE (Program of All-inclusive Care for the Elderly) is a joint Medicare–Medicaid program that helps individuals meet their healthcare needs in the community instead of going to a nursing home or other care facility.

"Dual eligible" individuals meet eligibility requirements for both Medicare and Medicaid. Like other beneficiaries, they may choose between traditional Medicare and a Medicare Advantage plan. Their Part D prescription drug coverage comes through Medicare, and they may qualify for assistance in paying Part D premiums if their incomes and resources are below thresholds set by CMS. Such individuals also may qualify for assistance from Medicaid in paying the premiums for Part B Medicare coverage. Medicaid in some states also may cover some drugs and other care that Medicare does not cover.

# ACKNOWLEDGMENTS

A coedited volume with many authors is, by definition, a complex undertaking, and *Medicare and Medicaid at 50* is no exception. What began in late 2012 as a project to commemorate the fiftieth anniversary of the creation of the Medicare and Medicaid programs blossomed into a more expansive analysis of the programs' accomplishments, challenges, and future directions written for a general audience. The volume took shape from the insightful contributions of its authors and the collaborative team effort of its editors.

From the outset, this project was a joint venture between Alan Cohen of Boston University and the Robert Wood Johnson Foundation Investigator Awards in Health Policy Research Program and Keith Wailoo at Princeton University. They were quickly joined in this project by David Colby of the Robert Wood Johnson Foundation and Julian Zelizer of Princeton University. Many of the book's authors have a connection to the Investigator Awards Program or to another Foundation program, either as alumni or as members of the programs' national advisory committees. We are indebted to the Robert Wood Johnson Foundation, the Woodrow Wilson School of Public and International Affairs and the Center for Health and Wellbeing at Princeton University, and the National Institute on Aging for their generous support of this endeavor.

The editors wish to thank the authors for their steadfast dedication throughout the drafting and redrafting phases of the project. The final product benefited greatly from the stimulating and collegial dialogue among authors at a February 2014 conference held at Princeton University.

The project also benefited from the advice, input, and tireless efforts of numerous individuals. Bridget Gurtler of Princeton University and Jed Horwitt of Boston University played key roles in organizing the Princeton conference and in coordinating the work of four co-editors and 17 authors. We are deeply grateful to both for their hard work and perseverance throughout the project. We also wish to thank Stephen Somers and Jonathan Oberlander for their comments on an earlier draft of the conclusion, and Anne Case, Janet Currie, Susan Rizzo, Pamela Garber, Katie Player, and Christine Halbig for their assistance in administrative matters related to the Princeton conference.

Finally, we wish to thank Audra Wolfe for her magnificent editorial insights and skills, Chad Zimmerman of Oxford University Press for his editorial advice, guidance, and encouragement, and members of the editorial and marketing staff at Oxford for bringing the project to a successful conclusion.

Alan B. Cohen
David C. Colby
Keith A. Wailoo
Julian E. Zelizer

# ABOUT THE CONTRIBUTORS

**Andrea Louise Campbell, PhD**, is a Professor of Political Science at the Massachusetts Institute of Technology.

**Alan B. Cohen, ScD**, is a Professor of Health Policy and Management at Boston University's School of Management, and National Program Director of the Robert Wood Johnson Foundation Investigator Awards in Health Policy Research Program.

**David C. Colby, PhD**, was Vice President of Policy at the Robert Wood Johnson Foundation.

**Elisabeth Fauquert** is a former École Normale Supérieure de Cachan student, PhD student at Université Lumière–Lyon 2, teacher at Institut d' Études Politiques de Lyon (IEP de Lyon), and Visiting Scholar at Brown University (2013 and 2014).

**Judith Feder, PhD**, is a Professor of Public Policy in the McCourt School of Public Policy at Georgetown University and an Urban Institute Fellow in Washington, D.C.

**Rashi Fein, PhD**, was Professor of the Economics of Medicine, *Emeritus*, at Harvard Medical School's Department of Global Health and Social Medicine.

**Jacob S. Hacker, PhD**, is Stanley Resor Professor of Political Science and Director of the Institution for Social and Policy Studies at Yale University.

**Theodore R. Marmor, PhD**, is Professor *Emeritus* of Political Science, Public Policy and Management at Yale University's School of Management.

**James Morone, PhD**, is the John Hazen White Professor of Political Science and Public Policy in the Department of Political Science at Brown University.

**Jonathan Oberlander, PhD**, is Professor and Vice Chair of Social Medicine and Professor of Health Policy and Management at the University of North Carolina at Chapel Hill.

**Mark A. Peterson, PhD**, is Professor of Public Policy, Political Science, and Law, and Chair of the Department of Public Policy at the Luskin School of Public Affairs, University of California, Los Angeles.

**Jill Quadagno, PhD**, is a Professor of Sociology and the Mildred and Claude Pepper Eminent Scholar in Social Gerontology in the Pepper Institute on Aging and Public Policy at Florida State University.

**Uwe E. Reinhardt, PhD**, is the James Madison Professor of Political Economy and Professor of Economics and Public Affairs at the Woodrow Wilson School of Public and International Affairs, Princeton University.

**Sara Rosenbaum, JD**, is the Harold and Jane Hirsh Professor of Health Law and Policy and Founding Chair of the Department of Health Policy, Milken Institute School of Public Health, The George Washington University.

**Mark Schlesinger, PhD**, is Professor of Health Policy and a Fellow of the Institution for Social and Policy Studies at Yale University and past editor of the *Journal of Health Politics, Policy and Law*.

**David Barton Smith, PhD**, is Research Professor in the Center for Health Equality and the Department of Health Management and Policy (and *Emeritus* Professor in the Risk, Insurance and Healthcare Management Department in the Fox School of Business and Management) at Temple University.

**Paul Starr, PhD**, is Professor of Sociology and Public Affairs at Princeton University and co-editor of *The American Prospect*.

**Frank J. Thompson, PhD**, is a Distinguished Professor in the School of Public Affairs and Administration, Rutgers-Newark, and the Center for State Health Policy at Rutgers University.

**Keith A. Wailoo, PhD**, is the Townsend Martin Professor of History and Public Affairs and Vice Dean of the Woodrow Wilson School of Public and International Affairs at Princeton University.

**Julian E. Zelizer, PhD**, is the Malcolm S. Forbes, Class of 1941 Professor of History and Public Affairs at Princeton University and a Fellow at New America. He writes a column for CNN.com.

# INDEX

big government (*continued*)
party affiliations, 233–234, 245–247
political rhetoric *vs.* pragmatics of governance, 234
under Ronald Reagan, 234, 237–239
Bipartisan Commission on Comprehensive Health
and Long-term Care Coverage, 263
Blacks
health care before the Civil Rights Act, 22–24
Jim Crow healthcare, 24
separate but equal health care, 24
*See also* civil rights; desegregation; racial
division; segregated healthcare
the blind
Aid to the Blind, 44, 78
cash assistance to, 194
blood supply, segregated, 31
books and publications
"Killing Medicaid the California Way," 202
*Medicine and Health*, 42
"The New Property," 101
*The Political Life of Medicare*, 151
*Redefining Health Care*, 170
*Remedy and Reaction*, 321
"Socialized Medicine and You," 12
*Yale Law Review*, 101
Boren Amendment, 109
Bow, Frank, 15
Bowen, Otis, 239
Breaux, John, 160–162
Brewer, Jan, 246
Brown, Lawrence, xiv, 336
*Brown v. Board of Ed*, 302
Bush, George H. W.
defeat by Clinton, 66
HCBS waivers, 198
healthcare reform, 68
means-testing Medicare Part B, 148
Medicaid expansion, 194–195
Medicare cost controls, 174, 178, 289
Medicare initiatives, 147–148
Bush, George W.
big government, 233, 243–247
campaign finance support, 162
CHIP proposal, 242
compassionate conservatism, 68
HIFA (Health Insurance Flexibility and
Accountability) Demonstration Initiative, 80
Medicaid expansion, 196–198
Medicare Modernization Act of 2003, 265
Medicare reform, 196–198, 310–311
prescription drug benefits, 243–247, 265
private accounts proposal, 326
support for Medicare Part D, xv
waivers, 198
Byrnes, John, 16

Cadillac tax on health plans, 329
California, 12, 13, 79, 111–112, 162, 170–171, 193,
201–203, 237, 304
Campbell, Andrea, 133–134
capped entitlements, 268
Carter, Jimmy
avoiding the third rail of politics, 157
big government, 235–237
electoral demographics, 313
on health reform, 65
history of social insurance, 311
Medicare cost controls, 175
national elections of 1988, 305
case-based costing systems, 176
cash-and-counseling model of home care, 136–137
catastrophic coverage. *See* MCCA (Medicare
Catastrophic Coverage Act).
*Catch 22*, 275
categorically needy
Medicaid coverage for, 78
*vs.* medically needy, 44
CBO (Congressional Budget Office), 281
CEA (Council of Economic Advisers), 39–40
Centers for Medicare and Medicaid Services
(CMS). *See* CMS (Centers for Medicare and
Medicaid Services).
Chaffee, John, 312
children, care for
Aid to Dependent Children, 100
Children's Health Insurance Program
(1997), 197
EPSDT (Early and Periodic Screening,
Diagnosis, and Treatment) Program, 106
expanding Medicaid eligibility, 195
Kiddycare, 59–61
Medicaid expansion, 239–243
Medicaid for pregnant women and infants, 79
*See also* AFDC (Aid to Families with Dependent
Children); CHIP (State Children's Health
Insurance Program)
Children's Health Insurance Program (1997),
80–83, 98, 107, 197, 200, 209
CHIP (State Children's Health Insurance Program)
combining with Medicaid, 81
cost, 242
enactment of, 67–68
increased federal funding, 80
Medicaid expansion, 239–243
Civil Rights Act of 1964
desegregating health care, 25–35
Hill-Burton program, 24
and the history of social insurance, 302
Johnson administration, 24–27
Kennedy administration, 24
passage of, 15–16